SENSORY GUIDANCE
OF MOVEMENT

The Novartis Foundation is an international scientific and educational charity (UK Registered Charity No. 313574). Known until September 1997 as the Ciba Foundation, it was established in 1947 by the CIBA company of Basle, which merged with Sandoz in 1996, to form Novartis. The Foundation operates independently in London under English trust law. It was formally opened on 22 June 1949.

The Foundation promotes the study and general knowledge of science and in particular encourages international co-operation in scientific research. To this end, it organizes internationally acclaimed meetings (typically eight symposia and allied open meetings, 15–20 discussion meetings, a public lecture and a public debate each year) and publishes eight books per year featuring the presented papers and discussions from the symposia. Although primarily an operational rather than a grant-making foundation, it awards bursaries to young scientists to attend the symposia and afterwards work for up to three months with one of the other participants.

The Foundation's headquarters at 41 Portland Place, London W1N 4BN, provide library facilities, open every weekday, to graduates in science and allied disciplines. The library is home to the Media Resource Service which offers journalists access to expertise on any scientific topic. Media relations are also strengthened by regular press conferences and book launches, and by articles prepared by the Foundation's Science Writer in Residence. The Foundation offers accommodation and meeting facilities to visiting scientists and their societies.

Information on all Foundation activities can be found at http://www.novartisfound.demon.co.uk

Novartis Foundation Symposium 218

SENSORY GUIDANCE OF MOVEMENT

1998

JOHN WILEY & SONS

Chichester · New York · Weinheim · Brisbane · Singapore · Toronto

Published in 1998 by John Wiley & Sons Ltd,
   Baffins Lane, Chichester,
   West Sussex PO19 1UD, England

   National 01243 779777
   International (+44) 1243 779777
   e-mail (for orders and customer service enquiries): cs-books@wiley.co.uk
   Visit our Home Page on http://www.wiley.co.uk
     or http://www.wiley.com

Other Wiley Editorial Offices

John Wiley & Sons, Inc., 605 Third Avenue,
New York, NY 10158-0012, USA

WILEY-VCH Verlag GmbH, Pappelallee 3,
D-69469 Weinheim, Germany

Jacaranda Wiley Ltd, 33 Park Road, Milton,
Queensland 4064, Australia

John Wiley & Sons (Asia) Pte Ltd, 2 Clementi Loop #02-01,
Jin Xing Distripark, Singapore 129809

John Wiley & Sons (Canada) Ltd, 22 Worcester Road,
Rexdale, Ontario M9W 1L1, Canada

Novartis Foundation Symposium 218
ix+344 pages, 62 figures, 6 tables

Library of Congress Cataloging-in-Publication Data

Sensory guidance of movement / [editors, Gregory R. Bock and Jamie A.
 Goode].
   p. cm. – (Novartis Foundation symposium ; 218)
   Symposium on Sensory Guidance of Movement, held at the Novartis
 Foundation, London, 20–22 January 1998.
   Includes bibliographical references and index.
   ISBN 0-471-98262-8 (alk. paper)
   1. Sensorimotor integration–Congresses. 2. Sensorimotor cortex-
-Congresses. 3. Cerebellum–Congresses. I. Bock, Gregory.
 II. Goode, Jamie. III. Symposium on Sensory Guidance of Movement
(1998 : London, England) IV. Series.
 QP454.S46 1998
 573.7′37–dc21   98-38056
                  CIP

British Library Cataloguing in Publication Data

A catalogue record for this book is available from the British Library

ISBN 0 471 98262 8

Typeset in 10½ on 12½ pt Garamond by Dobbie Typesetting Limited, Tavistock, Devon.
Printed and bound in Great Britain by Biddles Ltd, Guildford and King's Lynn.
This book is printed on acid-free paper responsibly manufactured from sustainable forestry,
in which at least two trees are planted for each one used for paper production.

Contents

Participants

Richard A. Andersen   Division of Biology 216-76, California Institute of Technology, 1200 E California Boulevard, Pasadena, CA 91125, USA

Timothy Ebner   University of Minnesota, Department of Neurosurgery, Lions Research Building, #421 2001 Sixth Street SE, Minneapolis, MN 55455, USA

Eberhard E. Fetz   Department of Physiology and Biophysics, University of Washington School of Medicine, Seattle, WA 98195-7290, USA

Apostolos P. Georgopoulos   Brain Sciences Center (11B), VAMC, One Veterans Drive, Minneapolis, MN 55417, USA

Alan R. Gibson   Division of Neurobiology, Barrow Neurological Institute, St Joseph's Hospital, 350 W. Thomas Road, Phoenix, AZ 85013, USA

Mitchell Glickstein   (*Chairman*) Department of Anatomy and Developmental Biology, Neuroscience and Behaviour Group, University College London, Gower Street, London WC1E 6BT, UK

Melvyn Goodale   Department of Psychology, Graduate Program in Neurosciences, University of Western Ontario, London, Ontario, Canada N6A 5C2

Klaus Peter Hoffmann   Lehrstuhl Allgemeine Zoologie und Neurobiologie, Fakultät Biologie, Ruhr-Universität Bochum, Universitätstrasse 150, Bochum D-44801, Germany

Marc Jeannerod   Institut des Sciences Cognitives, 67 Boulevard Pinel, F-69500 Bron, France

Roland S. Johansson   Department of Physiology, Umeå University, S-901 87 Umeå, Sweden

John F. Kalaska   Centre de Recherche en Sciences Neurologiques, Département de Physiologie, Faculté de Medécine, Université de Montréal, Case Postale 6128, Succursale Centre-ville, Montréal, Québec, Canada H3C 3J7

Mitsuo Kawato   ATR Human Information Processing Research Laboratories, 2-2 Hikaridai, Seika-cho, Soraku-gun, Kyoto 619-0288, Japan

Roger N. Lemon   Sobell Department of Neurophysiology, Institute of Neurology, Queen Square, London WC1N 3BG, UK

C. David Marsden   University Department of Clinical Neurology, Institute of Neurology, The National Hospital for Neurology and Neurosurgery, Queen Square, London WC1N 3BG, UK

Jason B. Mattingley   (*Novartis Foundation Bursar*) Department of Psychology, Monash University, Clayton, Victoria 3168, Australia

R. Chris Miall   University Laboratory of Physiology, Parks Road, Oxford OX1 3PT, UK

Fred A. Miles   Laboratory of Sensorimotor Research, National Eye Institute, NIH Building 49, Room 2A50, Bethesda, MD 20892, USA

Lee Miller   Department of Physiology, Northwestern University Medical School, 303 East Chicago Avenue, Chicago, IL 60611, USA

Richard E. Passingham   Department of Experimental Psychology, University of Oxford, South Parks Road, Oxford OX1 3UD, UK

Giacomo Rizzolatti   Istituto di Fisiologia Umana, Università di Parma, Via Gramsci, 14-43100 Parma, Italy

Helen E. Savaki   University of Crete, P.O. Box 1393, Medical School, 71110 Heraklion, Crete, Greece

John Stein   University Laboratory of Physiology, Parks Road, Oxford OX1 3PT, UK

Peter L. Strick   Research Service (151S), VA Medical Center, 800 Irving Avenue, Syracuse, NY 13210, USA

W. Thomas Thach Department of Anatomy & Neurobiology, Washington University School of Medicine, 660 S. Euclid Avenue, St Louis, MO 63110, USA

Peter Thier Neurol. Universitätsklinik, Hoppe-Seyler Str. 3, D-72076 Tübingen, Germany

Daniel Wolpert Sobell Department of Neurophysiology, Institute of Neurology, The National Hospital for Neurology and Neurosurgery, Queen Square, London WC1N 3BG, UK

Chairman's introduction

Mitchell Glickstein

Department of Anatomy and Developmental Biology, Neuroscience and Behaviour Group, University College London, Gower Street, London WC1E 6BT, UK

Most human and animal movements are under continuous sensory guidance. This symposium is organized to consider the way in which that sensory guidance is accomplished by the brain. Some general questions which can be addressed are as follows.

(1) **What are the relevant sensory cues in the sensory guidance of movement?**
Classical psychophysics has typically been concerned with analysis of the nature of sensory responses to specified physical stimuli. We will consider an equally important and related area of study, sensorimotor psychophysics.

Marc Jeannerod and his colleagues have studied the way in which motor responses are determined by visual stimuli. Their data form an essential basis for thinking about the role of the brain in the sensory guidance of movement.

Most attention has been paid to the study of visually controlled movement. Other sensory mechanisms may play an equally important role for some classes of movement.

Roland Johansson and his colleagues have shown how in addition to the visual properties of an object to be lifted, grip is highly influenced by tactile input from the digits.

(2) **Do all cortical visual areas contribute equally to the visual guidance of movement?**
The number of visual areas that are recognized has increased over time. Do all of these areas play an equal role in the visual guidance of movement?

Richard Andersen and colleagues have studied extensively the activity of cells in the posterior parietal cortex. It is clear that the response properties of cells in these areas are related to their function in control of the limbs as well as the eyes.

Melvyn Goodale and his colleagues have studied the differential effect of loss of the extrastriate visual areas on sensory guidance of movement. His evidence has helped to distinguish the differential function of visual recognition and visually guided action.

(3) How do cells in the primary motor cortex control movement?
Since Fritsch and Hitzig's work it has been clear that a specialized region of the cerebral cortex is involved in motor control. Stimulation of that region elicits movement; ablation makes people or animals clumsy in the use of that limb. Obviously, no single cell controls movement. How do neurons in the motor cortex act as an ensemble in motor control?

Apostolos Georgopoulos, John Kalaska and **Roger Lemon** and their co-workers have been among the major contributors to answering the question of the role of individual motor cortical cells in motor control. Their work forms an essential link in the study of sensory guided movement.

(4) What is the role of motor cortical areas beyond the primary motor cortex in the sensory guidance of movement?
There was an analogous increase in the number of recognized motor areas of the cerebral cortex. Initially motor, premotor and supplementary motor areas were recognized. In the past few years the number of cortical motor areas has increased further.

Giacomo Rizzolatti and **Peter Strick** and their colleagues have continued to explore the structure and function of cortical areas beyond the classical cortical motor areas in motor control. What is the function of these areas in the sensory guidance of movement?

(5) How are sensory areas of the brain connected to motor areas?
After the original discoveries of primary motor and sensory areas, it was often tacitly assumed that connections are by way of cortico-cortical fibres. But high level sensory motor guidance is still possible in animals in which all cortico-cortical links have been cut. A priori, connections could be still made by way of two massive subcortical routes; one via the basal ganglia, the other by way of the cerebellum.

Dick Passingham will discuss the evidence from PET and MRI studies of the differential role of these circuits in the sensory guidance of movement.

(6) What is the role of the cerebellum and its target structures in the sensory guidance of movement?

Tom Thach and **Alan Gibson** and their colleagues have recorded from cells in the cerebellar cortex and nuclei as well as the cerebellar targets and studied the activation of cells in those structures in movement.

(7) Are there underlying theoretical principles which help to organize the data from physiological, anatomical and behavioural studies on the role of the brain in the sensory guidance of movement?

Whether we make our theories explicit or not, all data are collected with some theoretical underpinning in mind. It will clearly be useful to have an explicit and well-defined theoretical framework to interpret experimental evidence and to suggest new avenues for research.

Mitsuo Kawato has been one of the major contributors to the theoretical understanding of motor control, particularly the role of internal models in sensorimotor transformations.

Chris Miall has proposed theoretical solutions to deal with the problems that latency of activation impose on input to sensorimotor control mechanisms in the cerebellum.

(8) Can the evidence on sensory control of movement help us to understand impairments in neurological patients?

David Marsden is a major contributor at the interface between clinical neurology and experimental neuroscience. Hopefully, he will be able to help evaluate the possible applications of these advances to the management of the problems of people with motor deficits.

I recognize that I have been guilty of cerebral cortical chauvinism. It is clear that the same questions about the sensory guidance of movement apply to subcortical sensory and motor structures.

The choice of who should speak and who should be a discussant was often rather arbitrary. I would hope that the discussants would have an equal contribution to make in addressing the questions posed by the symposium.

Tim Ebner has contributed to our understanding of the role of the cerebellum in movement, and to the study of the nature of the motor deficit in neurological patients.

Eb Fetz has been a major contributor to the study of neuronal activity in movement and particularly the development of spike-triggered averaging in that analysis.

Klaus Peter Hoffmann and his colleagues have shown that some of the control of simple reaching movements may be organized at the level of the superior colliculus.

Fred Miles has contributed to our understanding the role of individual cells in the cerebellum in the control of eye movements.

Lee Miller has contributed to analysis of the role of the red nucleus in the control of arm movements.

Helen Savaki has used 2-deoxyglucose to chart the activation of motor cortex and cerebellum in sensory guided movement.

John Stein has been a major contributor to the analysis of the role of cortical visual areas in visually guided movement and the possible role of dysfunction of these circuits in dyslexia.

Peter Thier has contributed to our understanding of the physiology and the anatomical circuitry of visual input to the cerebellum.

Dan Wolpert has contributed to our understanding of the nature of arm trajectories in simple reaching movements.

I am personally unhappy that **Shigeru Kitazawa** who was to have been a discussant at this symposium could not attend because of personal reasons.

The Novartis Foundation arranges for a young junior colleague to participate as a discussant in the meeting — I am pleased at the selection of **Jason Mattingley** for the Novartis Foundation bursary.

I look forward to an exciting symposium.

Grasping an object: one movement, several components

M. Jeannerod, Y. Paulignan* and P. Weiss†

*Institut des Sciences Cognitives, 67 Boulevard Pinel, *Vision et Mortricité, INSERM U94, F-69500 Bron, France and †Department of Neurology, Heinrich Heine Universität, Düsseldolf, Germany*

Abstract. The visuomotor transformations for producing a grasping movement imply simultaneous control of different visual mechanisms. The object size, orientation and 3D characteristics have to be encoded for the selection of the appropriate opposition space, within which the opposition forces will be applied on the object surface. These mechanisms also have to combine with those of the transport of the hand to the object location. Finally, biomechanical constraints impose categorical visuomotor decisions for positioning the opposition space according to object changes in size, orientation and spatial location. This paper examines possible interactions between the specialized structures for visuomotor transformation and the internal model that adapts prehension to its goals.

1998 Sensory guidance of movement. Wiley, Chichester (Novartis Foundation Symposium 218) p 5–20

The kinematic description of grasping, at first sight, seems to imply the concurrence of several submovements. Transporting the hand to the object, orienting the wrist and preshaping the fingers into an appropriate grip, each involve sets of muscles and joints characterized by different control modalities, both in terms of the neural structures involved and the underlying functional mechanisms. The fast, ballistic type of movement of the arm responsible for the reach contrasts with the ramp-like independent movements of the fingers during the grasp. These striking differences were the basis for the hypothesis of 'visuomotor channels' put forward in the early 1980s (Jeannerod 1981, Arbib 1981). This theory held that each of the components of the act of prehension behaves as an identifiable system, characterized by its own input and output and its own intrinsic mechanisms. The theory went as far as affecting each visuomotor channel to a specific mode of visuomotor transformation, such that the transport component related to the spatial (egocentric) aspects of the action — processing distance and direction — whereas the grasp processed intrinsic aspects of the object such as shape or size. Following earlier work by Brinkman & Kuypers (1973), the visuomotor channel hypothesis received its main support from physiological and anatomical studies in the monkey, which convincingly showed that reaching and grasping are subserved by different neural pathways (for a review, see Jeannerod 1997). In humans, posterior parietal lesions can affect the grasp without altering the reach (Jeannerod et al 1994), and PET studies reveal areas activated by the grasp but not by the reach (Faillenot et al 1997). Although this view has now evolved and is challenged by new interpretations of the planning of prehension (see below), it still remains an influential one.

Covariation of prehension components

Although reach and grasp may differ widely in terms of their neural organization, the notion of separate systems does not capture all the aspects of prehension. In addition to the specific visuomotor transformation effected by each channel, one has to consider the fact that all the channels concur to the same final goal of achieving a stable grasp for holding and manipulating an object. In the next two sections, we explore the issue of integration of the components of prehension into a single goal-directed action.

In an experiment where subjects grasped cylindrical objects, we had noticed that the variability of the spatial paths of index finger and thumb tended to decrease sharply while the fingers approached the object (Fig. 1) (Paulignan et al 1991a), suggesting that the fingers were aiming at a predetermined locus on the object surface. This observation can be interpreted as evidence for a planning of the action of prehension in terms of a single goal for the upper limb, rather than as the addition of several components with different goals. If this interpretation is correct, however, one should be able to find some evidence for a covariation of the spatial and/or temporal parameters of the two submovements. The search for this covariation has led to mixed results. Studies in the early 1990s stressed the fact that the two main components were far from independent from each other, because the movements at the different joints tended to covary during the action of prehension. For example, it was observed that altering the reaching movement (e.g. by varying the distance of the object) also affected the formation of the grip (Jakobson & Goodale 1991, Chieffi & Gentilucci 1993). Conversely, altering the grip (e.g. by varying the size of the object) affected the kinematics of the reach (Marteniuk et al 1990, Gentilucci et al 1991, Jakobson & Goodale 1991, Zaal & Bootsma 1993, Bootsma et al 1994). Although they were of a relatively small amplitude, these changes were considered to reflect a single mechanism for prehension, where the processing of distance and size of the object could not be separated from each other.

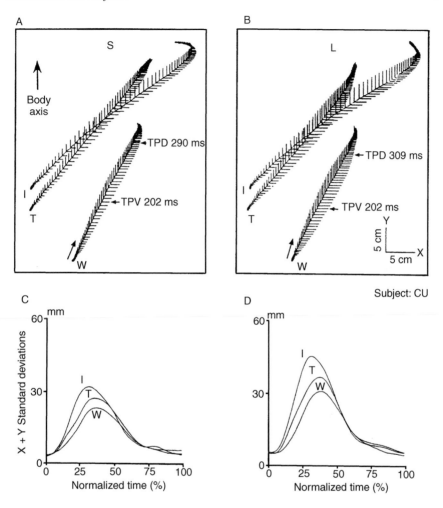

FIG. 1.   Variability of prehension movements. (*Upper part*) Normalized spatial paths of the wrist (W), tip of the thumb (T) and tip of the index finger (I) in two blocks of 10 trials directed at a small (S, 1.5 cm) object (A) and a large (L, 6 cm) object (B), respectively. Movements are shown in two dimensions (X and Y) as if seen from above. The starting position of the hand is at the bottom of the drawings, with the arrow indicating the direction of the wrist. Numbers on the wrist spatial path represent the mean values of time to peak velocity (TPV) and the time to peak deceleration (TPD). Horizontal and vertical bars on the averaged spatial paths represent the amplitude of one standard deviation in the X and Y spatial dimensions, respectively. (*Lower part*) Resultant variability as a function of time for wrist, thumb and index spatial paths, for the movements to the small object (C) and to the large object (D). From Paulignan et al (1991b).

In a recent study, Kudoh et al (1997) held a more balanced view. They confirmed that variability of movement parameters was not evenly distributed across movement time. In addition, they found that the peak of variability of the wrist was higher when object distance (but not object size) increased, whereas the peak of variability in grip aperture was affected by both distance and size of the object. Furthermore, the time occurrence of the peak variability of the wrist remained scaled to movement time, whereas for grip aperture the peak occurrence varied over movement time according to object size. Thus the two curves of variability appeared to vary independently from each other. Together with the fact that the kinematics of wrist and grip aperture were found to correlate poorly with each other in at least some subjects (see also Paulignan et al 1991a), Kudoh et al's (1997) results do not contradict a relative independence of the two components.

As a matter of fact, the above covariations speak in favour, not of a global planning of prehension, but of a cross-talk between the two components, reflecting a coordination mechanism. One of the most robust findings in prehension is that maximum grip aperture is consistently achieved after the occurrence of the peak deceleration of the wrist. This also holds true when the course of the movement is perturbed (e.g. by changing object position at movement onset): in this situation, the initial sequence of peak deceleration and maximum grip aperture is followed by a second one, in the same order (Paulignan et al 1991a; see also Haggard & Wing 1991). By contrast, if perturbations in object position affect the grasp, perturbations in object size have little effect on the transport (Paulignan et al 1991b). Thus, the coordination between the components could rely on an information flow from transport to grip, not the reverse. Following these considerations, the most likely organization for prehension would be that the transport component is controlled by a single feedforward controller, terminal error in transport being compensated for by a larger grip aperture when distance or velocity increase. The grasp component would also be controlled by a feedforward controller up to the time of maximum aperture, and then the closure would be feedback regulated. If this model is correct, one should predict that the absence of visual feedback should not affect transport, nor should it affect the grip up to the time of maximum grip aperture, but it should definitely affect the closure phase. This remains to be fully verified (see Jeannerod 1984).

Modes of planning goal-oriented actions

The issue of partly independent visuomotor components now merges with the modern concepts about the coordination between joints within a limb. The question of how the motor system controls the multiple degrees of freedom of the arm, which allow for a potentially infinite number of solutions for a particular motor task (the redundancy problem), was approached by postulating that the motor system might not control all the degrees of freedom, but only a few critical variables, hence reducing its computational load. One of these variables is the limb endpoint trajectory in space. In an influential paper, Morasso (1981) reported that the planar displacements of a hand-held lever toward visual targets had bell-shaped velocity profiles and followed approximately straight spatial paths. These characteristics fit those one would expect for a movement planned in Cartesian coordinates and where the only parameter controlled by the central nervous system is the spatial path of the hand (see Hogan & Flash 1987).

This view, however, is in conflict with other models that postulate that the motor system plans movements in joint coordinates and controls the position of each of the joints contributing to the movement (Soechting & Flanders 1992). By contrast with the spatial path model, the joint-space model predicts curved movement trajectories, a type of trajectory which is observed in many natural movements. The apparent discrepancy with Morasso's (1981) observations (where the trajectories were straight) was recently resolved by Desmurget et al (1997). They measured pointing movements in two conditions: in the 'constrained' condition, the subjects held in their hand a cursor that they displaced toward the target; in the 'unrestrained' condition, they moved their hand freely to the target. Whereas in the first condition, movements had a straight spatial path, in the second condition, the trajectory was curved and the degree of curvature depended on the eccentricity of the target. This result demonstrates that control strategies for goal-directed movements (and the resulting coordination between joints) differ according to the task in which the subject is involved. Prehension movements as considered here obviously pertain to the category of the unrestrained movements and should therefore fit the joint-space model. This point is discussed in the next two sections.

Planning the final arm posture

A variant of the joint-space model is that of planning a final arm posture. The general idea is that the motor control system plans actions by using optimization principles, such as minimizing the number of joints involved, avoiding biomechanical discomfort or preserving an optimal final posture when the goal of the movement is achieved. Several results with prehension indicate that, whenever possible, the final arm posture tends to remain invariant. Desmurget et al (1995) recorded the final arm posture when a subject reached to grasp a bar placed at different orientations. On some occasions, the orientation of the bar was changed at the onset of the reaching movement. The configuration of the arm was rapidly altered so as to match the new orientation; that is, the arm moved to the final posture that was assumed during unperturbed movements directed at a bar with the same orientation. In other words, each orientation of the bar determined a unique final posture of the whole limb. This idea of final posture coding can also be used for explaining recent data on visuomotor control of prehension obtained by Paulignan et al (1997). The main hypothesis of the experiment was that, because the fingers that contribute to the grasp represent the effector of the movement, their position on the object at the end of the movement should be the main parameter to be controlled for achieving an efficient grasp. Finger positions on the object determine the opposition axis, the axis along which the opposing grip forces are exerted on the object, such that a stable grasp will be obtained (Napier 1955, Iberall et al 1986). In most real-life situations, object properties such as shape and size clearly define an opposition axis: the task of the motor system in the prehensile act is to bring the fingers in the adequate positions and to choose the optimal configuration of the arm corresponding to these positions. The experiment of Stelmach et al (1994) shows that a relatively small change in orientation of an object which affords only one possible opposition axis results in a major reconfiguration of the arm, including wrist pronation and shoulder abduction.

To better understand the processes involved in selecting the adequate opposition axis, however, it is more helpful to employ objects which allow for more than one opposition axis, e.g. cylinders. By analysing prehension movements to cylindrical objects at different positions in the workspace, the limb configuration for a given object at a given position can reveal on which information the motor system predominantly relies. Will the motor system use a preferential opposition axis for all object positions, resulting in different limb postures, although other opposition axes are feasible as well? Or, alternatively, will the motor system minimize the changes in limb configuration by using different opposition axes depending on the position of the object? An experiment was performed where the position of vertical cylinders of different sizes was systematically varied across the workspace. The first result was that the spatial paths of the two fingertips over repeated movements directed at the same object tended to converge on the points of contact, as indicated by the sharp decrease in variability during the final part of the trajectory. This strongly suggests that the final finger position (and therefore the orientation of the opposition axis) is the controlled variable of prehension.

The second result was that this position is determined, not with respect to external (visual) coordinates, but with respect to body-centred coordinates. Although the orientation of the opposition axis apparently varied for each position of the object in the workspace, it remained invariant with respect to a reference attached to the body (e.g. the line connecting the centre of the head and the centre of the object). This result is shown in Fig. 2, which represents a plot of finger positions on the object placed at different spatial locations. When finger positions are plotted in head coordinates, they appear to be aligned for all object

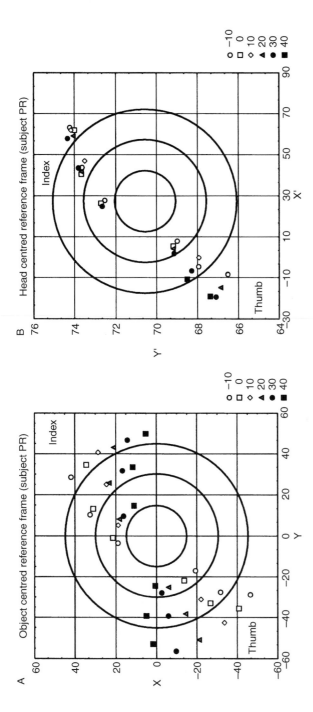

FIG. 2.   Effect of object position and size on final finger position. Final finger position was plotted in two different reference frames: object-centred (A) and head-centred (B). Note that in *A* finger position changes with object location (see symbols on the right side of the drawings) and size (the three concentric circles each represent one object size). In *B*, finger positions are superimposed for different object locations. From Paulignan et al (1997).

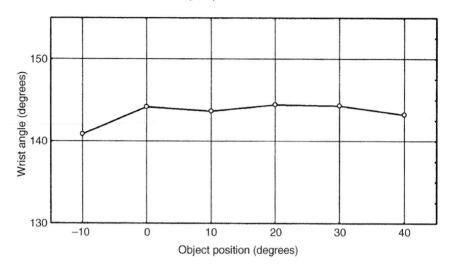

FIG. 3.   Effect of object position on the wrist angle during prehension movements. Objects of different sizes (3, 6 and 9 cm) were placed in the workspace at different positions with respect to subject's sagittal axis (object position, in degrees). Note lack of significant change in wrist angle. Objects of the three sizes have pooled together for each object position.

locations. In addition, and most importantly for the present purpose, this invariant angle of the opposition axis did not involve a different configuration of the forearm for each object position: as shown in Fig. 3, the wrist angle remained identical for different object positions, which implies that the forearm and the hand were displaced as a whole, irrespective of object location. Because of this, the main changes had to occur at the level of the elbow and the shoulder joints for keeping the orientation of the opposition axis invariant.

Visual and motor factors thus compete for orienting the opposition axis. Whenever possible, the final arm posture tends to remain invariant and it is only when required by object shape that new degrees of freedom are recruited. In addition, behavioural strategies can be used for preserving an invariant forearm posture in spite of constraining object shapes: this is the case when the subject rotates his body around the object until the orientation of the opposition axis afforded by the object becomes compatible with the optimal arm posture. The fact that the opposition axis is computed with respect to a body reference makes this possibility (which is excluded in most laboratory situations where a fixed position of the body with respect to the workspace is imposed) an economical one in terms of the number of degrees of freedom involved. In conclusion, the fact that when no visual constraints are present (as with cylindrical objects), the position of the fingertips on the object reflects the selection of an invariant final posture of the arm, not an invariant visual landmark on the object, validates the idea of a global planning of prehension. This idea would be compatible with Rosenbaum et al's (1990) finding of spontaneous grasping preferences (e.g. overhand vs. underhand) when grasping a bar that has to be placed on a support. In this case, the initial discomfort of the arm posture is tolerated for the sake of final comfort, because the end-state comfort is critical for the future task demands.

Control of final arm posture and visuomotor channels

The problem here is to know to what extent the concept of visuomotor channels can still account for the aspects of prehension which are described in Paulignan et al's (1997) experiment. Indeed, the results of this experiment tend to show that the position of the fingers on the object is not independent from the proximal (transport) component of prehension. In other words, the mechanisms that determine the selection of an appropriate opposition axis would not be separate from those that determine the hand position in the workspace. A possible explanation for this fact is that, among the visual parameters that contribute to the final pattern of grasping, orientation of the object has a special status. This interpretation was used by Soechting & Flanders (1993) to explain the errors in matching the orientation of an object with a hand-held rod, in the absence of visual control of one's hand. As these errors depended both on the slant of the object and on its location in the workspace, they concluded that the neural transformation from target orientation to hand orientation is influenced by both visual spatial and arm posture parameters. In fact, a more general explanation should be looked for, as orientation is not the only object parameter to affect distal as well as proximal degrees of freedom: increase in object size, to mention only one other, at first requires a change in grip aperture and, beyond a critical size, requires intervention of the two hands.

Although the notion of holistic programming does seem to contradict that of visuomotor channels, a hypothesis can be proposed for integrating the two. Adapting the configuration of the upper limb to the grasping situation requires taking a number of appropriate visuomotor decisions (e.g. pronation vs. supination of the forearm, one or two hands, etc.). This process cannot be achieved only through a direct visuomotor transformation, because it must take into account the fact that any given decision may simultaneously involve several channels. For this reason, it would be better achieved by an internal model where the consequences of the decision could be fully represented. Thus, our hypothesis suggests that an action such as prehension is organized on several levels. At one level, visuomotor transformation requires the activation of specific channels characterized by their own input–output relationships. At another level, these channels are embedded into a distinct mechanism which represents the internal model of the action. A strong argument in favour of this mode of functioning is the temporal organization of prehension movements. Several temporal landmarks can be described for prehension. First, the two components are synchronized at movement onset: the opening of the grip and the projection of the arm toward the object start within less than 50 ms as a consequence of nearly simultaneous contraction of the muscle groups involved (Jeannerod & Biguer 1982). Second, as already mentioned, the two components are phased near the end of the deceleration of the reach. Finally, the two components simultaneously stop at the time of contact with the object. An internal model for such a movement could thus be conceived as a temporal frame with a few critical points on the time axis (Jeannerod 1981). This view was taken up more recently by Hoff & Arbib (1993) in their time-based coordination model. They postulated the existence of a 'coordinating schema' which receives from each of the constituent schemas (the visuomotor channels) an estimate of the time it needs to move from its current state to the desired final state. Whichever channel is going to take longer is given the full time it needs, while the others will be slowed down. The time needed by each channel is regulated by optimality criteria which are embedded in feedback controllers. This model has been found to account for the rapid corrections generated in response to sudden displacement of the target object at the onset of a reaching movement (see Paulignan et al 1991a).

The previously mentioned visuomotor decisions (such as the Rosenbaum et al [1990] grasping preferences or the Stelmach et al [1994] intrusion of pronation) represent a rationale for the existence of a postural counterpart in the internal model of prehension (see Gomi & Kawato 1996, Wolpert et al 1995). The interaction between the visuomotor channels and the internal model could thus explain both the processing of the relevant object-related visual information by the specialized structures and the temporal and postural organization of the whole action.

References

Arbib MA 1981 Perceptual structures and distributed motor control. In: Brooks VB (ed) Handbook of physiology, section 1: The nervous system, vol II: Motor control. Williams & Wilkins, Baltimore, p 1449–1480

Bootsma RJ, Marteniuk RG, MacKenzie CL, Zaal FT 1994 The speed-accuracy trade-off in manual prehension: effect of movement amplitude, object size and object width on kinematic characteristics. Exp Brain Res 98:535–541

Brinkman J, Kuypers HG JM 1973 Cerebral control of contralateral and ipsilateral arm, hand and finger movements in the split-brain rhesus monkey. Brain 96:663–674

Chieffi S, Gentilucci M 1993 Coordination between the transport and the grasp component during prehension movements. Exp Brain Res 94:471–477

Desmurget M, Prablanc C, Rossetti Y et al 1995 Postural and synergic control for three-dimensional movements of reaching and grasping. J Neurophysiol 74:905–910

Desmurget M, Jordan M, Prablanc C, Jeannerod M 1997 Constrained and unconstrained movements involve different control strategies. J Neurophysiol 77:1644–1650

Faillenot I, Toni I, Decety J, Gregoire M-C, Jeannerod M 1997 Visual pathways for object-oriented action and for object recognition: functional anatomy with PET. Cereb Cortex 7:77–85

Gentilucci M, Castiello U, Colladini ML, Scarpa M, Ulmita C, Rizzolatti G 1991 Influence of different types of grasping on the transport component of prehension movements. Neuropsychologia 29:361–378

Gomi H, Kawato M 1996 Equilibrium-point control hypothesis examined by measured arm stiffness during multijoint movement. Science 272:117–120

Haggard P, Wing AM 1991 Remote responses to perturbation in human prehension. Neurosci Lett 122:103–108

Hoff B, Arbib MA 1993 Models of trajectory formation and temporal interaction of reach and grasp. J Mot Behav 25:175–192

Hogan N, Flash T 1987 Moving gracefully: quantitative theories of motor coordination. Trends Neurosci 10:170–174

Iberall T, Bingham G, Arbib MA 1986 Opposition space as a structuring concept for the analysis of skilled hand movements. Exp Brain Res Suppl 15:158–173

Jakobson LS, Goodale MA 1991 Factors affecting higher-order movement planning: a kinematic analysis of human prehension. Exp Brain Res 86:199–208

Jeannerod M 1981 Intersegmental coordination during reaching at natural visual objects. In: Long J, Baddeley A (eds) Attention and performance IX. Lawrence Erlbaum Associates Inc, Hillsdale, NJ, p 153–168

Jeannerod M 1984 The timing of natural prehension movements. J Mot Behav 16:235–254

Jeannerod M 1997 The cognitive neuroscience of action. Blackwell, Oxford

Jeannerod M, Biguer B 1982 Visuomotor mechanisms in reaching within extrapersonal space. In: Ingle D, Goodale MA, Mansfield R (eds) Advances in the analysis of visual behavior. MIT Press, Cambridge, p 387–409

Jeannerod M, Decety J, Michel F 1994 Impairment of grasping movements following a bilateral posterior parietal lesion. Neuropsychologia 32:369–380

Kudoh N, Hattori M, Numata N, Maruyama K 1997 An analysis of spatiotemporal variability during prehension movements: effects of object size and distance. Exp Brain Res 117:457–464

Marteniuk RG, Leavitt JL, MacKenzie CL, Athenes S 1990 Functional relationships between grasp and transport components in a prehension task. Hum Mov Sci 9:149–176

Morasso P 1981 Spatial control of arm movements. Exp Brain Res 42:223–227

Napier JR 1955 Form and function of the carpo-metacarpal joint of the thumb. J Anat 89:362–369

Paulignan Y, MacKenzie CL, Marteniuk RG, Jeannerod M 1991a Selective perturbation of visual input during prehension movements. 1. The effects of changing object position. Exp Brain Res 83:502–512

Paulignan Y, Jeannerod M, MacKenzie C, Marteniuk R 1991b Selective perturbation of visual input during prehension movements. 2. The effects of changing object size. Exp Brain Res 87:407–420

Paulignan Y, Frak VG, Toni I, Jeannerod M 1997 Influence of object position and size on human prehension movements. Exp Brain Res 114:226–234

Rosenbaum DA, Marchak F, Barnes HJ, Vaughan J, Slotta JD, Jorgensen MJ 1990 Constraints for action selection. Overhand versus underhand grips. In: Jeannerod M (ed) Motor representation and control. Attention and performance XIII. Lawrence Erlbaum Associates Inc, Hillsdale, NJ, p 321–342

Soechting JF, Flanders M 1992 Moving in three-dimensional space: frames of reference, vectors and coordinate systems. Annu Rev Neurosci 15:167–191

Soechting JF, Flanders M 1993 Parallel, interdependent channels for location and orientation in sensorimotor transformations for reaching and grasping. J Neurophysiol 70:1137–1150

Stelmach GE, Castiello U, Jeannerod M 1994 Orienting the finger opposition space during prehension movements. J Mot Behav 26:178–186

Wolpert DM, Ghahramani Z, Jordan MI 1995 An internal model for sensorimotor integration. Science 269:1880–1882

Zaal FT, Bootsma RJ 1993 Accuracy demands in natural prehension. Hum Mov Sci 12:339–345

DISCUSSION

Andersen: Using your channel idea, have you looked at errors that might arise from the perceptual system to see whether there is a separate perceptual apparatus for grasp and for reach? If you make a mis-estimation of distance, for instance, does that cause you to reach too short and have a grasp that's too small, or do both have independent errors, thus suggesting the same distance might be computed twice by two separate systems?

Jeannerod: This question raises a number of issues. The first relates to visual control of the ongoing movement. Several investigators have carried out experiments in which the hand is masked during reaching and grasping. Although this does affect the movement to some extent, it hardly changes the pattern of the movement as it develops. There is perhaps a slight change to the peak velocity and the duration is a little longer. The shaping of the fingers will be appropriate, with maybe a slightly larger maximum grip aperture. Some people have conjectured that the faster or the further the movement goes, the task difficulty increases, with a tendency to open the fingers more in order to get a larger safety margin. To answer your question specifically, I don't think there is any experiment trying to analyse separately the reach or the grasp.

Thach: Three years ago, Bastian studied a question of coordination of pinch and reach in my laboratory (Bastian & Thach 1995). We looked at patients who had lesions of the lateral cerebellum and dentate (superior cerebellar artery territory infarcts). They were unable to coordinate fingers and arm segments in a pinch and a reach: they would overshoot the target and fail to close thumb and index finger on the target simultaneously. We contrasted that result with those patients who had small infarcts of the cerebellar thalamus, which receives the output of dentate and projects to the cerebral motor cortex. These thalamic patients could not coordinate the pinch but had a normal reach. We interpreted this as showing that the coordination mechanisms for pinch were expressed at the dentate to thalamic projection, whereas those for reach projected from dentate through brainstem mechanisms to the spinal cord. Nevertheless, the level of organization for reach *and* pinch was in the lateral cerebellum.

Jeannerod: We have seen only one patient out of many patients with parietal lesions who had a specific grasp deficit. She was not able to make the appropriate opening of the fingers and to close them at the right time, even though her reach was very good. This is one case where the two components can be separated out. The people working with monkeys could probably add a great deal to this because they have made specific small lesions.

Rizzolatti: In monkeys a selective deficit of grasping movements is obtained by inactivating parietal area AIP (Gallese et al 1994). Reaching is not affected. Recently, we found a similar selective grasping deficit following muscimol injection in monkey premotor area F5 that is heavily connected with area AIP (for a preliminary account see Gallese et al 1997).

Savaki: Dr Jeannerod, in your introduction you suggested that the anatomical substrate of reaching and grasping movements is lateralized. You mentioned that reaching pathways have been reported to be located in the ipsilateral cerebral hemisphere, in contrast to grasping pathways which are located in the hemisphere contralateral to the active forelimb. In a study using the quantitative [^{14}C]deoxyglucose method (Sokoloff et al 1977), we demonstrated that it is always the motor cortex in the cerebral hemisphere contralateral to the moving forelimb which is active during visually guided unimanual reaching movements (Savaki et al 1993). In contrast to Brinkman & Kuypers' (1972) early suggestion about ipsilateral cerebral control of the reaching forelimb, we have demonstrated that M1 in the cerebral hemisphere contralateral to the moving forelimb leads the limb reaching to visual targets even when this hemisphere is surgically 'blinded' after optic tract section combined with forebrain commissuorotomy (Savaki et al 1993). We have also demonstrated that M1 cortex in the 'blind' contralateral cerebral hemisphere which leads the forelimb reaching to visual targets is activated simultaneously with a pontocerebellar pathway, which includes the ipsilateral cerebellar paravermal and lateral hemispheric extensions of lobules V, VI and VIII (Savaki et al 1996).

Jeannerod: I only used the Brinkman and Kuypers experiment to show that the control of the reach includes both ipsilateral and contralateral pathways. This is different from the control of the grasp, which is exclusively contralateral. This was the main idea.

Goodale: I want to return to the question that Richard Andersen raised about the possible differential contribution of vision to grasp and reach. There are at least two pieces of evidence on this, each of which contradicts the other — one piece of evidence suggests that there is some shared processing in the visual control of the reach and grasp components, and another suggests that the visual processing for grasp may be separate from the visual processing for reach. When people are tested monocularly, they typically underestimate the distance of the object they are trying to pick up, and they also end up with a smaller grip — suggesting that there is some coupling of the visual analysis of distance for both grasp and reach (Servos et al 1992). On the other hand, patient DF, who has problems recognizing the shapes and sizes of objects, does not scale her grasp to the size of the goal object when tested monocularly (Marotta et al 1997). It appears as if her retinal image of the goal is unscaled for distance when binocular vision is not available. Therefore, she reaches with a larger grip to things that are closer to her. But not all her behaviour has been uncoupled from the appropriate distance scaling. Surprisingly, she continues to reach to the right place under monocular testing. Thus, even though she's not using distance properly to scale her retinal image size, she's reaching the correct distance to the object. It looks as though at some level there's shared visual processing, but at some other level the two computations involve some different levels of analysis.

Andersen: The lesion would take out most of the parietal cortex.

Goodale: This woman is a visual form agnosic — presumably because of damage to the ventral stream. She has no problems reaching, except monocularly. This suggests that the visuomotor system controlling grasp prefers to use binocular vision, falling back on things like pictorial cues only as a back-up. Pictorial cues would have to be supplied by the ventral stream.

Jeannerod: Maybe we shouldn't concentrate only on this aspect of correlation between reach and grasp. There is another set of arguments, which I didn't have time to develop, which comes from the timing of an action. If we look at the timing, there are more arguments in favour of some sort of holistic or global programming than for separate processing.

For example, if one measures the time of activation of the extensor of the finger (grasping) and of the biceps (reaching), one finds that the two muscles are activated at almost the same time, within a few milliseconds. Of course, due to inertia of the segments, the first movement to appear is the finger movement and then the onset of the reach. There is also an almost constant relationship between peak velocity of the reach and maximum grip aperture. If one considers that the two components stop at the same time at the object location, all these temporal landmarks speak in favour of global programming.

Glickstein: The question of whether reaching and grasping are independently controlled and the extent to which they are linked is a problem which several people in this room have been concerned with for a number of years. The point that Helen Savaki raises is that, curiously enough, even though the left hemisphere has no cortical visual input, it is still used in guiding the right arm in a rapid visuomotor task.

Johansson: I understand that the control goal in the reach-to-grasp task that we are discussing is to position the digits onto the object for a stable grasp. To that end, the subject has to exploit various degrees of freedom. The constraints regarding the location of grasp axis in your experiment were rather generous from a control point of view, whereas if you would put harder constraints on the possible grasp axes the outcome may be different. However, I was particularly interested in the 'demonstration' you did during your talk, and your comment 'sometimes I may even recruit a lot of degrees of freedom, I even move my body to another position'. Indeed, I can imagine in many situations in real life that we, instead of using the primary hand, shift when we grasp objects. You mentioned in your talk that subjects prefer to select 'biomechanically more comfortable positions', implicitly suggesting that there is a trade-off between biomechanics and to which degree you recruit more or fewer degrees of freedom — some sort of cost function may be involved. I would like you to comment on this recruitment of additional behaviours in more complex situations. For instance, in difficult plumbing situations the plumber may need to use quite strange postures and movements to grasp the relevant object. Would you please comment on this increased capacity we have to recruit additional behaviours in reach-to-grasp tasks in relation to the standard reach studies in our laboratories.

Jeannerod: Of course, in our laboratory situations, we constrain the subjects. They are obliged to stay in front of the table, etc. In other situations where one has to use tools, the whole body posture must be changed to maintain mechanical efficiency. It appears that there is a tendency to use degrees of freedom that are as proximal as possible.

Marsden: In everyday life, this is the way one plays sport with a bat and ball. You bring the bat to a position to hit the ball and rotate the whole of your body to get the bat at exactly the right position at the right time.

References

Bastian AJ, Thach WT 1995 Cerebellar outflow lesions: a comparison of movement deficits resulting from lesions at the levels of the cerebellum and thalamus. Ann Neurol 38:881–892

Brinkman J, Kuypers HGJM 1972 Split brain monkeys: cerebral control of ipsilateral and contralateral arm, hand, and finger movements. Science 176:536–539

Gallese V, Murata A, Kaseda M, Niki N, Sakata H 1994 Deficit of hand preshaping after muscimol injection in monkey parietal cortex. Neuroreport 5:1525–1529

Gallese V, Fadiga L, Fogassi L, Luppino G, Murata A 1997 A parietal–frontal circuit for hand grasping movements in the monkey: evidence from reversible inactivation experiments. In: Thier P, Karnath O (eds) Parital lobe contribution to orientation in 3D space. Springer-Verlag, Heidelberg, p 256–270

Marotta JJ, Behrmann M, Goodale MA 1997 Binocular but not pictorial cues calibrate grasp in visual form agnosia. Exp Brain Res 116:113–121

Savaki HE, Kennedy C, Sokoloff M, Mishkin M 1993 Visually guided reaching with the forelimb contralateral to a 'blind' hemisphere: a metabolic mapping study in monkeys. J Neurosci 13:2772–2789

Savaki HE, Kennedy C, Sokoloff M, Mishkin M 1996 Visually guided reaching with the forelimb contralateral to a 'blind' hemisphere in the monkey: contribution of the cerebellum. Neuroscience 75:143–159

Servos P, Goodale MA, Jakobson LS 1992 The role of binocular vision in prehension: a kinematic analysis. Vision Res 32:1513–1521

Sokoloff L, Reivich M, Kennedy C et al 1977 The [^{14}C]-deoxyglucose method for the measurement of local cerebral glucose utilization: theory, procedure, and normal values in the conscious and anaesthetised albino rat. J Neurochem 28:879–916

Vision for perception and vision for action in the primate brain

Melvyn A. Goodale

Department of Psychology, Graduate Program in Neuroscience, University of Western Ontario, London, Ontario, Canada N6A 5C2

Abstract. Visual systems first evolved not to enable animals to see, but to provide distal sensory control of their movements. Vision as 'sight' is a relative newcomer to the evolutionary landscape, but its emergence has enabled animals to carry out complex cognitive operations on perceptual representations of the world. The two streams of visual processing that have been identified in the primate cerebral cortex are a reflection of these two functions of vision. The dorsal 'action' stream projecting from primary visual cortex to the posterior parietal cortex provides flexible control of more ancient subcortical visuomotor modules for the production of motor acts. The ventral 'perceptual' stream projecting from the primary visual cortex to the temporal lobe provides the rich and detailed representation of the world required for cognitive operations. Both streams process information about the structure of objects and about their spatial locations—and both are subject to the modulatory influences of attention. Each stream, however, uses visual information in different ways. Transformations carried out in the ventral stream permit the formation of perceptual representations that embody the enduring characteristics of objects and their relations; those carried out in the dorsal stream which utilize moment-to-moment information about objects within egocentric frames of reference, mediate the control of skilled actions. Both streams work together in the production of goal-directed behaviour.

1998 Sensory guidance of movement. Wiley, Chichester (Novartis Foundation Symposium 218) p 21–39

The human hand is a remarkable piece of natural engineering — an instrument that is capable of plucking a delicate flower from a branch or wielding a heavy axe to topple a tree. Control of the hand depends on a complex interplay between incoming sensory information and motor signals. The most important source of distal information for controlling the hand, particularly for directing movements at objects out there in the world, is vision. Evidence for this control can be seen as soon as we reach out to pick up an object placed before us. Not only is our arm directed towards the object but the opening between our fingers and thumb reflects the size, shape, and orientation of the object well before our hand makes contact. In this chapter, I will explore some of the routes whereby visual input is transformed into a skilled motor act, such as grasping an object. I will argue that the mechanisms involved in transforming vision into action are quite distinct from those mediating our visual experience of the world and that — contrary to our impressions about what might be going on — what we 'see' is not always what guides our actions.

Separate visual mechanisms for perception and action: evidence from neurological patients

The assertion that the visual perception of objects and the visual control of skilled actions depend on different mechanisms might appear counterintuitive. After all, it seems self-evident that the actions we direct at objects are controlled by the perceptions that we have of those objects. Evidence from neurological patients tells us otherwise however. Consider the case of DF, a young woman who developed a profound visual form agnosia following carbon monoxide-induced anoxia (Milner et al 1991). Even though DF's basic visual abilities (e.g. her visual fields, contrast sensitivity, and flicker fusion) are reasonably intact, she can no longer recognize common objects on the basis of their form or even the faces of her friends and relatives; nor can she identify even the simplest of geometric shapes. (If an object is placed in her hand, of course, she has no trouble identifying it by touch, and she can recognize people from their voices.) Remarkably, however, DF continues to show strikingly accurate guidance of her hand and finger movements when she attempts to pick up the very objects she cannot identify. Thus, when she reaches out to grasp objects of different sizes, her hand opens wider mid-flight for larger objects than it does for smaller ones, just as it does in people with normal vision (Goodale et al 1991). Similarly, she rotates her hand and wrist quite normally when she reaches out to grasp objects in different orientations. At the same time, she is quite unable to describe or distinguish between the size, orientation, and shape of different objects when they are presented to her in simple discrimination tests. In fact, this is true even when DF is asked to indicate the size or orientation of an object manually. Thus, she cannot indicate the size of an object by opening her index finger and thumb a matching amount; nor can she rotate a hand-held card to match the orientation of a visual stimulus placed in front of her (see Fig. 1). Yet, when she directs more 'automatic' visuomotor responses to these same stimuli, her grip and her wrist rotation are well calibrated (see Fig. 1). Similar dissociations can be seen in her sensitivity to object shape (Goodale et al 1994a). Even though she cannot distinguish between different objects on the basis of their outline shape, she can use this same information to guide the placement of her fingers on stable grasp points on the boundary of the object.

DF's preserved visuomotor abilities are not limited to manual prehension. In a recent study (Patla & Goodale 1997), it became clear that DF is able to negotiate obstacles as well as control subjects when she walks through a room. Thus, when

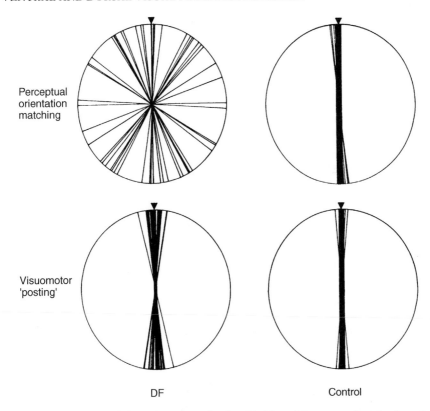

Perceptual
orientation
matching

Visuomotor
'posting'

DF   Control

FIG. 1.   Polar plots of the orientation of a hand-held card in two tasks of orientation
discrimination for the patient DF with visual agnosia and an age-matched control subject. In
the perceptual matching task (A) DF and the control subject were required to rotate the card
(without moving the card forward) until it matched the orientation of a vertically oriented slot
placed in different orientations in front of them. In the 'posting' task (B), they were required to
reach out and insert the card into the slot. In all the plots, the actual orientation of the slot has
been normalized to vertical. Adapted with permission from Goodale et al (1991).

obstacles of different heights were randomly placed in her path on different trials,
she stepped over these obstacles quite efficiently and the elevation of her toe
increased linearly as a function of obstacle height, just as it does in neurologically
intact individuals. Yet when she was asked to give verbal estimates of the height of
the obstacles, the slope of the line relating estimated and actual obstacle height was
much shallower in her case than it was in normal subjects. Similar dissociations
between perceptual judgements about the pitch of the visual field and its effect on
eye position have also been observed in DF (Servos et al 1995).

    In summary, although DF's visual system is no longer able to deliver any
perceptual information about the size, orientation, and shape of objects in the

world, the visuomotor systems in DF's brain that control the programming and execution of visually guided actions remain quite sensitive to these same object features. But what kind of brain lesion would produce such a dissociation? Although the damage in DF's brain is quite diffuse, the ventrolateral regions of her occipital lobe are particularly compromised; primary visual cortex, however, appears to be largely spared — as are the projections to the posterior parietal cortex.

But what about patients who have damage in the superior regions of the posterior parietal cortex — the visual areas that appear to be spared in DF? As it turns out, there is a long history of work showing that these patients present with a pattern of deficits and spared visual abilities that is essentially the mirror image of that seen in DF. Thus, such patients cannot use visual information about an object's location to direct a reaching movement towards it or information about its size, shape, or orientation to rotate their hand or to scale the opening of their fingers to pick up an object — even though they have no difficulty describing the size, shape, orientation, or relative location of objects in that part of the visual field (Bálint 1909, Goodale et al 1994a, Jakobson et al 1991, Jeannerod 1988, Perenin & Vighetto 1988).

Two visual systems in the primate cerebral cortex

The double dissociation of deficits in patients with different brain lesions outlined in the previous section provides compelling evidence that the human visual system does not construct a single representation of the world. Instead, vision for perception and vision for action appear to depend on separate neural mechanisms that can be differentially affected by neurological damage. Some years ago, David Milner and I (Goodale & Milner 1992) proposed that this distinction could be mapped onto the two prominent pathways or 'streams' of visual projections that were identified in the cerebral cortex of the monkey over 15 years ago by Ungerleider & Mishkin (1982): a ventral stream, which arises from primary visual cortex and projects to inferotemporal cortex, and a dorsal stream, which also arises from primary visual cortex but projects instead to the posterior parietal cortex (see Fig. 2). Additional support for this proposal comes from electrophysiological, anatomical and behavioural studies in the monkey (see following section below). Although some caution must be exercised in generalizing from monkey to human, it seems likely that the visual projections from primary visual cortex to the temporal and parietal lobes in the human brain may involve a separation into ventral and dorsal streams similar to that seen in the monkey.

Ungerleider & Mishkin (1982) originally proposed that the ventral stream plays a special role in the identification of objects, whereas the dorsal stream is responsible for localizing objects in visual space. Our re-interpretation of this

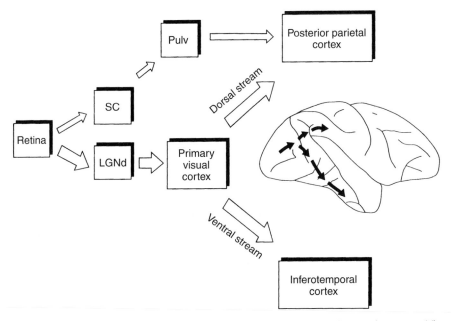

FIG. 2. Major routes whereby retinal input reaches the dorsal and ventral streams. The diagram of the macaque brain (right hemisphere) on the right of the figure shows the approximate routes of the cortico-cortical projections from primary visual cortex to the posterior parietal and the inferotemporal cortex, respectively. LGNd, lateral geniculate nucleus, pars dorsalis; Pulv, pulvinar; SC, superior colliculus. Adapted with permission from Goodale et al (1994a).

story places less emphasis on the differences in the visual information that is received by the two streams (object features versus spatial location) than it does on the differences in the transformations that the streams perform upon that information (Goodale 1993, Goodale & Milner 1992, Milner & Goodale 1993, 1995). According to our account, both streams process information about object features and about their spatial locations, but each stream uses this visual information in different ways. In the ventral stream, the transformations deliver the enduring characteristics of objects and their relations, permitting the formation of long-term perceptual representations. Such representations play an essential role in the identification of objects and enable us to classify objects and events, attach meaning and significance to them, and establish their causal relations. Such operations are essential for accumulating a knowledge base about the world. In contrast, the transformations carried out by the dorsal stream deal with moment-to-moment information about the location and disposition of objects in egocentric coordinates and thereby mediate the visual control of skilled actions, such as manual prehension, directed at those objects. In some ways then, the dorsal stream can be regarded as a cortical extension of the subcortical visual structures, such as the superior colliculus, the pretectal nuclei, and the accessory optic system, which mediate different visually guided movements in vertebrates from frogs to humans. Of course, the dorsal and ventral streams work together in controlling the rich stream of behaviour that we produce in living our complex lives. Their respective roles in this control differ however. The perceptual representations constructed by the ventral stream are part of a high-level cognitive network that enables an organism to select a particular course of action with respect to objects in the world; the visuomotor networks in the dorsal stream (and associated cortical and subcortical pathways) are responsible for the programming and online control of the particular movements that the selected action entails.

This division of labour in visual processing requires that different transformations be carried out on incoming visual information by the two streams. Consider first the task of the perceptual mechanisms in the ventral stream. To generate long-term representations of objects and their relations, perceptual mechanisms must be 'object based' so that constancies of size, shape, colour, lightness and relative location can be maintained across different viewing conditions. Some of these mechanisms might use an array of viewer-centred representations of the same object (e.g. Bülthoff & Edelman 1992); others might use a set of canonical representations (e.g. Palmer et al 1981); still others might generate representations that are truly 'object-centred' (Marr 1982). But whatever the particular coding might be, it is the identity of the object, not its disposition with respect to the observer that is of primary concern to the perceptual system. This is not the case for the visuomotor mechanisms in the dorsal stream, and other related structures, that support actions directed at that object. Here the underlying visuomotor transformations must be viewer-centred; in other words, both the location of the object and its disposition and motion must be encoded relative to the observer in egocentric coordinates, that is in retinocentric, head-centred, torso-centred, or shoulder-centred coordinates. Some object-based computations, such as those related to size, must be carried out, but even here the computations must reflect the nature of the effector system to be used. Finally, because the position and disposition of a goal object in the action space of an observer is rarely constant, such computations must be carried out on each occasion an action is performed (for a discussion of this issue, see Goodale et al 1994b). To use a computer metaphor, the action systems of the dorsal stream do most of their work online; only the perception systems of the ventral stream can afford to work offline. To summarize then, while similar (but not identical) visual information about object shape, size, local orientation, and location is available to both systems, the transformational algorithms that are applied to these inputs are uniquely tailored to the function of each system. It is the nature of the functional requirements of perception and action that lies at the root of the division of labour in the ventral and dorsal visual projection systems of the primate cerebral cortex.

Evidence from monkey studies

Electrophysiological, anatomical, and behavioural studies of the dorsal and ventral streams in the monkey lend considerable support to the distinction outlined above (for a detailed account of this work, see Milner & Goodale 1995). For example, monkeys with lesions of inferotemporal cortex, who show profound deficits in object recognition, are nevertheless as capable as normal animals at picking up small objects (Klüver & Bucy 1939), at catching flying insects (Pribram 1967), and at orienting their fingers to extract morsels of food embedded in small slots (Buchbinder et al 1980). Like DF, these monkeys are unable to discriminate between objects on the basis of the same visual features that they apparently use to direct their grasping movements. In addition to the lesion studies, there is a long history of electrophysiological work showing that cells in inferotemporal cortex and neighbouring regions of the superior temporal sulcus are tuned to specific objects and object features—and some of them maintain their selectivity irrespective of viewpoint, retinal image size and even colour (for review, see Milner & Goodale 1995). Moreover, the responses of these cells are not affected by the animal's motor behaviour but are instead sensitive to the reinforcement history and significance of the visual stimuli that drive them. It has been suggested that cells in this region might play a role in comparing current visual inputs with internal representations of recalled images (e.g. Eskandar et al 1992), which are themselves presumably stored in other regions, such as neighbouring regions of the medial temporal lobe and related limbic areas (Fahy et al 1993, Nishijo et al 1993). In fact, sensitivity to particular objects can be created in ensembles of cells in inferotemporal cortex simply by training the animals to discriminate between different objects (Logothetis et al 1995). These and other studies too numerous to cite here lend considerable support to the suggestion that the object-based descriptions provided by the ventral stream form the basic raw material for recognition memory and other long-term representations of the visual world.

In sharp contrast to the activity of cells in the ventral stream, the responses of cells in the dorsal stream are greatly dependent on the concurrent motor behaviour of the animal. Thus, separate subsets of visual cells in the posterior parietal cortex, the major terminal zone for the dorsal stream, have been shown to be implicated in visual fixation, pursuit and saccadic eye movements, visually guided reaching, and the manipulation of objects (Hyvärinen & Poranen 1974, Mountcastle et al 1975). In reviewing these studies, Andersen (1987) has pointed out that most neurons in these areas exhibit both sensory-related and movement-related activity. Moreover, the motor modulation is quite specific. Recent work in Andersen's laboratory, for example, has shown that visual cells in the posterior parietal cortex that code the location of a target for a saccadic eye movement are quite separate from cells in this region that code the location for a manual aiming movement to the same target (Snyder et al 1997). In other experiments (Taira et al 1990), cells in the posterior parietal region that fire when the monkey manipulates an object have also been shown to be sensitive to the intrinsic object features, such as size and orientation, that determine the posture of the hand and fingers during a grasping movement. Lesions in this region of the posterior parietal cortex produce deficits in the visual control of reaching and grasping similar in many respects to those seen in humans following damage to the homologous region (e.g. Ettlinger 1977). The posterior parietal cortex is also intimately linked with premotor cortex, the superior colliculus and pontine nuclei — brain areas that have also been implicated in various aspects of the visual control of eye, limb, and body movements (for review, see Goodale et al 1996). In short, the networks in the dorsal stream have the functional properties and interconnections that one might expect to see in systems concerned with the moment-to-moment control of visually guided actions. (Of necessity, this review of the monkey literature is far from complete. Interested readers are directed to Milner & Goodale [1995] and Jeannerod [1997].)

Dissociations between perception and action in normal observers

I began this paper by suggesting that the visual control of a skilled movement such as grasping depends on visual mechanisms that are quite distinct from those mediating our visual perception of the world. I went on to review evidence from both neurological patients and monkeys that supports the idea of a dorsal 'action' system and a ventral 'perception' system in the primate brain. But if visual perception and the visual control of action depend on different neural mechanisms in the human cerebral cortex, then it should be possible to demonstrate a dissociation between these two kinds of visual processing, even in neurologically intact individuals, with the right kind of task. In other words, the visual information underlying the calibration and control of a skilled motor act directed at an object might not always match the perceptual judgements made about that object.

Although there are numerous examples of such dissociations in the literature, particularly with respect to the spatial location of visual stimuli (for review, see Goodale & Haffenden 1998), some of the most compelling demonstrations have involved the use of pictorial illusions. Take the Ebbinghaus Illusion, for example. In this familiar illusion, two target circles of equal size, each surrounded by a circular array of either smaller or larger circles, are presented side by side (see Fig. 3). Subjects typically report that the target circle surrounded by the array of smaller

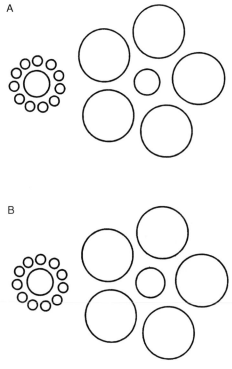

FIG. 3.   The 'Ebbinghaus' Illusion. Panel A shows the standard version of the illusion in which physically identical target circles appear perceptually different. Most people judge the target circle surrounded by the annulus of smaller circles to be larger than the other target circle. Panel B shows a version of the illusion in which the target circle surrounded by the annulus of larger circles has been made physically larger than the other target, compensating for the effect of the illusion. Most people now see the two target circles as equivalent in size. Adapted with permission from Aglioti et al (1995).

circles appears larger than the one surrounded by the array of larger circles, presumably because of the of the difference in the contrast in size between the target circles and the surrounding circles. In another version of the illusion, the target circles can be made to appear identical in size by increasing the actual size of the target circle surrounded by the larger circles (see Fig. 3).

Although our perceptual judgements are clearly affected by these manipulations of the stimulus array, there is good reason to believe that the calibration of size-dependent motor outputs, such as grip aperture during grasping, would not be. When we reach out to pick up an object, we must compute its real size if we are to pick it up efficiently; it is not enough to know that it is larger or smaller than surrounding objects. One might expect, therefore, that grip scaling would be

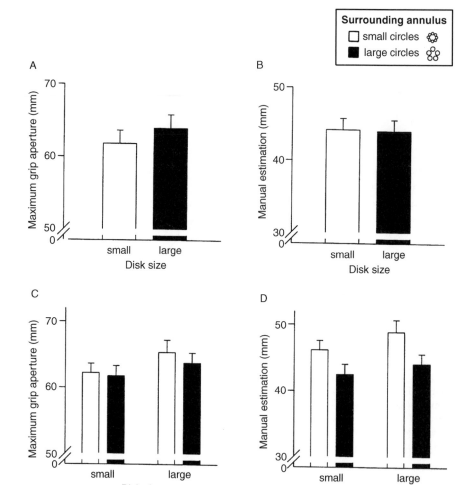

insensitive to size-contrast illusions such as the Ebbinghaus Illusion. Such a result was recently found in two experiments carried out in my laboratory (Aglioti et al 1995, Haffenden & Goodale 1998). We tested subjects with a three-dimensional version of the Ebbinghaus Illusion in which two thin 'poker-chip' disks were arranged as pairs on a standard Ebbinghaus annular circle display. Trials in which the two disks appeared perceptually identical but were physically different in size were randomly alternated with trials in which the disks appeared perceptually different but were physically identical. We found that even though subjects showed robust perceptual illusions (either by indicating whether or not the two disks appeared identical or by opening between their index finger and thumb until it matched the size of one of the disks), their grip aperture was correlated with the real size of the disk as they reached out to pick one of them up (see Fig. 4).

That perception is sensitive to pictorial illusions such as the Ebbinghaus Illusion is not surprising. Perception is by its very nature relative. Relations between objects in the visual array play a crucial role in scene interpretation and are central to the operation of the perception system. As we look out across a landscape, we cannot help but see some objects as larger or closer than others. In contrast, the execution of a goal-directed act such as grasping depends on computations that are centred on the target itself and must take into account the actual size and distance of that target — and transform that information into the coordinates of the relevant effectors.

FIG. 4. Calibration of the grasp (A and C) and manual estimations (B and D) for disks surrounded by the illusory annuli in perceptually identical but physically different conditions (A and B), and perceptually different but physically identical conditions (C and D). The difference between the maximum grip aperture achieved during a grasping movement was significantly greater for large disks than the maximum grip aperture for small disks ($P < 0.05$) independent of whether or not the subject perceived the disks to be the same or different sizes (A and C, respectively). There was no difference in maximum grip aperture between grasping movements made to the two small disks or between grasping movements made to the two large disks in the perceptual different but physically identical conditions (C). In contrast, manual estimations were influenced by the illusory display. The difference between manual estimations of the large and small disks in the perceptually identical but physically different condition (B) was not significant ($P > 0.05$). Perceptually different but physically identical disk pairs (D) produced significantly different manual estimations. The small disk surrounded by the small circle annulus was estimated to be larger than the small disk surrounded by the large circle annulus ($P < 0.01$). Manual estimations of the pair of large disks produced a similar result. The large disk surrounded by the small circle annulus was estimated to be larger than the large disk surrounded by the large circle annulus ($P < 0.05$). Error bars indicate the standard error of the mean averaged within each condition for all subjects. Adapted with permission from Haffenden & Goodale (1998).

Perception and action: complementary visual systems in the production of adaptive behaviour

Throughout this paper, I have made the point that there are two separate visual systems within the cerebral cortex of the primate brain: a ventral system that constructs our experiential visual perception of the world and a dorsal system that mediates the visual control of actions within that world. Of course, it is clear that the two systems interact and cooperate, even though they play complementary roles in the in the production of adaptive behaviour.

Consider for example the simple act of picking up a ripe pear from a basket of fruit. Your perceptual system, with its rich and detailed representation of the visual array, would enable you to discriminate the pears from the apples and other fruit in the bowl — and to select the most appealing of the several pears available. But once your perceptual system had 'flagged' a particular pear, dedicated visuomotor systems in the dorsal stream (in conjunction with related circuits in premotor cortex, the brainstem and other brain areas) would carry out the required computations to get your hand onto the pear to pick it up. Both systems are required for purposive behaviour — one system to select the goal object from the visual array, the other to carry out the required metrical computations for the goal-directed action. One of the most important questions yet to be addressed is the exact nature of the interactions between these two systems in the production of adaptive behaviour.

References

Aglioti S, DeSouza JFX, Goodale MA 1995 Size-contrast illusions deceive the eye but not the hand. Curr Biol 5:679–685
Andersen RA 1987 The role of the inferior parietal lobule function in spatial perception and visuomotor integration. In: Plum F, Mountcastle VB, Geiger SR (eds) Handbook of physiology, section 1: The nervous system, vol V: Higher functions of the brain, part 2. American Physiology Association, Bethesda, MD, p 483–518
Bálint R 1909 Seelenlähmung des 'Schauens', optische Ataxie, räumliche Störung der Aufmerksamkeit. Monatsschr Psychiatr Neurol 25:51–81
Buchbinder S, Dixon B, Hyang Y-W, May JG, Glickstein M 1980 The effects of cortical lesions on visual guidance of the hand. Soc Neurosci Abstr 6:675
Bülthoff HH, Edelman S 1992 Psychophysical support for a two-dimensional view interpolation theory of object recognition. Proc Natl Acad Sci USA 89:60–64
Eskandar EM, Richmond BJ, Optican LM 1992 Role of inferior temporal neurons in visual memory: I. Temporal encoding of information about visual images, recalled images and behavioral context. J Neurophysiol 68:1277–1295
Ettlinger G 1977 Parietal cortex in visual orientation. In: Rose FC (ed) Physiological aspects of clinical neurology. Blackwell, Oxford, p 93–100
Fahy FL, Riches IP, Brown MW 1993 Neuronal signals of importance to the performance of visual recognition memory tasks: evidence from recordings of single neurones in the medial thalamus of primates. In: Hicks TP, Molotchnikoff S, Ono T (eds) Progress in brain research,

vol 95: The visually responsive neuron: from basic physiology to behavior. Elsevier Science BV, Amsterdam, p 401–416

Goodale MA 1993 Visual pathways supporting perception and action in the primate cerebral cortex. Curr Opin Neurobiol 3:578–585

Goodale MA, Haffenden A 1998 Frames of reference for perception and action in the human visual system. Neurosci Biobehav Rev 22:161–172

Goodale MA, Milner AD 1992 Separate visual pathways for perception and action. Trends Neurosci 15:20–25

Goodale MA, Milner AD, Jakobson LS, Carey DP 1991 A neurological dissociation between perceiving objects and grasping them. Nature 349:154–156

Goodale MA, Meenan JP, Bülthoff HH, Nicolle DA, Murphy KJ, Racicot CI 1994a Separate neural pathways for the visual analysis of object shape in perception and prehension. Curr Biol 4:604–610

Goodale MA, Jakobson LS, Keillor JM 1994b Differences in the visual control of pantomimed and natural grasping movements. Neuropsychology 32:1159–1178

Goodale MA, Jakobson LS, Servos P 1996 The visual pathways mediating perception and prehension. In: Flanagan R, Haggard P, Wing A (eds) Sensorimotor control of the hand. Academic Press, New York, p 15–31

Haffenden AM, Goodale MA 1998 The effect of pictorial illusion on prehension and perception. J Cogn Neurosci 10:122–136

Hyvärinen J, Poranen A 1974 Function of the parietal associative area 7 as revealed from cellular discharges in alert monkeys. Brain 97:673–692

Jakobson LS, Archibald YM, Carey DP, Goodale MA 1991 A kinematic analysis of reaching and grasping movements in a patient recovering from optic ataxia. Neuropsychology 29:803–809

Jeannerod M 1988 The neural and behavioral organization of goal-directed movements. Oxford University Press, Oxford

Jeannerod M 1997 The cognitive neuroscience of action. Blackwell, Oxford

Klüver H, Bucy PC 1939 Preliminary analysis of functions of the temporal lobes of monkeys. Arch Neurol Psychiatr 42:979–1000

Logothetis NK, Pauls J, Poggio T 1995 Shape representation in the inferior temporal cortex of monkeys. Curr Biol 5:552–563

Marr D 1982 Vision. Freeman, San Francisco

Milner AD, Goodale MA 1993 Visual pathways to perception and action. In: Hicks TP, Molotchnikoff S, Ono T (eds) Progress in brain research, vol 95: The visually responsive neuron: from basic physiology to behavior. Elsevier Science BV, Amsterdam, p 317–338

Milner AD, Goodale MA 1995 The visual brain in action. Oxford University Press, Oxford

Milner AD, Perrett DI, Johnston RS et al 1991 Perception and action in "visual form agnosia". Brain 114:405–428

Mountcastle VB, Lynch JC, Georgopoulos A, Sakata H, Acuna C 1975 Posterior parietal association cortex of the monkey: command functions for operations within extrapersonal space. J Neurophysiol 38:871–908

Nishijo H, Ono T, Tamura R, Nakamura K 1993 Amygdalar and hippocampal neuron responses related to recognition and memory in monkey. In: Hicks TP, Molotchnikoff S, Ono T (eds) Progress in brain research, vol 95: The visually responsive neuron: from basic physiology to behavior. Elsevier Science BV, Amsterdam, p 339–358

Palmer S, Rosch E, Chase P 1981 Canonical perspective and the perception of objects. In: Long J, Baddeley A (eds) Attention and performance, vol IX. Lawrence Erlbaum, Hillsdale, NJ, p 135–151

Patla A, Goodale MA 1997 Visuomotor transformation required for obstacle avoidance during locomotion is unaffected in a patient with visual form agnosia. Neuroreport 8:165–168

Perenin M-T, Vighetto A 1988 Optic ataxia: a specific disruption in visuomotor mechanisms, I.
    Different aspects of the deficit in reaching for objects. Brain 111:643–674
Pribram KH 1967 Memory and the organization of attention. In: Lindsley DB, Lumsdaine AA
    (eds) Brain function and learning. University of California Press, Berkeley (UCLA Forum
    Med Sci 6), p 79–122
Servos P, Matin L, Goodale MA 1995 Dissociations between two forms of spatial processing by
    a visual form agnosic. Neuroreport 6:1893–1896
Snyder LH, Batista AP, Andersen RA 1997 Coding of intention in the posterior parietal cortex.
    Nature 386:167–170
Taira M, Mine S, Georgopoulos AP, Murata A, Sakata H 1990 Parietal cortex neurons of the
    monkey related to the visual guidance of hand movement. Exp Brain Res 83:29–36
Ungerleider LG, Mishkin M 1982 Two cortical visual systems. In: Ingle DJ, Goodale MA,
    Mansfield RJW (eds) Analysis of visual behavior. MIT Press, Cambridge, MA, p 549–586

DISCUSSION

Rizzolatti: I found your observation that DF has problems in copying the order of coloured targets very interesting (Murphy et al 1998). This indicates — I think for the first time — that DF has some spatial deficits. Yet DF's spatial behaviour is basically normal. She uses space as normal people do, she describes correctly what is on her right and on her left, and so on. In other words she perceives space. It seems to me, therefore, that the dichotomy that you and David Milner suggested between perception and action as functions of different brain 'streams' needs specification. Space perception is, basically, a function of the dorsal stream (the action stream) and not of the ventral stream.

Goodale: It depends on what you mean by perception of space. Space is one of the only commodities the nervous system uses. Another one is time. You have to act in space.

Rizzolatti: Would you therefore put space outside the domain of perception?

Goodale: No, I'm suggesting that the computations for the visual control of eye movements or hand movements eventually all require different frames of reference with respect to particular aspects of space. Similarly, in order to recognize an object, you would have to appreciate something about the spatial relationship between the elements that make up that object. Clearly, people with severe posterior parietal damage can recognize objects, so some appreciation of the spatial relationship amongst the components of an object must remain in order for them to do that.

Thier: You have followed this patient for many years. Is there any evidence of some sort of recovery of function in the sense that one system might take over the function of another?

Goodale: Not exactly. On some of our perception tests, however, she is able to use her visuomotor system to perform the task correctly. I'm not suggesting that she perceives things with her visuomotor system, but she can perform better on the perception test by using a visuomotor strategy. For example, we can no longer test her on the orientation-matching task, where she is asked to rotate her hand in place to match the orientation of a slot placed in front of her. When she was first tested 10 years ago, DF couldn't match her hand to the orientation of the slot, but now she can — by using an intention movement. She makes a slight 'posting' movement toward the slot which presumably captures some of the motor programming required, and then she uses the resulting position of her hand as her matching response (Murphy et al 1996).

Mattingley: You gave evidence for an apparent double dissociation between two kinds of neurological patient: your visual form agnosic DF, who apparently has impaired perception but reasonable action, and an optic ataxic patient with the opposite pattern. They obviously fit neatly into the ventral/dorsal distinction. But you didn't mention a third group of neurological patients: those who have visuospatial neglect. These neglect patients have what you might think is dorsal stream damage — posterior parietal damage in the classic 'textbook' kind of case. Such individuals clearly have impaired awareness and impaired perception for objects and events on their contralesional side of space. How do you think that visuospatial neglect patients fit into your dorsal/ventral distinction?

Goodale: David Milner and I have grappled with that question. The first pass at an answer is that optic ataxia and visual neglect are neurologically dissociable. Although they often occur together, because nature doesn't respect functional boundaries, one can find patients who have optic ataxia who don't have visual neglect, and vice versa. Therefore, there's clearly some functional modularity. The optic ataxia patients are those who have damage to the human homologue of the monkey dorsal stream, and the patients with visual neglect have damage to more ventral regions of the parietal cortex that are as yet poorly specified in terms of function. There is evidence for an interaction between object-based and egocentric coordinates in some cases of neglect following damage to this region of the parietal cortex. Perhaps it represents an interaction of sorts between the dorsal and ventral streams. Neglect (unlike optic ataxia) tends to arise more from damage to the right than the left hemisphere — as does visuospatial memory loss from damage to the temporal lobe, presumably because of damage to mesial structures in the temporal lobe that are linked with the ventral stream. In other words, the association of neglect with damage to the right hemisphere may have something to do with the lateralization of visual functions in the human ventral stream and may have nothing at all to do with what is happening in the dorsal stream.

Miles: I have a comment concerning your view that signals in the dorsal stream are not perceived. How do you account for the data from Bill Newsome's group (Newsome & Paré 1994, Salzman & Newsome 1994, Salzman et al 1992, Britten et al 1992), which show that MT neurons provide motor signals for perceptual judgements?

Goodale: MT is interesting, because it might be looked on as a kind of add-on to primary visual cortex. Perhaps it is a specialized system for doing motion processing. It feeds both dorsal and ventral streams, and although classically it is placed in the dorsal stream, it has lots of projections to the ventral stream. Presumably, it is via these projections to the ventral stream that MT plays a role in things like structure-from-motion (and even the perception of motion *per se*). At the same time, MT also clearly feeds into areas in the dorsal stream that are important for the guidance of limb movements.

Jeannerod: We must be careful when we infer dichotomies such as perception/action or conscious/unconscious from patients. Consider, for example, a positron emission tomography (PET) experiment in normal subjects where brain activity is compared during visuomotor transformation and during a task of matching shapes (a purely perceptual task without any motor demands). If one looks at the areas involved during the matching task, one finds areas which light up in the posterior parietal cortex (PPC). I don't think it would be true to say that the PPC is devoid of subjective experience and doesn't participate in perception. Patients with PPC lesions are also sometimes unable to draw objects, and may even have difficulty identifying objects when they are presented in a non-canonical orientation. Thus this whole dichotomy runs into difficulty.

Goodale: I may have over-emphasized the dichotomy between the two streams in developing my argument. I'm trying to sharpen some of the distinctions between the way in which people have regarded the nature of the operation of the dorsal and ventral streams. That is, I'm trying to move away from a purely perception-based account, towards an account that looks at the streams in terms of the output systems that they serve. Of course, both dorsal and ventral have to work in an integrated fashion. I also don't think that the parietal cortex is devoid of contact with subjective conscious experience; it's just a question of whether or not that experience is visual. That is, you might have all kinds of subjective experience about performing actions, and perhaps this requires some input from the parietal cortex and so on. But appreciating the visual cues that are actually used to calibrate your grasp is another matter. You do not have access to that visual input. Instead, your ventral stream provides you with perception of the goal object and your moving hand. But the actual visual information that is controlling your grasp is inaccessible to conscious experience.

Andersen: The results of your copying experiment appear similar to constructional apraxia, a deficit also found in parietal lobe lesions. Do you think this similarity is an example of space being used in both streams? How would you then reinterpret the constructional apraxia effect which occurs with parietal lesions? Do you think the parietal deficit is perhaps a visuomotor object ataxia?

Goodale: I think constructional apraxia, like visual neglect, is a bit of a rag bag.

Andersen: Have you tried your parietal lesioned patient with this particular task?

Goodale: No, we haven't been able to get her to come into the lab again. I don't have any great insights into the nature of constructional apraxia, because I don't understand it yet. I suspect that individuals with a number of different neurological problems could show deficits that might be described as constructional apraxia.

Lemon: I'm interested in seeing how far this model will go when you're dealing with having to act in a very complex environment. What we have seen so far involves extremely simple objects which you reach out and pick up, but there must be situations when you're having to guide your hand through various obstacles and where the object you're looking for is embedded in a very complex background in which both visual and metric discrimination is necessary.

Goodale: By using these simple situations, one can study the separate operation of the two streams. But you are correct: in a complex task such as looking in a kitchen drawer for a spatula, both streams are involved and there's a lot of interaction between them. Object information tells you that the object is a spatula and stored information about its function helps you to shape your hand appropriately. But at the same time, when you reach out to pick up the spatula you also have to scale your grasp for the size, shape and orientation of the particular spatula in the drawer. Thus, there is an interplay between information from the ventral and dorsal stream in the performance of everyday actions. Some of the time, however, the control of actions is 'handed off' completely to the dorsal stream and its attendant sensorimotor systems — and the actions are controlled quite autonomously. For example, you can continue to walk around the kitchen drying the dishes and having a conversation with your spouse without bumping into things.

Wolpert: The examples you've shown us are situations in which DF acts on the world. Is there any difference when the world acts on her? For example, if you move an object towards her and ask her to grasp it, does she show an appropriate grip?

Goodale: As far as we can see, yes. She can catch a ball, within limits, reasonably well. If you extend your hand towards her, and she is in a situation where she is anticipating this, she will extend her hand in the right direction.

Hoffmann: You have given interesting results about abolishing stereoopsis by covering one eye (Marotta et al 1997). Of course, one thing that is missing under such circumstances is a vergence signal. If you cover one eye the subject no longer makes vergence eye movements.

Goodale: I'm not suggesting it is stereo: I was careful to use the term binocular.

Hoffmann: My question is: do you have a special idea of how the true stereoscopic system acts in the dorsal versus the ventral stream of visual processing?

Passingham: Alan Cowey showed some time ago that inferotemporal lesions have a severe effect on global stereopsis as tested with random dot stereograms (Cowey & Porter 1979).

Stein: But that's because they affect vergence.

Andersen: There has been a lot of work on stereo processing in the dorsal stream, but Fujita and colleagues have recently shown that a substantial proportion of inferotemporal neurons also show disparity tuning (Uka et al 1997). Their results for IT look surprisingly similar to what is found in MT, for instance — there are a lot of near cells and far cells but not many excitatory tuned cells. It appears that the two pathways both use stereo.

Goodale: It might be interesting to see the nature of the stereo that they use, and in particular whether one is more concerned with relative stereo judgements while the other combines vertical disparities and/or vergence with horizontal disparities to deliver metrically accurate (or absolute) judgements about where things are. The latter is certainly what you would need for grasp. If you are going to use stereo, you have got to know where something is in real-world metrics.

Hoffmann: Your patients substitute something by stereopsis, because if you take stereopsis away, they can't perform the task.

Goodale: They perform the task in a way that shows that they're still using some information about the retinal image size, but it seems to be rather uncalibrated. When the object is closer to them, they open their hand wider.

Hoffmann: Is that when they use one eye only?

Goodale: Yes.

Hoffmann: But if they use both eyes they are fine. Therefore my guess would be that it is the vergence system which is providing the information.

Miles: So far as I am aware, all of the disparity-selective neurons in the neurophysiological literature pertain to *absolute* disparity, which is poorly perceived in depth. To date, there have been no convincing demonstrations of neuronal responses specifically selective for *relative* disparity, which is the basis for the perception of depth in most of the psychophysical literature. Thus the relevance of the disparity signals described in the dorsal and ventral streams for the perception of stereo is far from clear.

Goodale: I agree. This is true of so many psychophysical phenomena, where people have asked for perceptual judgements about objects or surfaces, but they have not always appreciated the fact that if they were to look at how someone reaches out to pick something up, they might get entirely different psychophysics.

Marsden: I'd like to broaden the discussion. In analysis of human patients we run into the problem of what are the human homologues of monkey parietal lobes. We are using terms such as superior parietal and inferior parietal for monkey brain. I would value some guidance as to what equivalent areas we are talking about in the human being.

Goodale: The degree of homology between the human and monkey parietal cortex is still an unresolved issue for many people.

Passingham: I have just reviewed the PET data for the human brain and single-unit data for monkeys (Passingham 1998). It seems to me that there is no reason to think that there is any difference in general layout of the parietal cortex in the human as opposed to the monkey brain. In the human brain there is visual activation dorsally in area 7, but in monkeys there are visually responsive cells in area MIP in the upper bank of the intraparietal sulcus. Even Brodmann identified an area 7 dorsally at the back of the intraparietal sulcus in the monkey brain. Furthermore, the distinction Brodmann drew between areas 40 and 39 in inferior parietal cortex probably corresponds to the distinction between areas 7b and 7a in the monkey brain.

Glickstein: A lesion of the posterior parietal areas of monkeys produces motor symptoms which are almost indistinguishable from those described by the classical neurologists for humans. David Ferrier's description of the deficit in monkeys is almost identical to that of Bálint and Holmes of their patients with parietal lobe lesions.

Rizzolatti: I fully agree with Dick Passingham. The layout of parietal lobe is very similar in humans and monkeys. The notion that there is a substantial difference in parietal cytoarchitecture between the two species is essentially due the use of Brodmann nomenclature. Since the work of von Bonin & Bailey (1947) it is clear that areas PE (superior parietal lobule), and PF and PG (inferior parietal lobule) constitute the main subdivisions of the posterior parietal lobe in humans and monkeys.

References

Britten KH, Shadlen MN, Newsome WT, Movshon JA 1992 The analysis of visual motion: a comparison of neuronal and psychophysical performance. J Neurosci 12:4745–4765

Cowey A, Porter J 1979 Brain damage and global stereopsis. Proc Roy Soc Lond B 204:399–407

Marotta JJ, Behrmann M, Goodale MA 1997 The removal of binocular cues disrupts the calibration of grasping in patients with visual form agnosia. Exp Brain Res 116:113–121

Murphy K, Racicot C, Goodale MA 1996 The use of visuomotor cues as a strategy for making perceptual judgements in a patient with visual form agnosia. Neuropsychology 10:396–401

Murphy K, Carey DP, Goodale MA 1998 The perception of spatial relations in a patient with visual form agnosia. Cogn Neuropsychol, in press

Newsome WT, Paré EB 1988 A selective impairment of motion perception following lesions of the middle temporal visual area (MT). J Neurosci 8:2201–2211

Passingham RE 1998 The specialization of the human cerebral cortex. In: Milner AD (ed) Brain and cognition in monkeys, apes and man. Oxford Univ Press, Oxford, p 271–298

Salzman CD, Newsome WT 1994 Neural mechanisms for forming a perceptual decision. Science 264:231–237

Salzman CD, Murasugi CM, Britten KH, Newsome WT 1992 Microstimulation in visual area MT: effects on direction discrimination performance. J Neurosci 12:2331–2355

Uka T, Tanaka H, Kato M, Fujita I 1997 Disparity sensitivity and representation of 3-dimensional surface structure in monkey inferior temporal cortex. Soc Neurosci Abstr 23:2063

von Bonin G, Bailey P 1947 The neocortex of *Macaca mulatta*. University of Illinois Press, Urbana

General discussion I

Glickstein: It is probably reasonable to believe that a particular region of cortex has a particular function. The cortex is a laminar structure with six to 14 layers, depending on which region of it you look at. The number six is arbitrary. In the posterior parietal cortex of a rat, layer 5 has a massive projection to subcortical structures: every single cell in the deeper sublayer 5B goes to the pontine nuclei and thus relays to the cerebellum. Every cell in 5A probably projects to the basal ganglia. The idea that a single cortical area has to be committed to either visual recognition or visually guiding movement is not necessarily true. It could be that the same structure is in fact providing an input to two or more totally different circuits.

Georgopoulos: How can we talk about the function of a given cortical area, if the projections from different layers can be so different? Could one, for example, suppose that a given area does serve one function, and that different projections subserve a different function? Is there any evidence that, for example, selective lesion of an area of layer 3 would produce a different effect from a lesion of layer 5? Do these differential layer projections serve a different function, or are they all part of the same function subserved by different layer-specific dynamical circuits?

Glickstein: Your comment makes me think about a magic machine which would allow me to make a laminar lesion! The first laminar lesion I would make would be in layer 6, because of the massive cortico-thalamic projection from lamina 6 back onto lateral geniculate or other thalamic relays.

Rizzolatti: I am not so sure that cortical functions are so specifically reflected in laminar subdivisions.

Glickstein: It is quite the reverse in the rat. Lamina 5 has two visible and clear subdivisions: 5A goes to the basal ganglia, 5B goes to the pons and hence to the cerebellum. There is a tiny tier of cells between 5A and 5B that probably projects to both. Monkeys (and doubtless humans) have at least 32 visual areas and the rat has seven. Have humans got 25 more visual areas than a rat or is each one of the rat's seven doing five or six jobs? I think that humans have 25 more.

Hoffmann: I have an example from another system. Even if you look at one functional complex such as slow eye movements, there are separate projections from the same cortical area by distinct populations of cells, i.e. one population subserving slow phases during OKN projects to the *accessory optic nuclei*, whereas another population, intermingled with the first, subserving smooth pursuit,

40

projects to the *pontine nuclei*. This argument, made by Mitchell Glickstein, is extremely important. The same area contributes to a whole set of functions with its different projections. The function you will see for an area is the one you test.

Kalaska: Following up on that, probably everyone in the room is aware of the work of Eb Fetz, Paul Cheney and Chris Fromm (Fetz et al 1996, Fromm 1983, Bauswein et al 1989) looking at the response properties of cells projecting to different targets. The work of Chris Fromm, in particular, suggests that even within primary motor cortex, the properties of cells that are projecting to a particular structure match the properties of the cells in that target structure. There will be more similarity between a particular output cell and its targets than with its neighbouring cells in the motor cortex which project to other structures. The function of the motor cortex, then, is not a product of a homogeneous set of response properties of the population of cells in that area, but rather how that entire ensemble of cells interacts with its targets, and how they then interact in turn. Function isn't defined just by a common response property across all the cells in a given area.

Glickstein: We recorded from cells in the visual cortex of the cat and identified those cells which project to the pontine nuclei. If you record from area 18 of a cat—an area well described by Hubel & Wiesel (1965)—the cells respond as Hubel and Wiesel described with complex and hypercomplex (receptive) fields and sharp orientation tuning. Deep in cortex you record from cells with different properties—there is no orientation tuning. All are directionally selective and all are responsive to the velocity of targets. These are the cells that project to the pontine nuclei. The receptive fields are indistinguishable from pontine visual cells except for their size. Whereas the receptive field of a cell in area 18 might be 3 by 4 degrees, in the pons it could be as big as 50 by 50 degrees or an entire hemifield. Thus the cells of this lamina are doing a different computation from the cells above.

Passingham: I agree that one can discuss the different functional properties of cell groups in different layers. But that does not mean that one cannot also discuss the functional properties of the whole cell population in an area. And the unique functions of an area are a function of its unique pattern of connections: it is because of its particular connections that an area can perform its specific operation. Conceptually, there is no problem in discussing the particular functions of a particular brain area.

Hoffmann: I think the point is that there are both intracortical and cortical–subcortical connections. In that respect one may discuss whether all these connections are subserving the same function or whether the area can be active in quite different functions depending on whether layer 5 or layer 3 is involved, for instance.

Passingham: What we must avoid is thinking that an area performs a behavioural task. Whatever an area does, the specific operation that it performs will be needed in a wide range of such tasks. And to perform that operation it will need to interact with other areas, both cortical and subcortical.

Ebner: There would be a computational problem if you wanted to have very specific functions for specific circuits. Circuits as well as cortical areas may be multifunctional, and to try to assign unique functions at the level of individual layers and circuits may be dangerous. We haven't talked about the temporal domain at all yet, and I think the information that flows across these circuits and areas changes dynamically with time and with task. Assigning function to architecture is going to be difficult.

Thach: If in a cortical area where there is an identified function there are systematic projections of one layer to one subcortical structure and also to another cortical structure, the presumption is that the subcortical is being brought in to somehow supplement the performance. But the cortical and subcortical contributions could be radically different. There could be reciprocal effects; the subcortical structure might be brought in when the cortical structure is not and vice versa. The functional consequence of this kind of anatomy is something that you can tell only with unit recording and human activation studies.

Glickstein: Let me make an analogy to the retinal ganglion cells. Cajal in 1892 showed that the inner plexiform zone was wonderfully stratified (Cajal 1892). The stratification is formed of dendritic extensions from the ganglion cells and the amacrine cells. The retina constructs at least five different classes of receptive fields, all going to different targets and all doing functionally different things. It is a wonderful analogy for what the cortex might be doing. Because they rely on graded conduction, retinas can't be very thick — the retina of a mouse is about the same thickness as the retina of a whale. All retinas have a laminated inner plexiform zone, constructing receptive fields that are appropriate for one or another target or task.

Fetz: The problem in trying to assign specific functions to anatomical regions is that nervous system operations are highly distributed and multiplexed. Although we are constantly tempted to try to determine what a particular region or circuit 'does', this approach has really had limited success. In light of the daunting complexities of connections and interactions, one could even conclude that this sort of functional phrenology is never likely to generate unequivocal answers. Instead, we need to understand better the rules of parallel and interleaved processing. Physiological and anatomical observations provide useful constraints but are ultimately insufficient, since so many of the essential variables remain unknown. A promising approach to investigating parallel distributed processing directly is with neural network simulations, in which the mechanisms can be analysed in detail.

Georgopoulos: I would like to raise the conceptual issue of what we mean by 'function'. We would agree that motor cortex serves a motor function and the visual cortex a visual function, but that doesn't help much. If we look more carefully at what Dr Passingham said, namely that the unique parallel connections of an area define its function (an idea to which I fully subscribe), then giving a name to that function is a different story, in that these connections may define a variety of subsets within a more general function; for example, subsets controlling movements parameters within 'movement control' in general. What I'm looking for is a conceptual framework to map what we usually mean by physiological functions to the pattern of unique connectivity that defines anatomically the uniqueness of a given area. It may be that this uniqueness in anatomical connectivity is a conceptual counterpart to the uniqueness of the way in which the family of processes define the specific function of a particular brain area.

Passingham: The problem is that functions can be identified at different levels. In PET studies, the function of an area is specified in psychological terms. In physiological studies, the function of an area is specified in computational terms. It is not clear from our discussion at what level we are trying to assign functions to areas.

Goodale: I'd like to pick up on a couple of points that were raised earlier about dynamics and distributed systems. If we say the problem is too complex, we're not going to get anywhere. At some point you have to start carving up the problem; you have to start making some distinctions, however crude or preliminary. I think we have gone a long way already: we understand a good deal about the brain. We know far more than we did a hundred years ago, and I think we got to this place doing what we're doing now—ascribing functions to particular areas.

Stein: I want to put a simplistic idea forward. We do know that lesions in certain parts of the brain cause specific symptoms. The argument is that the area affected has something to do with the function that it destroys. We know all the caveats, but surely that's something that we can rely on: there are specific neurological syndromes that are a consequence of lesions in particular areas.

Lemon: One of the excitements of the brain imaging work has been that many people who have been looking at brain activation maps are interpreting their results not only in terms of the movement itself, but also in the many other processes that are involved in the act. For example, when you change your limb position you have got to update all relevant parts of the brain as to your intention to move and the parameters of the intended movement. You have also got to be ready to cope with the sensory input that arises when you make the movement. This is an approach which was often missing from much of the early single-unit work where there was a very defined question (is this cell's firing related to this behaviour?) which rather sidelined all the other interesting features that are part of a family of sensorimotor functions.

Stein: Could we just have a comment from a clinical neurologist about whether the effects of lesions are reliable or not?

Marsden: It depends where they are — that's the problem. There are certainly some areas you can't do without, but this is a very small proportion of the human brain. Much more interesting is when you damage an area that ought to do something and it doesn't: this we see time and time again. There's no easy explanation for such discrepancies.

Glickstein: One of my hobbies is chasing down urban myths about the nervous system. One of these is that you can become a perfectly skilled machinist without a cerebellum! Another which I've heard is that children sometimes present with a tumour that requires excision of an entire cerebellar hemisphere, and yet they grow up essentially normally. I looked for the evidence in the literature and I had difficulty in finding it: I would be very grateful if you would lead me to any articles written on that problem.

Marsden: Before the advent of effective ways of shrinking the human brain in neurosurgery, surgeons sacrificed a third of the lateral lobe of the cerebellum with impunity.

Glickstein: I draw your attention back to the 1930s, when surgeons could cut the corpus callosum and reported that there was no effect whatsoever!

References

Bauswein E, Fromm C, Preuss A 1989 Corticostriatal cells in comparison with pyramidal tract neurons: contrasting properties in the behaving monkey. Brain Res 493:198–203

Cajal, Santiago Ramon y 1892 The structure of the retina. [Translated by Thorpe AS, Glickstein M 1972, Thomas, Springfield]

Fetz EE, Perlmutter SI, Maier MA, Flament D, Fortier PA 1996 Response patterns and postspike effects of premotor neurons in cervical spinal cord of behaving monkeys. Can J Physiol Pharmacol 74:531–546

Fromm C 1983 Contrasting properties of pyramidal tract neurons located in the precentral or postcentral areas and of cortical neurons in the behaving monkey. Adv Neurol 39:329–345

Hubel ED, Wiesel T 1965 Receptive fields and striate architecture in two non-striate visual areas (18 and 19) of the cat. J Neurophysiol 28:229–289

Sensory input and control of grip

Roland S. Johansson

Department of Physiology, Umeå University, S-901 87 Umeå, Sweden

Abstract. When we use our digits to manipulate objects the applied fingertip forces and torques tangential to the grip surfaces are a result of complex muscle activity. These patterns are acquired during our ontogenetic development and we select them according to the manipulative intent. But the basic force coordination expressed in these patterns has to be tuned to the physical properties of the current object, e.g. shape, surface friction and weight. This takes place primarily by parametric adjustments of the force output based on internal models of the target object, i.e. implicit memory systems that represent critical object properties. From visual or haptic information we identify objects and automatically retrieve the relevant models. These models are then used to adapt the motor commands prior to their execution. The formation of models and their swift updating with changes in object properties depend, however, on signals from tactile sensors in the fingertips.

1998 Sensory guidance of movement. Wiley, Chichester (Novartis Foundation Symposium 218) p 45–63

An appropriate control of contact forces between digits and objects in manipulative tasks is possible only if the subject is able to constrain the motor commands by the manipulative intent, the task and the physical properties of the manipulated objects. Most tasks, for instance, require *grasp stability*, i.e. to prevent slips and accidental loss of an object we have to apply large enough forces normal to the grip surfaces ('grip' forces) in relation to destabilizing load forces tangential to the grip surfaces. At the same time we typically avoid exceedingly large grip forces because they may crush fragile objects or injure the hand. The control problem that I will discuss specifically concerns how we adapt the fingertip forces to constraints imposed by objects' specific intrinsic properties for grasp stability. For instance, an object can be light or heavy, slippery or not, it may have a simple or a complex shape and have a distribution of mass that implies tangential torques (torsional loads) at the grip surfaces when we move it or use it as a tool. Such factors influence the magnitude, direction and points of application of feasible fingertip forces. Although vision may help when available, eventually humans adapt to such constraints by using sensory information provided by digital mechanoreceptors. Indeed, if one asks a person that suffers from impaired digital sensibility about her problems, she complains about disabilities to use the hand in manipulative tasks. For instance, she often drops objects, may easily crush fragile objects and has difficulties in dressing herself because she cannot complete such apparently simple tasks as buttoning a shirt. Thus, fundamental sensorimotor control processes used in manipulation are lost with impaired digital tactile sensibility.

Feedback control based on digital sensors

One way to use digital sensors to adjust the force output to object properties would be to engage them in closed feedback loops. But such loops imply large time delays. These time delays arise from, e.g. impulse conduction in peripheral nerves, conduction and processing time in the CNS, and, not least, the inherent sluggishness of muscles. In humans, these factors add up to at least 100 ms for the generation of a significant force response. Thus closed-loop feedback would be quite ineffective at frequencies above some 1 Hz (e.g. Hogan et al 1987). But, frequency components up to some 5 Hz occur in manipulation.

Despite these control issues, subjects rely on feedback control in certain types of manipulative tasks. This occurs in reactive tasks when we restrain 'active' objects that impose unpredictable loads tangential to the grip surfaces, e.g. when we hold a dog's leash. We have recently characterized sensorimotor transformations related to the precision grip when humans restrain an object subjected to trapezoidal load-force profiles with unpredictable onsets, amplitudes, rates and directions of loading and unloading (Fig. 1A) (for an overview see Johansson 1996). To

---

FIG. 1. Peripheral afferent and reactive grip force responses to unpredictable loading of the precision grip by a distal pull. (A) Schematic illustration of the experimental set up. The subject grasped the manipulandum between the tips of the thumb and index finger of the right hand. It consisted of two parallel grip surfaces (30 mm diameter; spaced 25 mm apart). The servo-controlled motor is able to deliver load forces in two opposite directions and the arrow indicates the direction of distal loading. The grip and load forces, perpendicular and tangential to the grip surfaces, respectively, and the position of the manipulandum in the loading directions were recorded. Afferent activity was recorded from the right median nerve with percutaneously inserted tungsten needle electrodes impaling the nerve about 10 cm proximal to the elbow. (B) Grip responses and average discharge rate of 10 FA I sensors to 2 N loads delivered to the receptor-bearing digit at 2 N/s (dashed lines) and 8 N/s (solid lines). The two traces of single-unit recordings above the load force signals are examples of responses in a single FA I sensor during load trials at 8 N/s (upper trace) and 2 N/s (lower trace). (C) Grip response and average discharge rate of 19 muscle afferents located in the long flexor muscles of the index, middle or ring finger to 2 N loads delivered at 4 N/s in the distal direction. The two traces of single unit recordings are examples of responses in two different muscle spindle afferents. In (B) and (C) the averages of forces and discharge rates are synchronized to the onset of the loading ramp; discharge rate represents average instantaneous frequency. Data in (B) are compiled from Macefield et al (1996) and those in (C) from Macefield & Johansson (1996).

Subject restrains an 'active' object

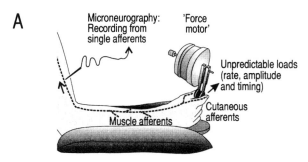

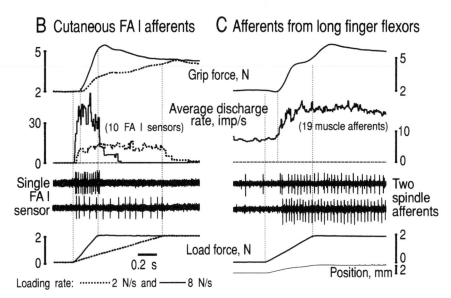

prevent the object from slipping, without specific instruction, subjects automatically respond to load changes by increasing and decreasing the grip force normal to the grip surfaces in parallel with the load force changes (see load and grip force signals in Figs 1B and C). But the changes in grip force lag those of the load force because they are reactively generated. A reactive grip response is initiated after some 100 ms delay that varies with the load force rate (Johansson et al 1992a). Because of this time lag, unless the background grip force prior to a load increase is strong enough the subject will lose the manipulandum. Indeed, following slips and trials with high rate of load force increases, subjects learn to increase the background grip force as an adaptation to the expected range of loadings.

We have used the technique of microneurography to record signals in single nerve fibres of the median nerve that supplies cutaneous, muscle and joint sensors (Fig. 1A) (Macefield & Johansson 1996, Macefield et al 1996). These experiments and collateral experiments with cutaneous anaesthesia (Häger-Ross & Johansson 1996) showed that the reactive responses are driven primarily by digital cutaneous inputs. Signals in rapidly adapting FA I afferents seems most important, but slowly adapting cutaneous afferents may also contribute. Note in Fig. 1B that the intensity of the cutaneous afferent responses is scaled by the rate of load force increase, and the afferent responses commence before the onset of the grip response. Furthermore, the size and duration of the grip force increase is scaled along with the intensity and duration of the afferent response, which is an attractive feature of a feedback-controlled behaviour.

In contrast to cutaneous afferents, afferents from intrinsic and extrinsic hand muscles and interphalangeal joints do not respond to load increases early enough to allow them to contribute to the initiation and the initial scaling of the grip responses. The muscle afferents respond reliably after the onset of the subject's grip with discharge rates related to changes in force output and, thus, to muscle activity (Fig. 1C) (Macefield & Johansson 1996). Thus, these afferents are primarily concerned with events in the muscle itself, rather than functioning as exteroceptors.

Feedforward control policies

Because of the long time delays with feedback control the swift coordination of fingertip forces during self-paced everyday manipulation of ordinary 'passive' objects must be explained by other mechanisms. Indeed, the brain relies on feedforward control mechanisms and takes advantage of the stable and predictable physical properties of these objects by parametrically adapting force motor commands to the relevant physical properties of the target object. Figure 2 illustrates principles for parametric adjustments of motor output to object weight (Johansson & Westling 1988a), friction in relation to the skin (Johansson & Westling 1984) and shape (Jenmalm & Johansson 1997).

The subject's task is to lift a test object from a support, hold it in the air and replace it. Note that the grip force in each instance is constrained by the active sensorimotor program to increase and decrease with no time delay in parallel with the vertical load force. This coordinative constraint ensures grasp stability, i.e. the grip force at any given load force exceeds the corresponding minimum grip force to prevent slippage by a certain safety margin (hatched areas in the lower graphs of Fig. 2). This parallel change in the grip force and linear load force is not specific to any particular task (e.g. Flanagan & Wing 1995) or grip configuration (e.g. grips by two or more digits and bimanual grips; Flanagan & Tresilian 1994, Kinoshita et al 1995, Burstedt et al 1997). Rather, this coordinative constraint is expressed during handling of inertial loads, but also when pushing or pulling against immovable objects (e.g. Johansson et al 1992b), when moving objects under viscous and elastic loads (Johansson & Westling 1984, Flanagan & Wing 1997), and in anticipatory adjustments of grip forces in complex bimanual actions (Johansson & Westling 1988b).

In most everyday tasks, however, the destabilizing loads of the grasp include not only linear load forces, but also torques tangential to the grasp surfaces. Such torsional loads occur whenever we tilt an object around a grip axis that does not intersect the vertical line through the object's centre of gravity. Importantly, the engaged sensorimotor program also accounts for such torsional loads. That is, rotational slips are prevented by the grip force which automatically increases in parallel with the tangential torque (Jenmalm et al 1997, Kinoshita et al 1997). The sensorimotor programs thus apparently model the effect of the total load in terms of linear forces, tangential torques and combinations thereof.

The coupling between grip force and load at the grip surfaces in self-paced manipulative tasks forms the basis for an efficient sensory control of the motor output to accommodate the physical properties of the object (Johansson 1996). With weight variations, the parallel change in grip and load forces ensures grasp stability when lifting objects of regardless of weights, i.e. with a heavier object both the grip and load forces reaches higher values before the weight is counterbalanced and the object is lifted than with a lighter one (Fig. 2A). Furthermore, with frictional variations, the balance between the grip and load force is a motor output parameter that is set to the current frictional limits (Fig. 2B). This also applies to object shape; the grip-to-load force ratio is higher with object tapered upwards than downwards (Fig. 2C).

*Internal models determining force coordination parameters
and their updating after changes in object properties*

As illustrated in Fig. 2A, with objects of different weights, subjects use a different
rate of force increase prior to lift-off, as if they know the final force. However, there
is no explicit information about object weight until lift-off. Likewise, with different
friction (Fig. 2B) and object shape (Fig. 2C) the force output reflects the object
features already at the initial force attack, i.e. before somatosensory cues derived

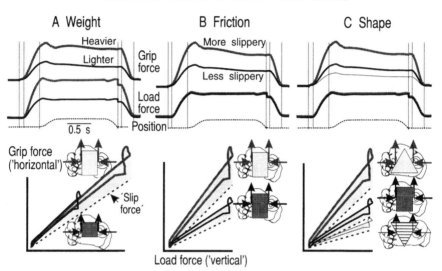

Parametric Control of Motor Commands

FIG. 2.   Principles for parametric adjustments of motor output to (A) object weight, (B)
friction in relation to the skin and (C) object shape. The subject lifts an instrumented test
object from a table, holds it in the air and then replaces it, using the precision grip. Upper
graphs show the horizontally oriented grip force, the vertically oriented load force ('lift force')
and the object's vertical position as a function of time for superimposed trials, indicated by
differently hatched curves. The lower graphs show the grip force as a function of the load for
in a phase-plane plot for the same trials. The dashed line indicates the minimum grip-to-load
force ratio to prevent slips and the safety margin against slips is indicated by hatching. After
contact with the object, demarcated by the far-left vertical line in the upper graphs, the grip
force increases for a short period while the grip is established before the command is released
for a parallel increase in grip and load force during isometric conditions (second vertical line).
This increase continues until the start of object movement when the load force overcomes the
force of gravity; the object lifts off at the third vertical line. After the replacement of the object
and table contact occurs (fourth line) there is a short delay before the two forces decline in parallel
(fifth line) until the object is released (sixth line). For more detailed information about the control
of this 'sequential coordination' see Johansson (1996), and for parametric adjustments of force
output to object weight, frictional condition and object shape see Johansson & Westling
(1988a), Johansson & Westling (1984) and Jenmalm & Johansson (1997), respectively.

from contact with the object could have exerted any influences. Thus, in each instance the neural controller operates in a feedforward fashion and uses motor command parameters somehow determined by internal models pertaining to the physical properties of the object. The question immediately arises about how such models are selected and updated for different objects and after changes in object properties.

Changes in object shape.   Figures 3A and B shows a sequences of trials from a lift series in which the surface angle was unpredictably changed between trials. The sequence is 30°, −30° and −30°, i.e. a transition from upward tapering to downward. When the subject sees the object there is no difference between the first and the second trial after the change (Fig. 3A). This indicates that visual geometric cues efficiently specify the force coordination for object shape already before the force output, i.e., in a feedforward manner. These cues appear to be used in a computational sense to parametrically determine the finger force coordination to objects' shape in anticipation of the upcoming force requirements. However, when subjects cannot see the target object they still adapt the force balance to changes in object shape — but it takes about 100 ms after contact with the object before the force coordination is tuned appropriately for the actual surface angle (see the first trial with −30° in Fig. 3B). That the grip force develops initially according to the force requirements in the previous trial indicates that memory of previous surface angle determines default force coordination in a feedforward manner. Indeed, in the second trial with −30° without vision, the force output is already adapted to the current surface angle by the onset of force application. Thus, an internal model related to object shape determines parametrically the force coordination in a feedforward manner, and somatosensory signals obtained at initial contact with the object mediate an updating of this model to changes in object shape (Jenmalm & Johansson 1997). Furthermore, a single trial is enough to update the relevant internal model.

Sensors in the digits are used to update the force coordination for object shape when subjects are blindfolded. Without vision and digital sensibility (digital anaesthesia) the adaptation is severely impaired, although the grip and load forces still change in parallel (Fig. 3D). Anaesthetized subjects learn to constantly apply strong grip forces regardless of surface angle. However, with vision, subjects still adapt the force coordination, with only some impairments with anaesthetized digits (Fig. 3C), reinforcing the notion of feedforward use of visual geometric cues.

The curvature of the grasp surfaces is another aspect of object shape. Surprisingly, the curvature of spherically curved symmetrical grasp surfaces has little effect on grip force requirements for grasp stability under linear force loads (Jenmalm et al 1998). However, it becomes acute in tasks involving torsional loads (Jenmalm et al 1997). The relationship between the grip force and tangential

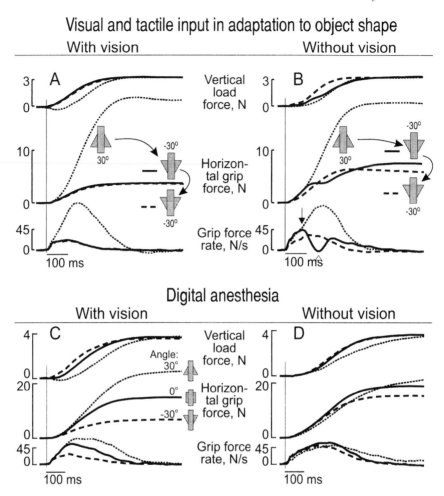

FIG. 3.   Changes in object shape. (A and B) Adjustments to changes in surface angle during lift series in which surface angle was unpredictably varied between lift trials. Vertical load force, horizontal grip force and grip force rate is shown as a function of time for trials with vision (A) and without vision (B) during normal digital sensibility. Object shape in the current and previous trials is illustrated by the hatched and hollow inset figures, respectively. Adjustment to a smaller angle is illustrated by trials with $-30°$ (solid line) that were preceded by trials with $30°$. Trials with $-30°$ (dashed line) and $30°$ (dotted line) not preceded by a change in surface angle are shown for comparison. Arrow in (B) indicates the point in time where the new surface angle was expressed in the motor output. (C and D) Adaptation to object shape during digital anaesthesia (C) with and (D) without vision. Vertical load force, horizontal grip force and grip force rate as a function of time are shown for trials with $30°$ (dotted), $0°$ (solid) and $-30°$ (dashed) surface angle. The object's shape is illustrated by the inset figures. Modified from Jenmalm & Johansson (1997).

torque is parametrically scaled by surface curvature: the grip force increases with increasing curvature. As with linear force loads, this parametric scaling of grip force is directly related to the minimum grip force required to prevent slippage, i.e. under torsional loads subjects keep a small but adequate safety margin against rotational slip. Finally, our preliminary evidence suggest that the parametric adaptation to surface curvature depends on tactile afferent cues (cf. Goodwin et al 1995).

Frictional changes.   So far there is no evidence that visual cues are useful for updating force coordination to friction, but tactile receptors in the fingertips are of crucial importance. As with object shape, after a change in friction the most important adjustment takes place shortly after the initial contact with the object and can be observed about 0.1 s after contact (Fig. 4A). Prior to this event there are burst responses in tactile afferents of different types and most reliably in the population of FA I (Meissner) afferents (Johansson & Westling 1987). The initial contact responses in subpopulations of excited FA I afferents are markedly influenced by the surface material, as shown in Fig. 4A with a single afferent. We believe that the adjustment of force coordination to the new frictional condition takes place on the basis of a detection of a mismatch between the actual and an expected sensory event. This adjustment involves a change in the grip-to-load force ratio (increase with a more slippery surface in Fig. 4A) along with an updating of the relevant internal model pertaining to the frictional condition between the object and the skin.

In a series of lifting trials with unpredictable variation of surface friction, sometimes this initial adjustment is inadequate and an unpredictable frictional slip occurs at a later point, typically at one digit only (Edin et al 1992). Burst responses to such slip events in dynamically sensitive tactile afferents promptly trigger an automatic upgrading of the grip-to-load force ratio to a higher maintained level (Johansson & Westling 1987). This restores the safety margin during subsequent manipulation by updating the internal model controlling the balance between grip and load force.

Weight changes.   During everyday manipulation, on the basis of visual identification of common objects we automatically select relevant internal models for appropriate parametric adjustment of force output to object weight. That is, during the very first lift of a common object, and before sensory information related to the object's weight becomes available, at lift-off the force development reflects the object's weight (Gordon et al 1993). Likewise, for classes of related objects, visually (and haptically) acquired object size cues influence the force development prior to lift off by size–weight associations (Gordon et al 1991). But, as we have all experienced, the force output may sometimes be erroneous. This may happen when the weight of an object has changed but not its visual appearance, and the lifting movement may be either jerky or slow (Johansson & Westling 1988a). For instance, if the object is lighter than expected from previous trials, the load and grip force drives are exceedingly strong when the load force overcomes the force of gravity and the lift-off takes place. Although somatosensory afferent events evoked by the unexpected lift-off trigger an abrupt termination of the drive, the delays in the control loop (some 100 ms) are still long enough to cause a pronounced position overshoot as everyone has experienced; burst responses in FA II (Pacinian) afferents that show an exquisite sensitivity to mechanical transients most quickly and reliably signal the moment of lift-off (Westling & Johansson 1987). Conversely, if the object is heavier than expected

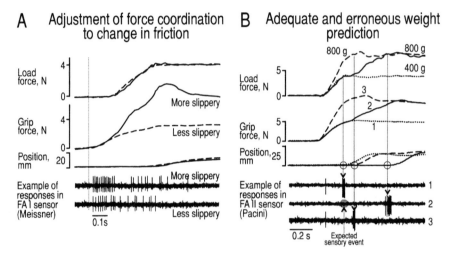

FIG. 4.   Single-unit tactile afferent responses and adjustments to changes in frictional condition between the object and the digits (A) and to object weight (B). Data from single lift trials. (A) The influence of the surface friction on the force output and examples of initial contact responses in a FA I unit. Two trials are superimposed, one with a fine grain sandpaper as grip surface (less slippery; dashed lines) and one subsequent trial with silk which represents a more slippery surface (solid lines). The sandpaper trial was preceded by a trial with sandpaper and therefore the force coordination is initially set for the higher friction. Vertical line indicates initial touch. (B) Initial parts of an adequately programmed lift with a 400 g weight (dotted; trial 1), a subsequent lift with 800 g (solid; trial 2) that was erroneously programmed for the lighter 400 g weight lifted in the previous trial, and the following lift with 800 g (dashed; trial 3). The vertical lines with arrowheads pointing downwards indicate the moment of lift-off for each of the trials and they point at the evoked sensory events exemplified by signals in a single FA II afferent. The absence of burst responses in FA II afferents at the expected point in time for the erroneously programmed 800 g trial (see 'expected sensory event') is used to initiate a new control mode. This involves a slow discontinuous parallel increase in grip and load forces, until terminated by the sensory input at the actual lift-off. (A) Modified from Johansson & Westling (1987) and (B) from Johansson & Cole (1992).

the force increase slows down when the load force has reached the level of the predicted lift-off but no sensory event is evoked confirming lift-off (Fig. 4B; solid curves). But this *absence* of a sensory event at the expected lift-off then causes the release of a 'new' set of muscle commands. These generate a slow discontinuous force increase, until terminated by a neural event at the true lift-off (Fig. 4B, afferent response during the 800 g lift preceded by 400 g). Taken together, these observations indicate that the absence of an expected sensory event may be as efficient as an unexpected sensory event in triggering compensatory motor commands. Moreover, whether the object's weight is correctly anticipated or not, somatosensory signals that represent the moment of lift-off are mandatory for the control of the force output. Finally, once an error occurs the internal model pertaining object's weight is updated, i.e. one lift is generally enough to update the internal model.

Summary of conclusions

Figure 5 schematically summarizes the properties of sensorimotor control in manipulation as they are emerging in studies focused on control of grasp stability. Both visual and somatosensory inputs are used in conjunction with sensorimotor memories (internal models) for parametric adjustment of fingertip forces to object properties. Common objects are identified by vision for automatic retrieval of relevant internal models used to parametrically adapt the motor commands prior to their execution, in anticipation of the upcoming force requirements. We have used the term *anticipatory parameter control* to denote these processes (e.g. Johansson 1996). In case of object shape and size, people may also use visual geometric cues in a computational sense for anticipatory control, relying on internal forward models representing relationships between visual geometric cues and force requirements. In general terms, there is plenty of evidence that in motor control the CNS entertains internal forward models of relevant limb mechanics, environmental objects and task properties to adapt motor commands according to task demands (e.g. Ghez et al 1991, Johansson & Cole 1992, Lacquaniti 1992, Miall & Wolpert 1996, Flanagan & Wing 1997).

In manipulation, the formation of models related to object properties and their updating with changes in these properties largely depend on signals from tactile sensors in the hand used according to a policy termed *discrete event, sensory-driven control* (e.g. Johansson 1996). At the heart of this control is the comparison of somatosensory inflow with an internal sensory signal that dynamically represents the predicted afferent input (cf. 'corollary discharge'). This internal signal is generated by the active sensorimotor program in conjunction with the efferent signals. Disturbances in task execution due to erroneous parameter specification of the sensorimotor program are reflected by a mismatch between predicted and

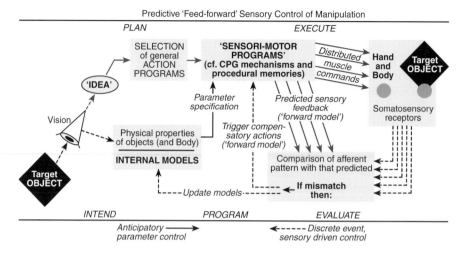

FIG. 5.   Some unfolding properties of sensorimotor control in manipulation with emphasis of the mechanism involved in control of grasp stability. Note that the same target object is represented at two sites. After being aware of the target object, from visual (or haptic) cues we decide about an action. From a set of general action programs acquired during ontogenetic development (e.g. Gordon 1994), we select and activate task-specific neural sensorimotor programs. These programs represent procedural memories that issue coordinated distributed muscle commands and dynamically specify the use of sensory information such as neural central pattern generators implied in the pacing of most self-generated motor behaviours. By vision (and haptics) we identify the object for automatic retrieval of relevant internal models of environmental objects and use these model to parametrically specify relevant aspects of the motor commands prior to their execution. We have termed this control policy *anticipatory parameter control,* (e.g. Johansson & Cole 1992, Johansson 1996). With novel objects, and with erroneous internal models, information from tactile sensors in the hand is used to update the model of the target object. This occurs if there is a mismatch between the predicted somatosensory input dynamically specified by the sensorimotor program and the actual input. In manipulation this takes generally takes place as 'single trial learning'. Such mismatches also trigger pre-programmed patterns of corrective motor responses. We have termed the control policy representing the use of somatosensory afferent information *discrete event, sensory-driven control* (e.g. Johansson & Cole 1992, Johansson 1996).

actual sensory input. For instance, discrete somatosensory events may occur while not expected, or alternatively, they do not occur while expected (cf. Fig. 4). Detection of such a mismatch triggers pre-programmed patterns of corrective responses (forward model) along with an update of the relevant internal model and thus a change in parameter specification. This updating typically takes place on a single trial basis. With regard to friction and aspects of object shape, the updating primarily occurs during the initial contact with the object. In trials erroneously programmed for object weight, the updating takes place at lift-off. Also, while restraining an object subjected to unpredictable destabilizing load forces (reactive control; Fig. 1) the task specific 'load-to-grip' sensorimotor transformation enabled by the selected sensorimotor program would exploit the discrete event, sensory-driven control policy. Indeed, rather than a continuously closed feedback loop, the transform appears to exploit short-term predictions based on somatosensory information related to the rate of load changes (Johansson et al 1992a, Cole & Johansson 1993, Johansson 1996). In general terms, the scheme outlined in Fig. 5 has several elements in common with aspects of recent schemes that have attempted to organize concepts of sensorimotor integration (e.g. Merfeld et al 1993, Prochazka 1993, Salinas & Abbott 1995, Miall & Wolpert 1996).

It is obvious that we are interested in how this proposed control scheme may be implemented in the CNS. In general terms, there is plenty of evidence around that the control of grasping and manipulation relies on distributed processes in the CNS, engaging most areas known to be involved in sensorimotor control. We have recently begun to study CNS processes engaged in object manipulation using magnetic brain stimulation (Johansson et al 1994, Lemon et al 1995) and positron emission tomography (PET). In the PET study we compared self-paced lifts with reactive control when the grasp was exposed to the same load profiles as previously generated during the lifting task (unpublished work in collaboration with R. Seitz, 1998). In the self-paced task the blindfolded subjects primarily relied on anticipatory parameter control for grip force regulation and in the matching reactive tasks they relied on sensory feedback, i.e. the discrete event-driven control policy. In the self-paced condition the regional blood flow substantially increased in the left primary motor, premotor and somatosensory cortex contralateral to the operating hand compared with when the subject just held the loaded object stationary in air. In contrast, during the matching reactive task there were small changes in cortical regional blood flow in these areas, although the force output was a bit stronger. This suggests that the anticipatory parameter control policy used in self-paced manipulative tasks put higher demands on cortical mechanisms than the feedback mechanisms supporting reactive tasks.

Acknowledgements

This study was supported by the Swedish Medical Research Council (project 08667), Department of Naval Research, Arlington, VA, USA (grant No. N00014-92-J-1919) and the Göran Gustafsson Foundation for Research in Natural Sciences and Medicine.

References

Burstedt MKO, Edin BB, Johansson RS 1997 Coordination of fingertip forces during human manipulation can emerge from independent neural networks controlling each engaged digit. Exp Brain Res 117:67–79

Cole KJ, Johansson RS 1993 Friction in the digit-object interface scales the sensorimotor transformation for grip responses to pulling loads. Exp Brain Res 95:523–532

Edin BB, Westling G, Johansson RS 1992 Independent control of fingertip forces at individual digits during precision lifting in humans. J Physiol (Lond) 450:547–564

Flanagan JR, Tresilian JR 1994 Grip load force coupling: a general control strategy for transporting objects. J Exp Psychol Hum Percept Perform 20:944–957

Flanagan JR, Wing AM 1995 The stability of precision grip forces during cyclic arm movements with a hand-held load. Exp Brain Res 105:455–464

Flanagan JR, Wing AM 1997 The role of internal models in motion planning and control: evidence from grip force adjustments during movements of hand-held loads. J Neurosci 17:1519–1528

Ghez C, Hening W, Gordon J 1991 Organization of voluntary movement. Curr Opin Neurobiol 1:664–671

Goodwin AW, Browning AS, Wheat HE 1995 Representation of curved surfaces in responses of mechanoreceptive afferent-fibers innervating the monkey's fingerpad. J Neurosci 15:798–810

Gordon AM 1994 Development of the reach to grasp movement. Adv Psychol 105:37–56

Gordon AM, Forssberg H, Johansson RS, Westling G 1991 Integration of sensory information during the programming of precision grip: comments on the contributions of size cues. Exp Brain Res 85:226–229

Gordon AM, Westling G, Cole KJ, Johansson RS 1993 Memory representations underlying motor commands used during manipulation of common and novel objects. J Neurophysiol 69:1789–1796

Häger-Ross C, Johansson RS 1996 Non-digital afferent input in reactive control of fingertip forces during precision grip. Exp Brain Res 110:131–141

Hogan N, Bizzi E, Mussa-Ivaldi FA, Flash T 1987 Controlling multijoint motor behavior. Exerc Sport Sci Rev 15:153–190

Jenmalm P, Johansson RS 1997 Visual and somatosensory information about object shape control manipulative finger tip forces. J Neurosci 17:4486–4499

Jenmalm P, Goodwin AW, Johansson RS 1997 Control of grasp stability when humans lift and tilt objects with different surface curvatures. Soc Neurosci Abstr 23:2092

Jenmalm P, Goodwin AW, Johansson RS 1998 Control of grasp stability when humans lift objects with different surface curvatures. J Neurophysiol 79:1643–1652

Johansson RS 1996 Sensory and memory information in the control of dextrous manipulation. In: Lacquaniti F, Viviani P (eds) Neural bases of motor behaviour. Kluwer Academic Publishers, Dordrecht, p 205–260

Johansson RS, Cole KJ 1992 Sensory-motor coordination during grasping and manipulative actions. Curr Opin Neurobiol 2:815–823

Johansson RS, Westling G 1984 Roles of glabrous skin receptors and sensorimotor memory in automatic control of precision grip when lifting rougher or more slippery objects. Exp Brain Res 56:550–564

Johansson RS, Westling G 1987 Signals in tactile afferents from the fingers eliciting adaptive motor responses during precision grip. Exp Brain Res 66:141–154

Johansson RS, Westling G 1988a Coordinated isometric muscle commands adequately and erroneously programmed for the weight during lifting task with precision grip. Exp Brain Res 71:59–71

Johansson RS, Westling G 1988b Programmed and triggered actions to rapid load changes during precision grip. Exp Brain Res 71:72–86

Johansson RS, Häger C, Riso R 1992a Somatosensory control of precision grip during unpredictable pulling loads. II. Changes in load force rate. Exp Brain Res 89:192–203

Johansson RS, Riso R, Häger C, Bäckström L 1992b Somatosensory control of precision grip during unpredictable pulling loads. I. Changes in load force amplitude. Exp Brain Res 89:181–191

Johansson RS, Lemon RN, Westling G 1994 Time varying enhancement of human cortical excitability mediated by cutaneous inputs during precision grip. J Physiol (Lond) 481:761–775

Kinoshita H, Kawai S, Ikuta K 1995 Contributions and coordination of individual fingers in multiple finger prehension. Ergonomics 38:1212–1230

Kinoshita H, Bäckström L, Flanagan JR, Johansson RS 1997 Tangential torque effects on the control of grip forces when holding objects with a precision grip. J Neurophysiol 78:1619–1630

Lacquaniti F 1992 Automatic control of limb movement and posture. Curr Opin Neurobiol 2:807–814

Lemon RN, Johansson RS, Westling G 1995 Corticospinal control during reach, grasp and precision lift in man. J Neurosci 15:6145–6156

Macefield VG, Johansson RS 1996 Control of grip force during restraint of an object held between finger and thumb: responses of muscle and joint afferents from the digits. Exp Brain Res 108:172–184

Macefield VG, Häger-Ross C, Johansson RS 1996 Control of grip force during restraint of an object held between finger and thumb: responses of cutaneous afferents from the digits. Exp Brain Res 108:155–171

Merfeld DM, Young LR, Oman CM, Shelhamer MJ 1993 A multidimensional model of the effect of gravity on the spatial orientation of the monkey. J Vestib Res 3:141–161

Miall RC, Wolpert DM 1996 Forward models for physiological motor control. Neural Networks 9:1265–1279

Prochazka A 1993 Comparison of natural and artificial control of movement. IEEE Trans Rehab Eng 1:7–17

Salinas E, Abbott LF 1995 Transfer of coded information from sensory to motor networks. J Neurosci 15:6461–6474

Westling G, Johansson RS 1987 Responses in glabrous skin mechanoreceptors during precision grip in humans. Exp Brain Res 66:128–140

DISCUSSION

Ebner: In the PET study, in the reactive test, how did the subcortical structures behave?

Johansson: There was some activity in basal ganglia. The left putamen was activated in the reactive condition with constant weight, but not in the self-paced task. However, these are preliminary data.

Lemon: The internal model gives the brain the opportunity of comparing the desired movement with what is going on in the real world. How big does the mismatch, the error signal, have to be before you update the program? Is that signal much larger than is needed for the subject to be aware that something has actually changed? In other words, is it on the same scale of magnitude as the sort of stimuli that psychophysicists would study, simply asking subjects whether anything has changed?

Johansson: First, we haven't thoroughly studied the absolute sensitivity of the system in terms of changing force coordination. In our studies we have used variations of the object properties to disclose effects, but we haven't examined, for example, how much of a weight difference is needed for an updating of the object-related internal models.

Concerning the second question, about how large the errors have to be to make the subject aware about changes, a striking finding is that a lot can happen on the motor output side that the subjects are completely unaware of. For instance, subjects may be unaware of changes in the surface friction, even though these changes result in robust changes in the grip force output. Likewise, with different surface material on the two grasped surfaces, subjects may not notice the difference, but they still adapt the fingertip forces to the local frictional condition. Finally, small accidental slips often occur when we hold an object. Such a slip triggers a response to increase the grip force and an updating of the coordination for future actions even though we are not aware of them.

Miall: In a slightly different context we've recently done some experiments asking people to adjust the size of their movements on the basis of visual feedback, and then providing them with noisy visual feedback (Ingram & Miall 1998). In these sorts of tasks people make quite a few errors anyway. It seems that as long as the artificial errors we introduce are of the same magnitude as the normal errors, the subjects never notice them. But as soon as we raise the errors a few percent above the normal errors, they suddenly interfere with learning. It is as if people can cope with the normal variance within their movements, and they can't tell that you are imposing similar variance, but beyond that the errors are noticeable.

Miller: Are you making a distinction between the subjects improving their behaviour versus noticing the errors?

Miall: We are looking for an adaptation to perturbed visual feedback; when the feedback is noisy it impairs learning but when it is about as noisy as their intrinsic variance they begin to learn.

Miller: Are the subjects aware of the fact that these errors are occurring?

Miall: No, there is often learning in the situation when they're not aware of what's going on.

Johansson: What is the task?

Miall: It is a pointing task in which we are trying to get subjects to adapt the amplitude of their reaching on the basis of a gain change in visual feedback, with or without added 'noise' in the visual feedback signal.

Goodale: I was pondering the different sources of visual information that would be used for different aspects of grasp. Factors such as the size, orientation and the shape of an object can be derived from first principles. You don't have to know anything about what happened before — you can get all of that right from the first glimpse of the object. You can imagine a fairly hard-wired system that could do that. On the other hand, to judge factors such as weight and friction you would have to have some experience with the object. I wonder if this could give you any clues as to the mechanisms that are used to compute grip aperture on the one hand and lift forces on the other.

Johansson: The weight of an object is an interesting issue. Density couples the size of an object with its weight: when you change the weight of an object without changing its visual appearance, you change the density. In trials where the density but not the appearance of an object is altered, if the new density is within the range of commonly experienced densities — between about 0.4 kg/l and 3 kg/l — one trial is typically enough for the subject to adapt and update the weight-related memory pertaining to the object. But with objects whose densities are more extreme, such as lead or styrofoam, then more trials are needed for the subjects to adapt, and the long term stability of the memory system seems to be rather weak. That is, if I present a novel object to a subject and the density is within this easily adjustable range, if they come back the day after they will apply the right force output. But with these extreme densities they tend to forget. In my own experience, I have a piece of lead tubing in my basement, and each time I move this tubing I am always caught out by its heaviness. I also have a block of styrofoam which I occasionally move around, and its lightness surprises me each time. This doesn't occur with objects of more common densities.

Goodale: I'm struck by the similarity between your data on grip forces and the recent observations of Brenner & Smeets (1996). They carried out an experiment in which they examined the effects of an illusion on grip aperture, just as we had done with the Ebbinghaus Illusion (Aglioti et al 1995, Haffenden & Goodale 1998). They used the Ponzo, or railway track, illusion and found (as we did earlier) that grip aperture to the target object was not affected by the illusion. But when they measured indirectly the lift forces that were applied to the target object, they found that these forces were affected by the context (i.e. the illusion), so that when the target appeared bigger, more force was applied. This would suggest that the systems that compute grip aperture use rather different sources of information than those that compute lift forces. I suspect that the former computations involve largely dorsal stream mechanisms while the latter involve largely ventral stream mechanisms (that have access to long-term memory).

Johansson: This is indeed an interesting observation. I would have guessed the opposite outcome of the experiment. Aperture relates to object size, whereas grip forces primarily relate to other factors such as weight and friction, which in some sense are even more intrinsic to the object than its size.

Goodale: It is likely to be quite contextual, because, for example, if you have taken the books out of a carton then clearly you are going to apply different lift forces than if you had left the books in.

Johansson: This brings us back to this density issue. If you have an empty box it will always feel light.

Goodale: I presume, however, that if you had just taken the books out of the box, then when you pick it up you would not apply the same forces that you would if you had left the books in. But if you had forgotten that you had taken out the books, you might have quite a surprise! Your knowledge about what is in the box is important here. In other words, there is a heavy cognitive modulation of the lift forces that are applied.

Georgopoulos: Did you record EMGs of the relevant muscles in these trials? I was curious whether you tried instructing the subjects to maintain the grip, or to 'not intervene' with it, and then look at the EMGs to see whether there are responses which would allow you to infer an automatic or voluntary control of the muscles concerned.

Johansson: Presumably you are asking about whether changing the instruction would influence the motor output. It does.

Georgopoulos: No, my question is, what happens to the muscles?

Johansson: If the muscles didn't respond, the subjects wouldn't increase the grip force and they would lose the object.

Georgopoulos: It is an interesting question, because in both cases the mechanoreceptors would be activated.

Johansson: The motor response to an afferent signal is certainly dependent on the subject's sensorimotor set. In the case of dextrous manipulation the sensorimotor transformations involved presumably reflect a more complex control than that studied, for instance, in the context of stretch reflexes.

Georgopoulos: That's why it's so interesting. When the object slips, even if you let it go, there is a dynamic change in the discharge of mechanoreceptors.

Johansson: With a slip, subjects react to it automatically: the shortest latency here is around 60 ms. If we are considering response latencies in the reactive grip restraint task that I discussed in my paper, the latency varies with the rate of tangential load force application.

Georgopoulos: Do you see many peaks in the EMG response, or is there usually just one?

Johansson: The response is a bit more complex than that. There are two basic elements. First, an initial 'catch-up response', which is like a unitary response lasting for some 0.25 s whose amplitude is modulated by the rate of increase in tangential load force. Then, if the load force continues to increase, the catch-up response is followed by a tracking response, i.e. the grip force changes track those of the time-varying load force.

Georgopoulos: That is not dissimilar from the short latency, stretch reflex response. There, the responses are 50–60 ms or so. Then there are EMG peaks with longer latencies.

Johansson: In the grip reactive tasks, the fastest grip responses are initiated about 60 ms after the load force increase. This latency corresponds to that of triggered actions people previously termed long-loop reflexes.

References

Aglioti S, DeSouza J, Goodale MA 1995 Size-contrast illusions deceive the eyes but not the hand. Curr Biol 5:679–685

Brenner E, Smeets JB 1996 Size illusion influences how we lift but not how we grasp an object. Exp Brain Res 111:473–476

Haffenden A, Goodale MA 1998 The effect of pictorial illusion on prehension and perception. J Cognit Neurosci 10:122–136

Ingram HA, Miall RC 1998 The effect of noisy visual feedback on adaptation to a visuomotor transformation. In: 8th Annual Conference, Neural Control of Movement Abstracts, Vol 3: B-5, Key West, Florida

Motor areas on the medial wall of the hemisphere

Peter L. Strick, Richard P. Dum and Nathalie Picard

Research Service, Veterans Administration Medical Center, and Departments of Neuroscience & Physiology and of Neurosurgery, State University of New York, Health Science Center at Syracuse, Syracuse, NY 13210, USA

Abstract. The primary motor cortex (M1) receives input from four premotor areas on the medial wall of the hemisphere: the supplementary motor area (SMA) and three cingulate motor areas located on the banks of the cingulate sulcus (CMAr, CMAd and CMAv). All four premotor areas have maps of the body containing distinct proximal and distal representations of the arm. Surprisingly, the size of the distal representation is comparable to or larger than the size of the proximal representation in each area. Thus, contrary to some previous hypotheses, the anatomical substrate exists for the premotor areas on the medial wall to be involved in the control of distal, as well as proximal arm movements. Each of the premotor areas on the medial wall also has substantial direct projections to the spinal cord. Corticospinal axons from these premotor areas terminate in the intermediate zone of the spinal cord. Some corticospinal axons from SMA, CMAd, and CMAv terminate around motoneurons. In this respect, these motor areas are like M1 and appear to have direct connections with spinal motoneurons, particularly those innervating muscles of the fingers and wrist. These results suggest that the premotor areas on the medial wall are an important source of descending commands for the generation and control of movement. In recent experiments we examined the pattern of functional activation in the premotor areas on the medial wall during the performance of sequences of pointing movements. The patterns of activation were then compared with the body maps revealed by our anatomical studies. Overall, our initial results indicate that the attributes of motor control are unequally represented across the premotor areas. For example, one of the areas on the medial wall, the CMAd, was strongly and selectively activated during the performance of highly practised, remembered sequences of movement. Further insights into the function of the premotor areas are likely to come from examining their participation in a broad range of behavioural paradigms. These initial results support our hypothesis that each premotor area makes some unique contribution to the planning, initiation and/or execution of movement.

1998 Sensory guidance of movement. Wiley, Chichester (Novartis Foundation Symposium 218) p 64–80

Overview

Our concepts about the organization and function of the cortical motor areas have changed dramatically in the last 15 years. Classically, the primary motor cortex

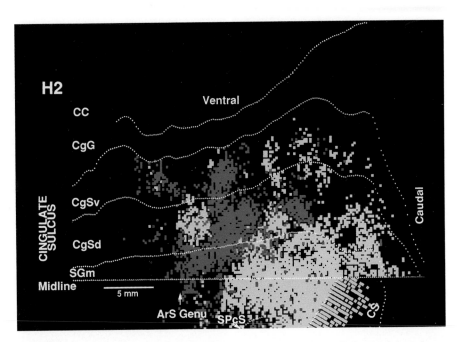

PLATE 1 Overlap map of corticospinal neurons on the medial wall that project to lower cervical and lower lumbar segments. Layer V of every fourth section was divided into bins (200 μm). *Blue bins* contain only neurons that project to cervical segments; *yellow bins* contain only neurons that project to lumbosacral segments; *red bins* contain two or more neurons projecting to cervical segments and two or more neurons projecting to lumbosacral segments ('overlap' bins). Note that few overlap bins are present in any of the medial wall premotor areas. See Fig. 1 for conventions and abbreviations. (From He et al 1995.)

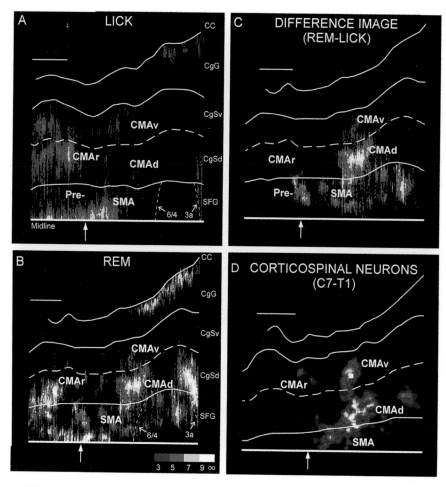

PLATE 2 Relative 2DG uptake in the medial wall during two different tasks. (A) The LICK task. (B) The REM task. Each map is from a single monkey. Local 2DG concentration is colour coded as a function of the number of standard deviations above the mean background uptake in each animal. *Arrows* indicate the level of the arcuate genu. (C) Motor areas activated exclusively during the REM task. This map was created by removing the activations present during the LICK task (A) from the activations generated by the REM task (B). (D) Density map of corticospinal neurons that project to the lower cervical segments (C7–T1). Colour scale = >1 neuron (blue) to >4.5 neurons (white) (fractions result from smoothing). See Fig. 1 for conventions and abbreviations. SFG, superior frontal gyrus. Scale bars = 5 mm. (From Picard & Strick 1997.)

(M1) had been viewed as the 'upper motoneuron' or the sole source of descending commands for the central generation of voluntary movement. The premotor areas were thought to be hierarchically superior to M1 and were seen as important 'links in the chain of command' from cortical areas in the prefrontal and parietal lobe to M1. The results of recent studies have led us to challenge this concept (Dum & Strick 1991a,b, 1993, 1996b, He et al 1993, 1995, Picard & Strick 1996, 1997).

We have used the presence of direct projections to M1 to define the premotor areas in the frontal lobe. On this basis, the frontal lobe contains at least six spatially separate premotor areas (Fig. 1; for review see Dum & Strick 1991a,b, 1996a). Two of these lie on the lateral surface of the hemisphere and four of them are located on the medial wall of the hemisphere. In the present paper, we will focus on the anatomy and function of the medial wall premotor areas (Figs 1–2 and Plate 1). These include the supplementary motor area (SMA) and three cingulate motor areas located in the banks of the cingulate sulcus (CMAr, CMAd and CMAv).

One major observation that has forced a re-evaluation of concepts about the premotor cortex is the finding that each premotor area projects not only to M1, but also directly to the spinal cord (Fig. 2; e.g. Dum & Strick 1991a,b, 1996b, He et al 1993,1995, Murray & Coulter 1981, Nudo & Masterton 1990, Toyoshima & Sakai 1982). In fact, the number of corticospinal neurons in the medial wall premotor areas is substantial and can comprise as much as 40% of the total number of corticospinal neurons in the frontal lobe. Thus, each premotor area provides a potential source of descending commands to the spinal cord that are independent from those that originate from M1. Furthermore, each premotor area appears to receive a unique pattern of inputs from prefrontal, parietal and motor areas as well as from subcortical motor nuclei such as the basal ganglia and cerebellum (Dum & Strick 1991a, 1993). These and other results have led us to propose that each premotor area should be considered a nodal point for a functionally distinct efferent system driven from largely separate afferent sources.

In the next three sections we will present the results of three recent sets of experiments on the structure and function of the premotor areas on the medial wall. The first set explored the body map in the premotor areas (He et al 1995). The second examined whether corticospinal efferents from the premotor areas gain access to the output mechanisms of the spinal cord (i.e. motoneurons and last-order interneurons) (Dum & Strick 1996b). With this anatomical framework as a basis, the third set of experiments examined functional activation of the premotor areas during different motor tasks (Picard & Strick 1997).

Topographic organization of the premotor areas on the medial wall

We used a double-labelling approach to explore the topographic organization of the premotor areas on the medial wall. To define the pattern of 'arm' and 'leg'

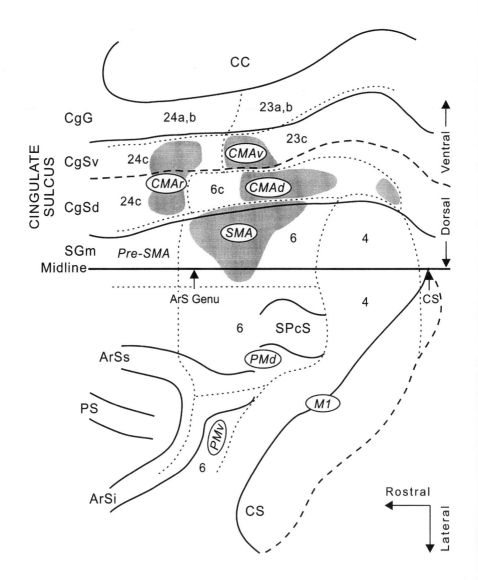

representation in each area, we injected one fluorescent tracer into lower cervical segments of the spinal cord and another fluorescent tracer into lower lumbosacral segments. In another set of animals, we explored the topographic organization of 'proximal' and 'distal' arm representation by injecting different tracers into upper cervical and lower cervical segments.

All four of the premotor areas on the medial wall project to cervical and lumbosacral segments of the spinal cord (He et al 1995). Three of these areas (SMA, CMAd and CMAv) are like M1 in having distinct arm and leg representations (Plate 1). Within the arm representation, each of the four motor areas on the medial wall contains separate regions that project densely to upper or to lower cervical segments. This observation suggests that each premotor area contains distinct proximal and distal representations of the arm. Surprisingly, the size of the distal representation is comparable to or larger than the size of the proximal representation in each premotor area. Thus, contrary to some previous hypotheses, the anatomical substrate exists for the premotor areas on the medial wall to be involved in the control of distal, as well as proximal arm movements. The maps of body representation produced by our double-labelling approach are fully consistent with those generated by other methods (e.g. Mitz & Wise 1987, Luppino et al 1991, Shima et al 1991, for review see Dum & Strick 1993). These maps provide the anatomical framework for interpreting sites of activation in functional imaging studies in trained primates (see below).

Spinal cord terminations of corticospinal efferents

In another set of experiments, we used anterograde transport of WGA-HRP to examine the pattern of spinal termination of efferents from the SMA, CMAd and CMAv. The termination patterns of these efferents were compared with those from

FIG. 1.   Location of the premotor areas and M1 in the frontal lobe. In this reconstruction of the frontal lobe of a macaque brain, the medial wall is unfolded and reflected upward to reveal the cingulate sulcus. The anterior bank of the central sulcus is also unfolded. A *dashed line* marks the fundus of each unfolded sulcus. The centres of the different cortical motor areas are designated by the *circled lettering*. The origin of corticospinal neurons that project from the medial wall premotor areas to the cervical segments of the spinal cord is indicated by *shading*. The boundaries between the motor areas and cytoarchitectonic areas (identified by *numbers*) are denoted with *dotted lines*. Abbreviations: ArS Genu (with arrow), the level of the genu of the arcuate sulcus; ArSi, inferior limb of the arcuate sulcus; ArSs, superior limb of the arcuate sulcus; CC, corpus callosum; CgG, cingulate gyrus; CgSd, dorsal bank of the cingulate sulcus; CgSv, ventral bank of the cingulate sulcus; CMAd, cingulate motor area on the dorsal bank of the cingulate sulcus; CMAr, rostral cingulate motor area; CMAv, cingulate motor area on the ventral bank of the cingulate sulcus; CS, central sulcus; PMd, dorsal premotor area; PMv, ventral premotor area; pre-SMA, pre-supplementary motor area; PS, principal sulcus; SGm, medial portion of the superior frontal gyrus; SPcS, superior precentral sulcus; SMA, supplementary motor area. (Adapted from Dum & Strick 1996b.)

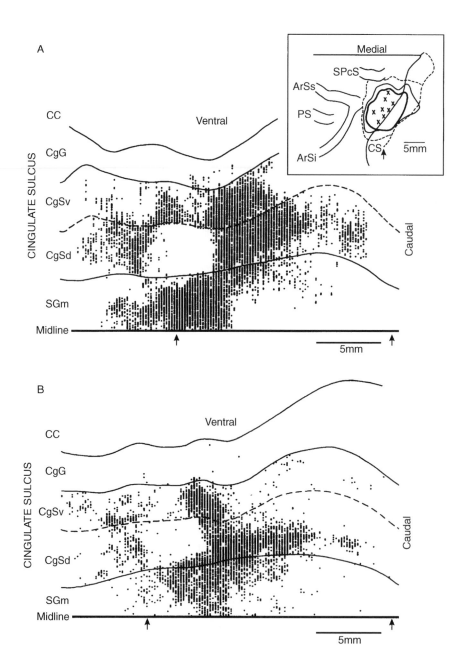

M1 (Dum & Strick 1996b). In general, the efferents from the premotor areas on the medial wall terminate in a pattern that is surprisingly similar to that of M1. Efferents from each of the premotor areas, like those from M1, terminate most densely in the intermediate zone of the cervical spinal cord (laminae V–VIII). For example, efferents from the SMA terminate densely in three regions: (1) dorsolaterally within laminae V–VII; (2) dorsomedially within lamina VI; and (3) ventromedially within lamina VII and adjacent lamina VIII (Fig. 3). Overall, the cingulate motor areas display a comparable pattern of laminar termination. However, efferents from the CMAd terminate most densely in the dorsolateral portion of the intermediate zone, whereas those from the CMAv are most concentrated in the dorsomedial region (Dum & Strick 1996b). Thus, the CMAd and CMAv may innervate separate sets of interneurons and, as a consequence, influence different aspects of segmental motor control.

One of our most important findings is that the efferents from the SMA, CMAd and CMAv terminate in the ventral horn (lamina IX). Although these terminations are not as dense as those from M1 (Fig. 3), they are like M1 terminations in that they are heaviest over the dorsolateral portions of the lower cervical segments where motoneurons that innervate distal forelimb muscles are located. Thus, the SMA, CMAd and CMAv appear to have direct connections with spinal motoneurons, particularly those innervating muscles of the fingers and wrist. Taken together, these results indicate that the anatomical substrate exists for each of these premotor areas on the medial wall to generate and control movement in a manner comparable to M1.

Functional activation of the premotor areas on the medial wall

We have proposed that each premotor area makes some unique contribution to the planning, preparation, initiation and/or execution of movement (Dum & Strick 1991a,b). To begin to test this concept, we used the 2-deoxyglucose (2DG) method to map functional activation of the medial wall in monkeys trained to perform remembered sequences of reaching movements (Picard & Strick 1997).

FIG. 2.   (A) Map of the cortical neurons that project from the premotor areas on the medial wall to M1. The WGA-HRP injection site in the arm area of M1 is indicated on a reconstruction of the frontal lobe (inset at upper right). The region of densest reaction product (*heavy line*) encircles the sites of needle penetration (X). A 'halo' of reaction product (*light line*) and a region of dense cells (*dashed line*) surround the core of the injection. In the reconstruction of the medial wall, every fourth section was unfolded as described in Fig. 1. Note that neurons (*dots*) projecting to the arm area of M1 are located in the same regions that project to cervical segments of the spinal cord in B. (B) Map of corticospinal neurons that project from the medial wall premotor areas to the cervical enlargement (C4–T2). See Fig. 1 for conventions and abbreviations. (Adapted from Dum & Strick 1991b.)

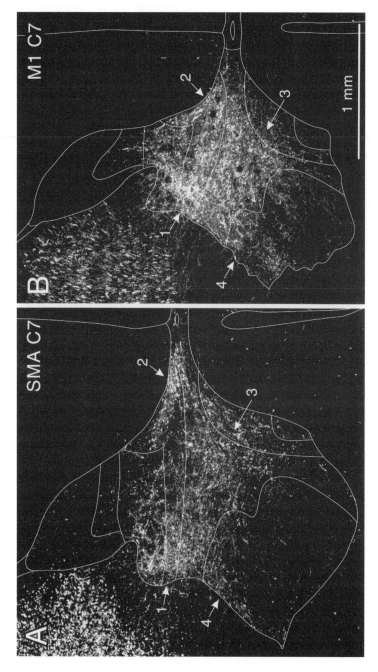

FIG. 3. Corticospinal terminations in contralateral C7 of the macaque. (A) Photomicrograph under dark-field/polarized light of TMB labelling after WGA-HRP injections into the SMA. SMA efferents terminate densely in four regions of the grey matter (*numbered arrows*, see text for further description). (B) TMB labelling after injection into M1. M1 efferents terminate densely in the same four regions of the grey matter as do SMA efferents. Laminar borders are indicated. (From Dum & Strick 1996b.)

The ability to perform sequences of movements is critical to many of the motor tasks we perform as part of our daily activities such as dressing, operating mechanical equipment, playing music or participating in sports. Early functional imaging studies in humans promoted the hypothesis that the SMA was preferentially involved in the generation of movement sequences, even when the sequences were not performed, but were imagined (Orgogozo & Larsen 1979, Roland et al 1980). Subsequent imaging studies have questioned these results in two respects. First, experiments using more sensitive imaging methods found activation in the SMA during the performance of even simple finger movements (Colebatch et al 1991, Fox et al 1985, Grafton et al 1993). Second, the area activated during the imagined performance of movement sequences was the rostrally located pre-SMA, and not the more caudally located SMA proper (for references and review see Picard & Strick 1996). However, the resolution of this controversy is difficult in humans because it is not possible to determine the cytoarchitecture of an activated area in each subject. The ability to correlate sites of activation with cytoarchitecture and well-defined body maps is one of the distinct advantages of conducting imaging studies in non-human primates.

We trained two animals to perform remembered sequences of reaching movements (REM task, Mushiake & Strick 1993, 1995). The monkeys faced a panel with five touch pads. The monkey initiated a trial by placing its hand on a hold key for 0.4–1.3 s. Then, three of five light emitting diodes (LEDs) located over each touch pad were illuminated sequentially. The LEDs remained illuminated until the end of the trial. After a delay of 1.25–2.15 s ('instructed delay' period), a 'Go' signal sounded. To receive a juice reward, the monkeys had to release the hold key and contact each of the three touch pads in the same order as the LEDs over them were illuminated. We presented the monkey with eight sequences which were varied pseudo-randomly between trials. Monkeys were given considerable practice on the REM task until they performed more than 90% of the trials correctly and inter-button intervals were relatively brief and regular.

To provide a baseline for comparison, another two animals performed a licking task (LICK task) in which they sat in the primate chair and licked juice delivered at a variable time interval (3.2–4.8 s). This interval approximated the rate of reward delivery for animals performing the REM task. The animals faced the same panel with five touch pads and were presented visual and auditory signals that were comparable to those of the REM task. However, these signals were behaviourally meaningless and the monkeys did not respond to them. Aside from licking, no movement was required. Conventional procedures were used to perform a semi-quantitative analysis of 2DG data from animals that performed either the REM or LICK task (e.g. Juliano et al 1981).

Activation on the medial wall in the animals that performed the LICK task was largely limited to the face representation of the SMA and a far rostral region in the banks of the cingulate sulcus (Plate 2). The monkeys that performed the REM task also displayed activation at these sites due to the licking movements they made to acquire the juice rewards. More importantly, several additional sites of activation were present on the medial wall of these monkeys. The most intense and extensive 2DG labelling was located in the dorsal bank of the cingulate sulcus, coincident with the arm representation in the CMAd. Weaker activations were present in the arm area of the SMA and in the pre-SMA. There was no significant 2DG incorporation in the ventral bank of the cingulate sulcus where the CMAv is located. These results indicate that the attributes of motor control are not represented equally across the motor areas on the medial wall. Specifically, the CMAd, more than any other area on the medial wall, appears to make a unique contribution to the preparation for and/or execution of highly practised sequences of movements.

The absence of focal activation in the SMA in the present study (Picard & Strick 1997) is surprising given the presence of sequence-specific neurons in this cortical area (Mushiake et al 1991, Tanji & Shima 1994). Several differences in the behavioural paradigms used in these studies may have contributed to this difference. For example, we overtrained our monkeys until the three elements of the movement sequence were performed as a stereotyped unit with invariant temporal characteristics. Mushiake et al (1991) did not train their animals to the same level of performance. Tanji & Shima (1994) used a fundamentally different task in which each movement in the sequence was triggered by an external stimulus. Thus, it is possible that the involvement of individual cortical areas depends on both the specific requirements of the task and the level of the animal's training on it.

Further support for the concept that participation of a motor area in a given task depends on the amount of training is provided by Aizawa et al's (1991) observations on the SMA. Normally, a large number of neurons in the SMA are related to the execution of a simple key press task. However, in an animal that was overtrained for more than a year, few task-related neurons could be found in the SMA. Following recovery from an ablation of M1, numerous movement-related neurons were again present in the SMA. This observation bolsters the view that the participation of specific cortical areas shifts with the level of task acquisition — particularly in the SMA.

Concluding remarks

There is growing evidence for the proposal that M1 is not the exclusive source of central commands for movement. It is now clear that the frontal lobe contains multiple premotor areas that project directly to M1 and to the spinal cord. Thus, each premotor area has the potential to influence motor output at both the cortical and spinal levels. In fact, some efferents from the premotor areas on the medial wall appear to project directly to motoneurons that innervate the distal limb. Thus, the anatomical substrate exists for the premotor areas to generate motor output independent of M1.

Each premotor area receives a unique mix of cortical and subcortical inputs. This implies that each motor area is differentially involved in specific aspects of motor behaviour. Physiological investigations provide some support for this conclusion. For example, some premotor areas appear to be particularly active during the preparation and generation of movement sequences, whereas others appear to be involved in the guidance of limb movement based on external cues (e.g. Mushiake et al 1991, Rizzolatti et al 1988). However, it is important to note that the field is at a relatively early phase in its examination of the functional contributions of these cortical areas. Indeed, several of the premotor areas on the medial wall have only recently been identified (for review see Picard & Strick 1996).

In this short presentation, we have reviewed some of the evidence concerning the pattern of body representation in each of the four premotor areas on the medial wall. One of the features of these maps deserves special emphasis. Each of these premotor areas, like M1, has a substantial part of their map devoted to the representation of the distal forelimb. Thus, these premotor areas appear to be involved in the control of distal as well as proximal limb movements.

On the basis of the insights derived from this structural framework, we have examined the functional activation of the premotor areas on the medial wall during the generation of sequential movements. This type of motor behaviour has long been thought to be within the province of the premotor cortex. Of the premotor areas on the medial wall, the CMAd was strongly and selectively activated during the performance of highly practised, remembered sequences of movement. This observation suggests that this premotor area plays some special role in the programming and/or execution of sequential movements. We believe that further insights into the function of the medial wall motor areas will come from examining patterns of functional activation during a broad range of behavioural paradigms. In every case, the interpretation of these patterns of activation will depend, in part, on a detailed knowledge of the body map within each premotor area. At present, such maps are only available for non-human primates. Thus, comparisons between imaging data in monkeys and humans will be essential for continued progress in this area.

References

Aizawa H, Inase M, Mushiake H, Shima K, Tanji J 1991 Reorganization of activity in the supplementary motor area associated with motor learning and functional recovery. Exp Brain Res 84:668–671

Colebatch JG, Deiber MP, Passingham RE, Friston KJ, Frackowiak RSJ 1991 Regional cerebral blood flow during voluntary arm and hand movements in human subjects. J Neurophysiol 65:1392–1401

Dum RP, Strick PL 1991a Premotor areas: nodal points for parallel efferent systems involved in the central control of movement. In: Humphrey DR, Freund H-J (eds) Motor control: concepts and issues. Wiley, Chichester, p 383–397

Dum RP, Strick PL 1991b The origin of corticospinal projections from the premotor areas in the frontal lobe. J Neurosci 11:667–689

Dum RP, Strick PL 1993 Cingulate motor areas. In: Vogt BA, Gabriel M (eds) Neurobiology of cingulate cortex and limbic thalamus. Birkhäuser, Boston, p 415–441

Dum RP, Strick PL 1996a The corticospinal system: a structural framework for the central control of movement. In: Rowell LB, Shepard JT (eds) Handbook of exercise physiology: integration of motor, circulatory, respiratory and metabolic control during exercise, section A: neural control of movement. Oxford University Press, New York, p 217–254

Dum RP, Strick PL 1996b Spinal cord terminations of the medial wall motor areas in macaque monkeys. J Neurosci 16:6513–6525

Fox PT, Fox JM, Raichle RM 1985 The role of cerebral cortex in the generation of voluntary saccades in a positron emission tomographic study. J Neurophysiol 54:348–369

Grafton ST, Woods RP, Mazziotta JC 1993 Within-arm somatotopy in human motor areas determined by positron emission tomography imaging of cerebral blood flow. Exp Brain Res 95:172–176

He SQ, Dum RP, Strick PL 1993 Topographic organization of corticospinal projections from the frontal lobe: motor areas on the lateral surface of the hemisphere. J Neurosci 13:952–980

He SQ, Dum RP, Strick PL 1995 Topographic organization of corticospinal projections from the frontal lobe: motor areas on the medial surface of the hemisphere. J Neurosci 15:3284–3306

Juliano SL, Hand PJ, Whitsel BL 1981 Patterns of increased metabolic activity in somatosensory cortex of monkeys *Macaca fascicularis*, subjected to controlled cutaneous stimulation: a 2-deoxyglucose study. J Neurophysiol 46:1260–1284

Luppino G, Matelli M, Camarda RM, Gallese V, Rizzolatti G 1991 Multiple representations of body movements in mesial area 6 and the adjacent cingulate cortex: an intracortical microstimulation study in the macaque monkey. J Comp Neurol 311:463–482

Mitz AR, Wise SP 1987 The somatotopic organization of the supplementary motor area: intracortical microstimulation mapping. J Neurosci 7:1010–1021

Murray EA, Coulter JD 1981 Organization of corticospinal neurons in the monkey. J Comp Neurol 195:339–365

Mushiake H, Inase M, Tanji J 1991 Neuronal activity in the primate premotor, supplementary, and precentral motor cortex during visually guided and internally determined sequential movements. J Neurophysiol 66:705–718

Mushiake H, Strick PL 1993 Preferential activity of dentate neurons during limb movements guided by vision. J Neurophysiol 70:2660–2664

Mushiake H, Strick PL 1995 Pallidal neuron activity during sequential arm movements. J Neurophysiol 74:2754–2758

Nudo RJ, Masterton RB 1990 Descending pathways to the spinal cord. III. Sites of origin of the corticospinal tract. J Comp Neurol 296:559–583

Orgogozo JM, Larsen B 1979 Activation of the supplementary motor area during voluntary movement in man suggests it works as a supramotor area. Science 206:847–850

Picard N, Strick PL 1996 Motor areas of the medial wall: a review of location and functional activation. Cerebral Cortex 6:342–353

Picard N, Strick PL 1997 Activation on the medial wall during remembered sequences of reaching movements in monkeys. J Neurophysiol 77:2197–2201

Rizzolatti G, Camarda R, Fogassi L, Gentilucci M, Luppino G, Matelli M 1988 Functional organization of inferior area 6 in the macaque monkey. II. Area F5 and the control of distal movements. Exp Brain Res 71:491–507

Roland PE, Larsen B, Lassen NA, Skinhoj E 1980 Supplementary motor area and other cortical areas in organization of voluntary movements in man. J Neurophysiol 43:118–136

Shima K, Aya K, Mushiake H, Inase M, Aizawa H, Tanji J 1991 Two movement-related foci in the primate cingulate cortex observed in signal-triggered and self-paced forelimb movements. J Neurophysiol 65:188–202

Tanji J, Shima K 1994 Role for supplementary motor area cells in planning several movements ahead. Nature 371:413–416

Toyoshima K, Sakai H 1982 Exact cortical extent of the origin of the corticospinal tract (CST) and the quantitative contribution to the CST in different cytoarchitectonic areas. A study with horseradish peroxidase in the monkey. J Hirnforsch 23:257–269

DISCUSSION

Fetz: These imaging studies are marvellous. They provide a great way to bypass all the time it would take to record neurons.

Strick: We are going to record as well.

Fetz: That would be useful. In the remembered sequencing task, I was surprised to see so little labelling in the pre-SMA and SMA, where Tanji's studies would predict that cells would be involved (Shima et al 1996, Tanji & Shima 1994).

Strick: Tanji's test is quite different from ours in one fundamental way: his animals perform one movement, then there is a pause. The second and third movements in the sequence are performed only after the second and third triggers. The organization of this task has been very useful for Tanji because it allows him to examine neuron activity during the delay period prior to the trigger signals. This activity may be related to the motor programming of movement sequences. We thought that our task is a more natural circumstance because the essence of a sequential movement is that one element of action is performed right after another. For instance, when you are tying your shoes, the movements form a continuous flow without a pause between each element. These task differences between Tanji's experiments and ours may be sufficient to explain why we don't see activation in the pre-SMA and see very little in the SMA during our REM task.

A second consideration is that the regions of cortex activated by a task may depend on the amount of practice that the animal has had on the task. Tanji has shown that neurons in the SMA were consistently active before movement onset during a simple key press task. However, in a monkey that was overtrained on that task for a year and a half, very little activity was present in the SMA (Aizawa et al 1991). Then, Tanji and his colleagues removed the primary motor cortex. Following recovery and some retraining, robust activity was again observed in the SMA. This result suggests that going from practiced to greatly over-practiced caused a shift in the regions of the cortex involved in generating the simple key press movement. The old adage that 'practice makes perfect' has to be translated in some way to changes in the nervous system. It may be that the reaching movements the monkeys used to perform our REM task were sufficiently over-practiced and gross (in terms of accuracy requirements), that they did not require intense activation of the primary motor cortex. On the other hand, it is likely that activation of the primary motor cortex and the SMA are necessary during the initial stages of learning the task.

Savaki: In your 2DG experiments, the values you report are not glucose consumption values but 2DG tissue concentration values — what you call '2DG uptake'.

Strick: No, what we do is a normalization procedure. We take the region where there is the peak 2DG uptake and set this to 100% activation. This happens to be in part of the face representation of SI. Then, we take a reading of background from a portion of the hindlimb representation of M1 and set this to 0%. With this procedure it is possible to normalize the activations from every animal to a common scale. We don't take blood samples because we don't want to disrupt the animals' behaviour.

Savaki: Normalization does not convert a qualitative to a quantitative study. The values which you report are not glucose consumption (local cerebral glucose utilization [LCGU]) values, but normalized 2DG tissue concentration values. The problem here is that the latter values depend not only on the local rate of glucose consumption but also on the blood glucose level of the monkey and the local blood flow. The original operational equation proposed by Sokoloff for the calculation of LCGU (Sokoloff et al 1977) takes care of these parameters and thus the quantitative 2DG method allows for comparisons within and between monkeys. The qualitative 2DG method, which you have been using, often leads to incorrect estimation of local metabolic activity in the brain and thus to misinterpretation of data.

Specifically, there is a problem with the 'background' which you have been using in your presentation as well as in your recent study (Picard & Strick 1997). You consider as 'background' the 'amount of labelling in a portion of the leg representation in M1'. Then, you express all the effects in reference to that value. In 1996, in a quantitative 2DG study, we reported maps of LCGU which demonstrate that the hindlimb–lower body representations in M1 are bilaterally activated by reaching movements, due to postural adjustment during reaching (Dalezios et al 1996, Savaki et al 1997). Thus, what you consider as background in the licking control monkey is lower than what you consider as background in the experimental monkeys. This means that you overestimate the background and you underestimate the effects in reaching monkeys. Consequently, all percentages and comparisons have been miscalculated in your study.

Strick: Let me address that precisely. Like you, we see 2DG activation in a part of the hindlimb region. However, we measure background in a different portion of the hindlimb region where there is low 2DG activation in *all* animals. This procedure does not lead to a miscalculation of background.

Savaki: Strictly speaking, if you have one region which displays increased labelling in your qualitative study and a second one which displays decreased labelling (let us call them dark and light regions), you can either say that the dark area is activated as compared with the light one which you may consider as the background, or that the light area is inhibited as compared with the dark one which you also may consider as the background. Only proper quantification could demonstrate which area is activated, which is inhibited and which is unaffected. Only glucose consumption values of unaffected regions should be considered as background values for further normalizations and intersubject comparisons.

Strick: We normalize our data because it allows us to put the results in a common framework that negates global sources of variation such as blood flow, glucose level, etc. For normalization to be valid, one must check that the patterns of activation observed in maps before normalization are comparable across animals. In every animal, we found the highest 2DG activity in the SI face representation and the lowest 2DG activity in a portion of the M1 hindlimb representation. This was true even though the raw values in the hindlimb region varied across animals.

Overall, I believe that the major difference between our results and yours is that your animals were performing a visually guided reaching task, whereas ours were performing an internally guided remembered sequence task. In fact, when we examined the patterns of cortical activation during a visually guided pointing task, our results look very similar to yours (Picard & Strick 1996, 1997, 1998). I don't believe one should underestimate the importance of task differences.

Lemon: The point is well taken about the multiplicity of these areas projecting to the cord. Let us assume that the execution component of the two tasks you have tested is absolutely identical. Then, let us make the further assumption that the 2DG results reflect, at least in part, a differential contribution of the corticospinal neurons in those different cortical motor areas (although the 2DG studies must reflect all of the cellular activity in those areas, not just the small proportion of cells that are going to the cord). The question we would all like to answer is what is different about the way in which those motoneurons and muscles are activated in the two tasks that requires a different cortical output to the spinal cord? Is the spinal cord interested in the 'context' of that movement?

Strick: Let me take the most extreme position. We have shown that there are a set of descending systems from the cortical motor areas that *appear* to have access to the same motoneurons and interneurons. One could imagine that a descending command from any one of these systems could produce an identical motor output. Thus, under these circumstances one would not be able to kinematically distinguish which system had generated a particular movement.

Thach: You see 'hotspots' alternating in each of these two different areas — each hotspot appropriate to each of two tasks. The 2DG and imaging wisdom is that a hotspot actually represents activity in the terminals coming into the area, rather than the cells themselves giving rise to the output. Since the inputs are often excitatory, it's reasonable to infer activation of the output of this area. This raises the question about what the activity is in the input areas, since you have shown that they receive differentially from basal ganglia and cerebellum. There have been various proposals as to differential roles of these structures in remembered sequences. I wonder whether you have seen differences in these structures in these events?

Strick: The answer to that is very complex. We've shown anatomically that there are multiple output channels in the basal ganglia. These channels target different cortical areas, and they are spatially separate within the output nuclei of the basal ganglia (Hoover & Strick 1993, Strick et al 1995). We have also shown that there are separate outputs from the basal ganglia to the face, arm and leg representations of M1 (Hoover & Strick 1998). In 2DG experiments where we have examined the pattern of activation in animals that are simply licking, we see activation in face M1, face SMA and some face pre-SMA. If, as our anatomical data suggest, each of these cortical areas is the target of a separate output channel in the globus pallidus, then one would expect to see multiple small patches of activation in the globus pallidus related to licking. Preliminary analysis of our data suggests that this is in fact the case. Differentiating these small patches related to licking from those associated with the performance of arm movements is very difficult because the two types of patches would be intermingled. The level of analysis that one must do to decipher patterns of activation in the basal ganglia is quite different from that required for the analysis of the cerebral cortex. Furthermore, more of the anatomical framework of basal ganglia organization is necessary before we undertake this task. For example, the location of the output channel in the globus pallidus that projects to the CMAd is unknown. The interpretation of patterns of activation in the basal ganglia and the relation of these to patterns of activation in the cortex depends critically on this type of information.

Andersen: Are there eye movement fields embedded within the multiple motor maps? Have you measured eye movements? Did you look at the currently known eye fields (frontal eye field and supplementary eye field) and is there differential activity in these eye fields in your tasks?

Strick: Eye movements were not the focus of our studies. In fact, we confined our analysis of the sites of activation to the cortical motor areas that we have shown in other studies project to cervical segments of the spinal cord.

We have done single neuron recordings in animals trained on these tasks (Mushiake & Strick 1993, 1995). Prior to neuron recording in the dentate and globus pallidus, we examined muscle activity and eye movements. During licking, animals make spontaneous eye movements, whereas during the remembered sequence task, animals make predictive eye movements — i.e. as the arm moves to the first target in the sequence, the eye begins to move to the next target in the sequence. Interestingly, we have seen marked activation in the supplementary eye field during the remembered sequence task, but not during the licking task.

References

Aizawa H, Inase M, Mushiake H, Shima K, Tanji J 1991 Reorganization of activity in the supplementary motor area associated with motor learning and functional recovery. Exp Brain Res 84:668–671

Dalezios Y, Raos VC, Savaki HE 1996 Metabolic activity pattern in the motor and somatosensory cortex of monkeys performing a visually guided reaching task with one forelimb. Neuroscience 72:325–333

Hoover JE, Strick PL 1993 Multiple output channels in the basal ganglia. Science 259:819–821

Hoover JE, Strick PL 1998 The organization of cerebellar and basal ganglia outputs to primary motor cortex as revealed by retrograde transneuronal transport of herpes simplex virus type 1. Submitted

Mushiake H, Strick PL 1993 Preferential activity of dentate neurons during limb movements guided by vision. J Neurophysiol 70:2660–2664

Mushiake H, Strick PL 1995 Pallidal neuron activity during sequential arm movements. J Neurophysiol 74:2754–2758

Picard N, Strick PL 1995 Differential involvement of M1 and a premotor area in a motor task. Soc Neurosci Abstr 21:2077

Picard N, Strick PL 1996 Comparison of 2DG uptake in medial wall motor areas during performance of visually guided and remembered sequences of movements. Soc Neurosci Abstr 22:2025

Picard N, Strick PL 1997 Activation on the medial wall during remembered sequences of reaching movements in monkeys. J Neurophysiol 77:2197–2201

Picard N, Strick PL 1998 Context dependent activation of arm M1 of the monkey in a sequential movement task. Soc Neurosci Abstr 24, in press

Savaki HE, Raos VC, Dalezios Y 1997 Spatial cortical patterns of metabolic activity in monkeys performing a visually guided reaching task with one forelimb. Neuroscience 76:1007–1034

Shima K, Mushiake H, Saito N, Tanji J 1996 Role for cells in the presupplementary motor area in updating motor plans. Proc Natl Acad Sci USA 93:8694–8698

Sokoloff L, Reivich M, Kennedy C et al 1977 The [14C]-deoxyglucose method for the measurement of local cerebral glucose utilization: theory, procedure, and normal values in the conscious and anaesthetised albino rat. J Neurochem 28:879–916

Strick PL, Dum RP, Mushiake H 1995 Basal ganglia 'loops' with the cerebral cortex. In: Kimura M, Graybiel AM (eds) Functions of the cortico-basal ganglia loop. Springer-Verlag, Tokyo, p 106–124

Tanji J, Shima K 1994 Role for supplementary motor area cells in planning several movements ahead. Nature 371:413–416

Grasping objects and grasping action meanings: the dual role of monkey rostroventral premotor cortex (area F5)

Giacomo Rizzolatti and Luciano Fadiga

Istituto di Fisiologia Umana, Università di Parma, Via Gramsci, 14-43100 Parma, Italy

Abstract. Monkey area F5 consists of two main histochemical sectors, one buried inside the arcuate sulcus, the other located on the cortical convexity. Neurons of both sectors discharge during hand movements. Many of them also fire in response to the presentation of visual stimuli. However, the visual stimuli effective for triggering the neurons in each sector are markedly different. Neurons located in the bank of the arcuate sulcus respond to the observation of 3D *objects*, provided that object size and shape is congruent with the prehension type coded by the neuron ('canonical' F5 neurons). Neurons of the convexity discharge when the monkey observes *hand actions* performed by another individual, provided that they are similar to the motor action coded by the neuron ('mirror' neurons). What do the canonical F5 neurons and the surprising mirror neurons have in common? The interpretation we propose is that these two categories of F5 neurons both generate an internal copy of a potential hand action. In the case of 'canonical' neurons, this copy gives a description of how to grasp an object; in the case of mirror neurons it gives a description of an action made by another person. Because the individuals know the consequences of their actions, we propose that the internal motor copies of the observed actions represent the neural basis for understanding the meaning of actions made by others.

1998 Sensory guidance of movement. Wiley, Chichester (Novartis Foundation Symposium 218) p 81–103

The view that the external reality cannot be understood without an active interaction between the perceiving agent and the world has been advanced by philosophers as diverse as Main de Biran (1802) and Schopenhauer (1819) in the last century and phenomenologists in the present. The role of motor system in semantics was, however, almost completely ignored by neurophysiologists (see, however, Varela et al 1992), the common view being that the motor system is a system that controls and executes movements. In this article we will review the functional characteristics of a premotor area (area F5; Matelli et al 1985), with the aim of showing that this area has a dual function: that of representing internally actions for programming hand movements and that of representing the same actions for understanding them when performed by another individual.

Area F5: motor properties

Studies in which the rostral part of inferior area 6 of the monkey (area F5) was electrically stimulated showed that in this sector of the premotor cortex there is a representation of hand and mouth movements (Rizzolatti et al 1988, Hepp-Reymond et al 1994). Single neuron studies confirmed this conclusion (Kurata & Tanji 1986, Rizzolatti et al 1988). Most importantly, they showed that the discharge of most F5 neurons correlates with the goal of an action much better than with that of the individual movements that form it (Rizzolatti et al 1988). A clear instance of this behaviour is represented by F5 neurons that discharge when the monkey grasps an object with its right hand or with its left hand or with its mouth. An example of such a neuron is illustrated in Fig. 1. It is obvious that in this case a description of neuron behaviour in terms of elementary movements makes little sense. Using the effective action as a classification criterion, we subdivided F5 neurons into a series of classes. Among them the most common are 'grasping' neurons, 'holding' neurons, 'tearing' neurons and 'manipulating' neurons.

Grasping neurons are the neurons most represented in F5. Many of them are selective for a particular type of prehension such as precision grip, finger prehension, or whole hand prehension. An example is shown in Fig. 2. This neuron discharges when the animal uses the finger and the thumb for grasping an object, but not all the fingers together. Some neurons show specificity for different finger configurations, even within the same grip type. Thus, the prehension of a large spherical object (whole hand prehension that requires the opposition of all fingers) is coded by neurons different from those that code the prehension of a cylinder (still whole hand prehension but performed with the opposition of the four last fingers and the palm of the hand).

The study of the temporal relation between the neural discharge and the grasping movement showed a variety of behaviours. Some F5 neurons discharge during the whole action that they code. Some are active during the opening of the fingers, some during finger closure, and some only after the contact with the object.

Taken together, the functional properties of F5 neurons suggest that this area stores a set of motor schemata (Arbib 1997) or, as we previously proposed, contains a 'vocabulary' of motor acts (Rizzolatti & Gentilucci 1988). The 'words' composing this vocabulary are constituted by populations of neurons. Some of them indicate the general category of an action (hold, grasp, tear, manipulate). Others specify the effectors that are appropriate for that action. Finally, a third group is concerned with the temporal segmentation of the actions. What differentiates F5 from the primary motor cortex (F1) is that its motor schemata

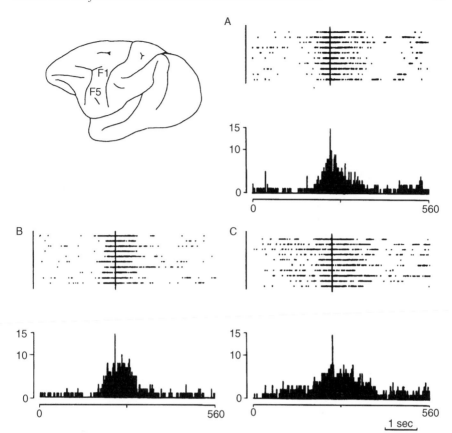

FIG. 1. 'Grasping with the hand and the mouth' neuron. In the upper-left panel a lateral view of the left hemisphere of the monkey brain is shown. Letters indicate the position of the precentral motor cortex (area F1) and the premotor area F5. (A) Discharge of neuron during grasping with the mouth. (B) Discharge of neuron during prehension with the contralateral hand. (C) Discharge of neuron during prehension with the ipsilateral hand. Histograms are aligned with the moment at which the animal touched the food. Individual trials are shown above each histogram. Bin width, 10 ms. Ordinates, spikes/bin; abscissas, ms.

are goal-directed actions (or fragments of specific actions), whereas F1 stores movements regardless of the action context in which they are used. In comparison with F5, F1 could be defined as a 'vocabulary of movements'.

The view that F5 contains a vocabulary of actions has important functional implications. Firstly, the presence of such a vocabulary strongly facilitates the execution of motor commands. The existence of preformed motor schemata which are anatomically strictly linked (hard-wired) with cortical (F1) and subcortical motor centres, facilitates the selection of the most appropriate

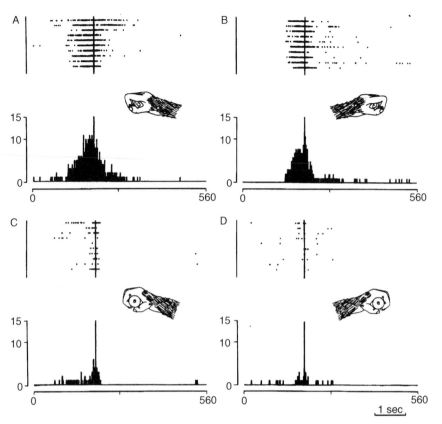

FIG. 2. 'Grasping with the hand' neuron. (A, B) Discharge of neuron during precision grip.
(C, D) Discharge of neuron during whole hand prehension. (A, C) Contralateral hand. (B, D)
Ipsilateral hand. Conventions as in Fig. 1.

combination of movements by reducing the number of variables that the motor
system has to control to achieve the action goal. Secondly, it simplifies the
association between a given stimulus (i.e. a visually presented object) and the
appropriate motor response toward it (see below). Thirdly, it gives the brain a
storage of 'action schemata' that, as we will show in the next sections, could be
used also for purposes other than strictly motor functions.

The motor properties of F5 we just described are possessed by all F5 neurons.
However, if one examines their responses to visual stimuli, it becomes apparent
that in F5 there are two radically different categories of visuomotor neurons.
Neurons of the first category discharge when the monkey observes graspable
objects. They appear to play a role in object-to-hand movement transformations
(see Jeannerod et al 1995, see also below for further evidence). Since visuomotor

transformation is one of the functions commonly attributed to ventral premotor cortex, we will refer to them as 'canonical F5 neurons'. Neurons of the second category discharge when the monkey observes another individual making an action in front of it. These neurons have been named 'mirror neurons' (Rizzolatti et al 1996a, Gallese et al 1996).

The two categories of F5 neurons are located in two different sub-regions of area F5: canonical neurons are mainly found in the posterior bank of arcuate sulcus, whereas mirror neurons are almost exclusively recorded from the cortical convexity of F5.

F5 canonical neurons

Visual responses and visuomotor transformation: electrophysiological recordings

Some years ago, in experiments in which we tested F5 neurons using food and other graspable objects, we found that many F5 neurons fired in response to object presentation (Rizzolatti et al 1988). Recently we re-examined the visual responses of F5 neurons using a formal behavioural paradigm, which allowed us to examine separately the responses to object presentation, the discharge during the delay between object presentation and movement onset, and the movement-related discharge (Murata et al 1997).

The results showed that about 20% of the tested neurons responded to 3D object presentation and two-thirds of them were selective to one specific object or to a cluster of similar objects. Figure 3 shows the responses of a visually selective neuron. Observation and grasping (Fig. 3A) of the ring produced strong responses. Responses to the other five objects were modest (sphere) or virtually absent.

Figures 3B and C show the behaviour of the same neuron in two other experimental conditions: object fixation and object grasping in the dark. In object fixation the objects were presented as before, but, at the 'go' signal, instead of grasping the object the monkey had to release a key. Grasping was not allowed. Note that in this condition the object is totally irrelevant for task solution which only requires the detection of the 'go' signal. Yet, the neuron strongly discharged at the presentation of the preferred object (Fig. 3B).

The behaviour of the neuron during object grasping in the dark is illustrated in Fig. 3C. In the absence of any visual stimulus the neuron discharged in association with ring grasping. The movement-related discharge was preceded by a preparatory discharge.

How can these findings be explained? It is obvious that the object-related visual responses were not due to non-specific factors such as attention or 'intention' (desire to grasp the object). If either of these explanations were true the neuron

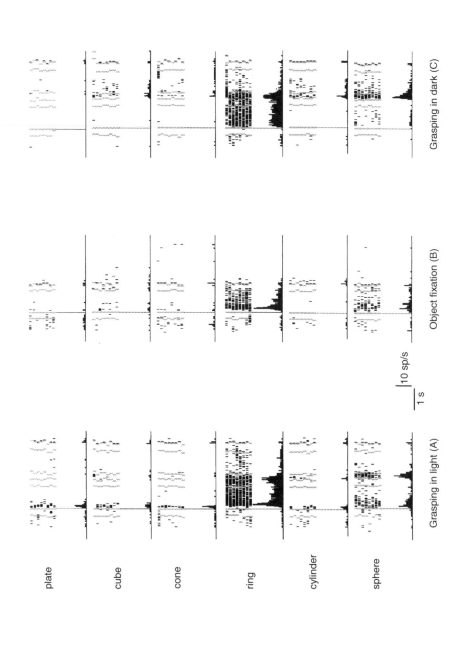

plate

cube

cone

ring

cylinder

sphere

10 sp/s

1 s

Grasping in light (A)

Object fixation (B)

Grasping in dark (C)

would have not shown object specificity. Attention and intention are the same regardless of the nature of the object presented. The interpretation we favour is that, in adult individuals, there is a close link between the most common 3D stimuli and the actions necessary to interact with them. Thus, every time a graspable object is presented, the related F5 neurons are addressed and the action is 'automatically' evoked.

Interestingly, recent brain imaging studies have demonstrated a similar phenomenon in humans (Perani et al 1995, Martin et al 1996, Grafton et al 1997). The presentation of tools or other graspable objects to normal human subjects activates the premotor cortex even when no motor response is required. Thus, object-related motor activation appears to represent in both monkeys and humans a 'potential' action — an 'idea' of how to act. Under certain circumstances, it guides the execution of the movement, under others, it remains an unexecuted representation of it.

Lesion experiments

The motor properties of F5 neurons and the visual properties of canonical F5 neurons just reviewed strongly suggest that F5 plays a crucial role in visuomotor transformations for grasping objects. In order to test directly this hypothesis we made reversible lesions of F5 (muscimol injections) in two monkeys trained to reach and grasp objects of different size and shape. Injection sites were chosen after stimulation and recording sessions in which the hand field of F1 and the region of F5 where canonical neurons are mostly located (posterior bank of the arcuate sulcus) were functionally identified.

Three different inactivation sessions were carried out for each monkey. They consisted of: (1) single injection in F5 bank, (2) multiple injections in F5 bank and, as a control, (3) single injection in F1 hand field.

After single injection in F5 bank, the monkeys showed a severe deficit in preshaping and execution of precision grip with the hand contralateral to the lesion. The hand was exaggeratedly opened during the transport phase and reached the object kept in an inappropriate way. Only after object contact was the hand posture corrected and the monkey able to grasp the object. Prehension

---

FIG. 3.   Example of a selective visuomotor neuron. Panels show neural activity (individual rasters and response histograms) recorded during grasping in light (A), object fixation (B) and grasping in dark (C) tasks. Rasters and histograms are aligned with the key press. In A and B the key press determined object presentation. The vertical grey bars across rasters indicate the different phases of the behavioural task. Their irregularity is due to the variability in task execution that changed from trial to trial. The fourth grey bar in each raster indicates the key release. In A and C the key release was followed by grasping. Bin width, 20 ms. For other details see Murata et al (1997).

of larger stimuli such as larger spheres and vertical and horizontal cylinders was preserved.

Following multiple injections in F5 bank, the observed deficit was much more severe than in the previous experiment. The hand *contralateral* to the injection side was used to grasp, usually incorrectly, only the largest objects, while it was not even moved to reach objects that required precision grip. The *ipsilateral* hand was also strongly affected. The deficit concerned grasping of most of the objects. As in the case of single injection, the final correct grip of the object was accomplished only after tactile exploration.

The inactivation of F1 (hand field) induced a severe deficit in the discrete finger movements of the contralateral hand. The monkey approached all objects with a stereotyped hand configuration keeping the fingers in a semi-flexed posture during the whole movement. Grasping of small objects could not be executed. Among large objects, only those (e.g. a large cylinder) which do not require discrete finger movement to be taken, were grasped, although with diminished force. Touching the object did not improve grasping performance.

Hand shaping during arm transport towards the target depends on the capacity to extract visual information on the intrinsic properties of the object and to transform it into hand movements. This capacity was lost following F5 inactivation. The deficit was not due to a paresis, as in the case of inactivation of F1. In fact, as soon as somatosensory information about the object was available, the monkey was able to grasp it.

Grasping deficits similar to those found after F5 inactivation were observed following muscimol injection in parietal area AIP (Gallese et al 1994), a parietal area connected with F5 bank region and involved in visual analysis of the intrinsic properties of objects (Taira et al 1990, Sakata et al 1995). Taken together, the data on inactivations of AIP and F5 provide direct evidence that the circuit formed by AIP and F5 plays a crucial role in visuomotor transformation for grasping.

F5 mirror neurons

Functional properties

Mirror neurons are a class of F5 neuron that become active when the *monkey acts* on an object *and* when the *monkey observes another monkey or the experimenter* making goal-directed actions (Rizzolatti et al 1996a, Gallese et al 1996). They appear, therefore, to be identical to canonical neurons in terms of motor properties, but to differ radically from them for visual properties.

The visual stimuli most effective in triggering mirror neurons are actions in which the experimenter's hand or mouth interacts with objects. The presentation of 3D objects, faces or gestures having emotional meaning is ineffective. Similarly, actions made using tools, even when identical to those made using hands, do not activate the neurons or only activate them very weakly. The distance from the monkey at which the effective action is made does not influence significantly the response intensity.

The observed actions which most commonly activate mirror neurons are grasping, placing and manipulating. Most mirror neurons respond selectively to one type of action (e.g. grasping). Some are highly specific, coding not only the action aim, but also how that action is executed. They fire, for example, during observation of grasping movements, but only when the object is grasped with the index finger and the thumb. Examples of mirror neurons are shown in Figs 4 and 5.

Typically, mirror neurons show congruence between the observed and executed action. This congruence can be extremely strict, i.e. the effective motor action (e.g. precision grip) coincides with the action that, when seen, triggers the neurons (e.g. precision grip). For other neurons the congruence is broader. For them the motor requirements (e.g. precision grip) are usually stricter than the visual ones (any type of hand grasping).

A possible functional role of mirror neurons

The first idea that comes to mind about mirror neurons is that their activity is preparatory to a impending movement or, even, that it depends on an abortive movements passed unnoticed to the experimenter. Both these hypotheses are incorrect. Control experiments showed that mirror neurons discharge in response to the appropriate stimulus both when the monkey is still (EMG recordings, single neuron recordings from F1) and when it performs movements that have no relation to the observed action. Furthermore, mirror neurons do not fire when an object (that when grasped or manipulated by the experimenter activate them) is moved towards the monkey and made, therefore, more available for an action on it (see Fig. 4). The 'motor preparation' hypothesis predicts exactly the contrary.

The most likely interpretation of mirror neurons is that their discharge generates an internal representation of the observed action (see Jeannerod 1994). We saw in the previous section that the same occurs in canonical neurons when an object is presented to the monkey. Thus, both categories of F5 neurons appear to generate 'ideas' on how to act, the difference being that in one case these ideas are generated by objects; in the second case by the sight of an action.

What is the purpose of a motor representation generated by the sight of actions of others? How may this representation be used? There are two likely possibilities: action imitation and action understanding (Jeannerod 1994, Rizzolatti et al 1996a,

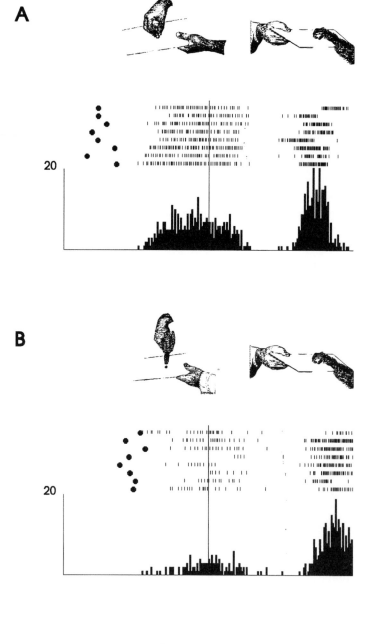

1 s

Gallese et al 1996, Carey et al 1997). These two possibilities are not in conflict with one another — rather, they are complementary.

Imitation is a fundamental ability of humans and apes, an ability which has played more than just a marginal role in human evolution (Donald 1991). PET data show that in humans observation of meaningful actions both for imitating and understanding activate the inferior frontal lobe, suggesting a common substrate for the two functions (Rizzolatti et al 1996b, Grafton et al 1996, Decety et al 1997). Whether monkeys, however, are able to imitate actions is not clear (see Byrne 1994, Galef 1988, Whiten & Ham 1992). If they really cannot do it, this would indicate that monkeys use the mirror system only for action recognition (see the next section), i.e. for a more basic function. In other words, monkeys, although endowed of a mechanism that generates internal copies of actions made by others, are unable to use them for replicating those actions. The intentional use of internal copies of actions developed only later in evolution.

Motor systems and the semantics of action

The studies of Perrett et al (1990) showed that in the anterior section of the superior temporal sulcus (STS), there is a variety of neurons that may contribute to visual recognition of actions. Some of them encode the form of body postures, others code specific body movements and still others discharge during goal-directed actions. The spectrum of body parts and body movements that are specified in the temporal lobe is wide and, at variance with F5, includes arbitrary postures and movements (Perrett et al 1990, Carey et al 1997).

Let us assume that this wide repertoire of neurons is present at birth and that each neuron fires when the appropriate stimulus appears in the field of vision signalling a given event. Is this sufficient? Can a new-born child give a meaning to this welter of information? How can it refer these signals to something it knows?

This problem can be solved theoretically if the motor system is endowed with an observation/execution matching system, such as that of mirror neurons. When an

---

FIG. 4. Visual and motor responses of a mirror neuron. Testing conditions are schematically represented above the rasters. Response histograms represent the sum of eight consecutive trials (raster display). (A) A tray with a piece of food is presented to the monkey (filled circles), the experimenter grasps the food, puts the food back onto the tray and then moves the tray towards the monkey who grasps the food. The phases when the food is presented and when it is moved towards the monkey are characterized by the absence of neuronal discharge. In contrast, a strong activation is present during grasping movements of both the experimenter and the monkey. (B) As above, except that the experimenter grasps the food with pliers. In both A and B, rasters and histograms are aligned with the moment at which the experimenter touched the food either with his hand or with the pliers (vertical line). Bin width, 20 ms. Ordinates, spikes/bin; abscissas, time.

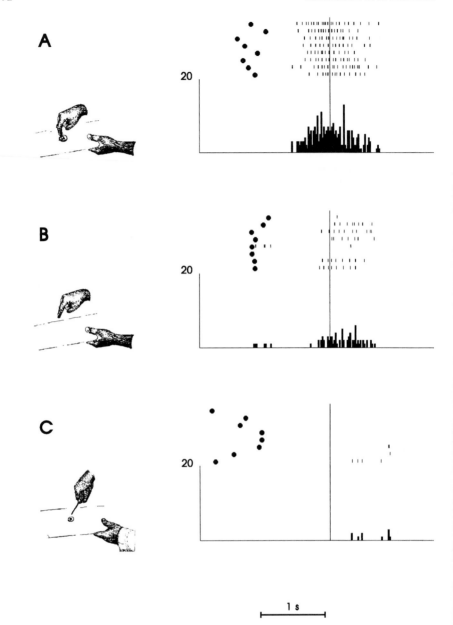

FIG. 5.   Visual responses of a mirror neuron. (A) The experimenter retrieves a piece of food placed in a well in a tray, using his index finger. This was the only action that activated the neuron when performed by the monkey. (B) The same action is mimed without food. (C) The food is retrieved using a tool. Conventions as in Fig. 4.

individual emits an action, he predicts ('knows') its consequences. This knowledge is most likely the result of an association between the 'idea' of movement, the potential action coded in the premotor cortex that we discussed above, and the consequences of this action. Mirror neurons are able to extend this knowledge to actions performed by others. When the observation of an action performed by another individual activates neurons that represent that action in the observer's premotor cortex, the observed action will be recognized because of the similarity (or even identity) of the evoked representation to that internally generated during its active programming.

It would take too long to review the theoretical reasons why we believe that mechanisms similar to those that render possible action understanding should be valid also for understanding object semantics (see Rizzolatti & Gallese 1997). What is important here is to note that having an internal copy of an action made by another individual makes it possible to give meaning not only to the observed action but also to other actions, movements and postures related to it. The parieto-frontal connections are reciprocal. The top-down output from premotor cortex to postrolandic cortices could serve therefore as a 'validating' input, not only for neurons coding actions but also for neurons that code action fragment or even postures. Through (for example) a coincident firing, 'assemblies' of neurons can be generated all 'marked' as elements of the same general action. This top-down action of premotor cortex should greatly enlarge the number of actions that have a meaning for the organism without putting the burden of detailed action coding on the premotor cortex.

Finally, it is important to stress that, although the considerations of this section are very speculative, they can be tested experimentally. Lesion studies of mirror neuron sites as well a simultaneous recording of F5 and 7b (or STS) neurons can assess empirically their validity.

Acknowledgements

The authors thank Marc Jeannerod for drawing their attention on the work of Main de Biran, and Jean-Luc Petit for his comments on the presented findings based on the latest work of Husserl. This work was supported by the EEC Contract Biomed/H4 CT95-0789 and by the Italian Consiglio Nazionale delle Ricerche (grants to G.R. and L.F.).

References

Arbib MA 1997 Modelling visuomotor transformations. In: Jeannerod M, Grafman J (eds) Handbook of neuropsychology, vol 11: Action and cognition. Elsevier Science BV, Amsterdam, p 65–90

Byrne R W 1994 The evolution of intelligence. In: Slater PGB, Halliday TR (eds) Behaviour and evolution. Cambridge University Press, Cambridge

Carey DP, Perrett DI, Oram MW 1997 Recognizing, understanding and reproducing actions. In: Jeannerod M, Grafman J (eds) Handbook of neuropsychology, vol 11: Action and cognition. Elsevier Science BV, Amsterdam, p 111–130

Decety J, Grezes J, Costes N et al 1997 Brain activity during observation of actions. Influence of action content and subject's strategy. Brain 120:1763–1777

Donald M 1991 Origins of the modern mind: three stages in the evolution of culture and cognition. Harvard University Press, Cambridge, MA

Galef BG 1988 Imitation in animals: field and laboratory analysis. In: Zental T, Galef BG (eds) Social learning: psychological and biological perspectives. Lawrence Erlbaum Associates, Hillsdale, NJ, p 1–28

Gallese V, Murata A, Kaseda M, Niki N, Sakata H 1994 Deficit of hand preshaping after muscimol injection in monkey parietal cortex. Neuroreport 5:1525–1529

Gallese V, Fadiga L, Fogassi L, Rizzolatti G 1996 Action recognition in the premotor cortex. Brain 119:593–609

Grafton ST, Arbib MA, Fadiga L, Rizzolatti G 1996 Localization of grasp representation in humans by PET: 2. Observation compared with imagination. Exp Brain Res 112:103–111

Grafton ST, Fadiga L, Arbib MA, Rizzolatti G 1997 Premotor cortex activation during observation and naming of familiar tools. Neuroimaging 6:231–236

Hepp-Reymond M-C, Husler EJ, Maier MA, Qi H-X 1994 Force-related neuronal activity in two regions of the primate ventral premotor cortex. Can J Physiol Pharmacol 72:571–579

Jeannerod M 1994 The representing brain: neural correlates of motor intention and imagery. Behav Brain Sci 17:187–245

Jeannerod M, Arbib MA, Rizzolatti G, Sakata H 1995 Grasping objects: the cortical mechanisms of visuomotor transformation. Trends Neurosci 18:314–320

Kurata K, Tanji J 1986 Premotor cortex neurons in macaques: activity before distal and proximal forelimb movements. J Neurosci 6:403–411

Main de Biran F-P 1802 Influence de l'habitude sur la faculte de penser. Oeuvres de Main de Biran. Tisserand edn, Alcan, 1930, Paris

Martin A, Wiggs CL, Ungerleider LG, Haxby JV 1996 Neural correlates of category-specific knowledge. Nature 379:649–652

Matelli M, Luppino G, Rizzolatti G 1985 Patterns of cytochrome oxidase activity in the frontal agranular cortex of macaque monkey. Behav Brain Res 18:125–137

Murata A, Fadiga L, Fogassi L, Gallese V, Raos V, Rizzolatti G 1997 Object representation in the ventral premotor cortex (area F5) of the monkey. J Neurophysiol 78:2226–2230

Perani D, Cappa SF, Bettinardi V et al 1995 Different neural systems for the recognition of animals and man-made tools. Neuroreport 6:1637–1641

Perrett DI, Mistlin AJ, Harries MH, Chitty AJ 1990 Understanding the visual appearance and consequence of actions. In: Goodale MA (ed) Vision and action. Ablex Publishing Corporation, Norwood, NJ, p 163–180

Rizzolatti G, Gallese V 1997 From action to meaning: a neurophysiological perspective. In: Petit J-L (ed) Le neurosciences et la philosophie de l'action. Vzin, Paris, p 217–229

Rizzolatti G, Gentilucci M 1988 Motor and visual-motor functions of the premotor cortex. In: Rakic P, Singer W (eds) Neurobiology of neocortex. Wiley, Chichester, p 269–284

Rizzolatti G, Camarda R, Fogassi L, Gentilucci M, Luppino G, Matelli M 1988 Functional organization of inferior area 6 in the macaque monkey: II. Area F5 and the control of distal movements. Exp Brain Res 71:491–507

Rizzolatti G, Fadiga L, Fogassi L, Gallese V 1996a Premotor cortex and the recognition of motor actions. Cogn Brain Res 3:131–141

Rizzolatti G, Fadiga L, Matelli M et al 1996b Localization of grasp representation in humans by PET: 1. Observation versus execution. Exp Brain Res 111:246–252

Sakata H, Taira M, Murata A, Mine S 1995 Neural mechanisms of visual guidance of hand actions in the parietal cortex of the monkey. Cereb Cortex 5:429–438

Schopenhauer A 1819 Die Welte as Will und Vorstellung. Italian edition, Vigliani ed. I Meridani, Mondadori, 1995, Milano

Taira M, Mine S, Georgopoulos AP, Murata A, Sakata H 1990 Parietal cortex neurons of the monkey related to the visual guidance of hand movement. Exp Brain Res 83:29–36

Varela F, Thompson E, Rosch E 1992 The embodied mind. MIT Press, Cambridge, MA

Whiten A, Ham R 1992 On the nature and evolution of imitation in the animal kingdom: reappraisal of a century of research. Adv Study Behav 21:239–283

DISCUSSION

Thach: Marc Jeannerod's (1994) paper on mental motor imagery was an eye-opener for me. From this paper and many of the human activation studies, it seemed at the time that there were a common set of neurons in premotor areas which were active in planning a movement, or in planning a movement without actually making the movement. The inference was that it was the same set of neurons that could either plan the move that is made, or think about the movement without moving. The results you have just described suggest to me that separate sets of neurons may be involved: one set which is planning movements and are associated with movement, and another set which is correlative of thinking about a movement that is not to be made.

Rizzolatti: Yes. There are two sets of movement-related neurons in F5: canonical neurons and mirror neurons. They are similar in their motor properties, but they differ in terms of stimuli that trigger them. I do not know which of the two sets (or their human equivalent) are active during mental imagery. It probably depends on the task. In the paper you mentioned, Marc Jeannerod suggested that mirror neurons are used for imitation learning. It seems, however, that monkeys are unable to learn by imitation. Yet the mirror system can be a preadaptative mechanism for this function. In monkeys this system is used for understanding the action made by others. In humans it could be used also for intentionally generating action previously observed.

Gibson: Perhaps due to my looks, our monkeys do imitate me! In training monkeys, we find that demonstrating the desired movement is often useful. They also imitate each other: in their home cages one monkey will start making a specific gesture, and, before long, the others will be making it.

Rizzolatti: There is a vast literature on this issue. The evidence is essentially against the view that monkeys can learn by imitation. What usually happens is the following: when a monkey notices that an another monkey interacts with an object, it pays attention to it and then tends to act on it. In doing this it uses gestures similar to those of the first monkey. This does not demonstrate at all that the second animal learned from the first one. It simply indicates that a certain object acquired salience because of the actions of the first animal and was then reacted to by using gestures common to the motor repertoire of the species.

Miller: You described these as grasp neurons, but it strikes me that there must be a pretty significant intention or expectation component as well. What would happen if instead of grasping a piece of fruit in front of the monkey, you grasped an inedible object such as a stone? Would you still see a similar response?

Rizzolatti: Yes; the only difference would be that after a while the monkey will stop looking at the stone, whereas it will continue to look at the piece of fruit. Therefore the neuron will fire during the stone's first presentation only.

Miller: After the monkey has figured out that this is a stone and he's not going to want to eat it, presumably there is no longer any discharge when it sees you grasping.

Rizzolatti: No, there is still a discharge. There is a discharge even when another monkey far away from the first one grasps food that, obviously, the first monkey will never get. What counts is action understanding, not its possible rewarding effects. Note that this action recognition occurs in the dorsal stream.

Goodale: Although when you get to imitation and recognition, akin to the motor theory for the perception of speech, at some point the process has to make contact with semantics.

Rizzolatti: In PET experiments on human subjects we found an activation of Broca's area during action observation (Rizzolatti et al 1996, Grafton et al 1996). It is possible that the semantics of actions is mediated by this area.

Goodale: Some years ago, in an entirely different context, we were interested in the idea that the visual perception of the actions of others might involve processing that takes place in a manner analogous to that proposed in the motor theory of speech recognition. We ran a rather simple-minded study in which we used 'point-light walker' displays to show people doing either complex movements, such as playing the violin, or simple axial movements, such as walking. We presented these displays to the left and right visual fields. We got the typically left visual field/right hemisphere advantage for recognition of the axial movements but with the complex movements we got a shift to a right visual field/left hemisphere advantage. This left hemisphere advantage for the recognition of complex movements suggests that something analogous to Broca's area might be invoked for the processing of this kind of visual information.

Jeannerod: In our PET experiments during mental stimulation, one area was consistently found to be involved, in the lower part of the prefrontal cortex, corresponding to areas 44–45. This would be one possibility for the mirror neurons in human. At least we are beginning to find some correspondence between humans and monkeys.

Georgopoulos: Have you seen any difference in the activity of cells in different layers?

Rizzolatti: We haven't studied this properly, but our impression is that mirror neurons are located superficially, probably in layers 2 and 3. This is however is only our impression, not a fact.

Goodale: Have you done any reversible lesion studies, looking at recognition?

Rizzolatti: We did one study, which was not completely successful. We inactivated that sector of F5 where mirror neurons are located. The inactivation was unilateral. In one monkey we found a specific deficit in action recognition. The effect was not very strong but significant. Colour and pattern discriminations were normal. A second monkey did not show, however, any deficit. We have to repeat the experiment making bilateral lesions.

Gibson: When recording in the thalamus, we have seen neurons similar to the ones that you have described. However, the neurons only fire if you grasp the raisin within the monkey's reach. Do you see this?

Rizzolatti: No, usually the distance doesn't matter, except where it affects the monkeys' attention.

Andersen: Are these cells in the same region where you and Graziano et al (1994) have reported cells that are body centric?

Rizzolatti: Body-centred neurons are common in F4 (Gentilucci et al 1988, Fogassi et al 1996), while mirror neurons are located in F5, a ventral premotor area rostral to F4. As far as F4 neurons are concerned, our data are in full agreement with those of Graziano et al (1997).

Lemon: A question that fascinates me about these sorts of neurons is what determines when the information they encode is applied to the individual's own action, and when it is used to calibrate or identify someone else doing the same action? Are these co-extensive with corticospinal neurons?

Rizzolatti: This is a very interesting issue. I can answer, however, only the last question, that concerning the F5 anatomy. Mirror neurons are mostly located on the cortical convexity. This is a sector of F5 devoid of corticospinal neurons. Corticospinal neurons are present in the part of F5 where neurons have 'canonical' properties.

Goodale: Do you intend to do any psychophysics on the visual input, to work out exactly what it is that constitutes sufficient visual impact for a cell to decide that it has seen a grasp? For example, if a person put on a funny glove that changes the appearance of the hand and did the same movement, would it have the same effect on the cells? Or if one had a video recording of a grasping action and played with the parameters, would this work?

Rizzolatti: We have a project in which we intend to videotape grasping and other monkey movements and to digitize the tapes. In this way we will be able to test monkeys with artificial or 'impossible' movements and to find out which are the crucial movement parameters for triggering mirror neurons.

Wolpert: Is there something special about the grasp? If you look hard enough, would you find neurons that respond to your elbows bending, for instance?

Rizzolatti: There is nothing of this kind in F5. Neurons respond there only to goal-directed actions. However, neurons that respond to the observation of isolated body part movements were found by Perrett and his co-workers in the superior temporal sulcus region (Carey et al 1997).

Marsden: What are the attributes of the gesture that fires these neurons? You showed the experimenter picking up a piece of fruit with a pair of pliers, and there was little or no response.

Rizzolatti: A description of the hand, I suppose.

Marsden: Is it? Did you have the experiment repeating that action, but actually putting the food in his mouth with the pliers?

Rizzolatti: This is an interesting question. We frequently give food to the monkeys using pliers. What we found is that initially there is no response but, after months of recordings and testing, some neurons also start to respond to the tool. It seems, therefore, that some mirror neurons can be conditioned to non-biological stimuli. The learning issue, however, should be addressed more formally.

Marsden: A fun experiment might be to get the experimenter to put a puppet on their hand and use the puppet's hand to grasp the food!

Georgopoulos: Do we know anything about the subcortical projections from F5? Do they go to the spinal cord?

Strick: We know that the portion of F5 (PMv) that is located in the posterior bank of the arcuate sulcus has corticospinal projections to upper cervical segments of the spinal cord (see Dum & Strick 1991, He et al 1993).

Georgopoulos: It is fine to think of it as a cortical circuit but there is always a subcortical output. It would be very interesting to learn about the patterns of activity in layer 5, for example.

Jeannerod: You briefly mentioned that you found similar types of activity in area 7b. Is this in that part of 7b which connects with area F5?

Rizzolatti: At the moment we have evidence that there are mirror neurons in the rostral part of area 7b. This 7b sector sends projection to F5, especially to the part of it located on the cortical convexity. This projection differs from that from AIP which mostly goes to the part of F5 buried in the arcuate sulcus.

Jeannerod: Isn't F5 convexity where you find the main focus?

Rizzolatti: Yes, in its most anterior part, rostral to F4.

Stein: Does F5 project back to motor cortex proper? I imagine it would project back to the hand area. And does it receive projections from the homologous place that 7b projects to in cingulate gyrus?

Rizzolatti: F5 projects backs to F1 hand area. We have not studied yet the precise cortical connections of the sector of 7b where mirror neurons are located.

Strick: F5 does not receive input from the cingulate gyrus. However, it is interconnected with the various cingulate motor areas that are buried in the cingulate sulcus. In fact, in recent experiments we have found that digit representation in F5 is interconnected with the digit representations in M1 and in the premotor areas including the PMd (R. P. Dum & P. L. Strick, unpublished results).

Johansson: There were two experimenters involved — one that put the food on the tray and the other who took it. Also, the first experimenter grasped the object, but there was no neural response. Likewise, there was no neural response in the monkey when the object was released. My question is, how context-sensitive is the neural activity that you record?

Rizzolatti: Some mirror neurons fire both when the experimenter places an object on a surface and when he grasps it. Other mirror neurons fire only when the object is grasped. The neuron in the film I showed — that with the high spontaneous discharge — fired both during grasping and placing. I am not aware of mirror neurons that fire during particular placing–grasping sequences, but I must say also that we never examined this aspect specifically.

Lemon: Do these cells fire when the monkeys reach in the dark for the objects?

Rizzolatti: Yes, they do.

Strick: One of the substantial inputs to the PMv (F5) is from SII. Thus, in terms of conceptualizing the function of the PMv, one must consider that it receives major inputs from at least two areas in the parietal lobe, area 7B or AIP into the intraparietal sulcus, and SII. I don't think we have given enough thought to what the input from SII might contribute, but given the density of this input, it certainly should have an impact on PMv function.

Rizzolatti: You are right. The input from SII ought to be important, but at the moment we do not know what its role might be.

Hoffmann: The key question seems to be whether or not the monkey has to see the whole sequence for the neurons to fire. Earlier you mentioned the effects of conditioning: you could present a tone to the monkey every time you reach for the target. What are these neurons doing after conditioning if you present the tone alone? Is the response internally generated, or does the monkey have to see what is going on?

Rizzolatti: Our interpretation is that the discharge of mirror neurons represents an internal copy of an action. When the neuron fires in the dark, the action copy is internally generated.

Jeannerod: In this case, is the monkey relying on some internal image?

Rizzolatti: Yes.

Jeannerod: This is a good paradigm for studying mental imagery in the monkey.

Rizzolatti: Yes.

Marsden: You introduced the concept that neurons with these sorts of properties might contribute to conscious recognition of gesture. Can you explain why humans with ideomotor apraxia (failure of gesture production) scarcely ever have lesions anterior to the central sulcus?

Rizzolatti: PET studies showed that in humans the mirror system is lateralized to the left hemisphere (Rizzolatti et al 1996, Grafton et al 1996). Lesions to the left hemisphere and in particular those to the inferior frontal gyrus very frequently produce aphasia. Now, many aphasic patients show deficit in action recognition. The conventional interpretation of this observation was that since these patients are aphasic, they have no capacity to describe what they see or have deficits in symbolic thinking. This is not necessarily true. An alternative possibility is that they are indeed impaired in gesture recognition. A recent neuropsychological study reports evidence in favour of such a view (Bell 1994).

Marsden: Five to ten percent of those with a failure of gesture recognition or production are not aphasics, but most have lesions in the dominant hemisphere posterior to the central sulcus.

Rizzolatti: It would take too long to speculate here on the relation between the frontal and the parietal lobe. My view, however, is that the matching system of the frontal lobe is fundamental for gesture recognition. During development the frontal lobe 'instructs' the parietal lobe. Thus, in adults a series of representations coded in parietal lobe acquires meaning because of their connections with frontal lobe. At this point a new and richer vocabulary of gestures is created in areas posterior to the central sulcus (see Rizzolatti & Gallese 1997). Its lesion may produce a failure in gesture recognition.

Goodale: Would you predict that Broca's aphasics would have difficulty in the visual recognition of gesture?

Rizzolatti: Yes.

Passingham: Basso et al (1985) reported that some patients with apraxia have frontal lesions, presumably including the premotor cortex. Of course, in such cases it is necessary to test the hand ipsilateral to the lesion.

Marsden: Then you get into the problem of callosal apraxias with the ipsilateral hand. The overwhelming majority of lesions causing ideomotor apraxia for gesture production and recognition are posterior to the central sulcus.

Andersen: When you talk about the symbolic coding here, are there a number of symbols besides grasp? Is there a columnar organization for some of these? Also, is there some space in which each gesture is tuned?

Rizzolatti: When I speak of vocabularies of actions I imply that neurons of these vocabularies represent actions. Our evidence, at the moment, concerns only hand movements, but my guess is that reaching movements are organized in a similar 'symbolic' way. In this case the firing of a neuron would code what is the appropriate arm-hand posture to reach an object.

Stein: Is there any evidence for positional cells coding for position or direction of reach, as opposed to grasp cells?

Rizzolatti: Nobody has addressed this point specifically. The studies of F4 mostly concern the sensory responses of F4 neurons.

Lemon: There are some old studies on this (Godschalk et al 1981, 1985). There are some cells in post-arcuate premotor cortex that are selective for the position of the target. These cells respond to particular targets in space providing that target is of interest to the monkey and he subsequently makes a reaching movement towards it. However, what one didn't know is whether they would have worked equally well in the sort of way that you have tested.

Stein: Correct me if I'm wrong, but I thought that was meant to be a visual response as opposed to a motor response.

Lemon: These cells fired for a particular position of a target in the delay phase of a delayed-response task. Their behaviour is truly visuomotor because they do fire on presentation of a visual stimulus but this discharge is contingent on an upcoming movement.

Miller: It seems to me that a cell which responds during grasping with either the hand or the mouth represents a very different level of behaviour than a cell which encodes a particular arm posture. I would not expect 'parietal positional' cells to encode a particular limb posture, which is a rather specific motor act. The grasp cells that you described encode a very general sort of goal achievement.

Rizzolatti: It may seem so. However, if you consider the notion of Jeannerod of two independent channels for reaching and grasping, it is possible that the different computational requests of the two channels justify the different levels of representation between arm and hand movements that you rightly noticed. For hand movements the goal is to grasp an object. Where it is located in space is immaterial. For reaching the arm should be placed in a well determined spatial position. The level of abstraction is less in the second case, but the goal of action is present in both cases.

Miller: I might expect that getting either hand to some point in space might fire the cell and, furthermore, since the limb is redundant, getting to this point in space by any configuration of the limb might fire the cell.

Rizzolatti: You are right. There is such a discrepancy between distal and proximal movement representations.

Marsden: I'm still battling with the concept of whether these cells in F5 are on the motor imagery side or the motor action side of the whole system. They showed the characteristics of double firing, the second burst being concerned with movement. Do you ever get that second burst from the animal if it doesn't actually move?

Rizzolatti: No.

Passingham: When you talk of a ventral premotor cortex containing a vocabulary of movements, I am concerned that you only test a very limited set of movements. One hypothesis is that you are looking at a specialized system for reaching and grasping in which the shape of the object determines the shape of the hand. Because much of a monkey's day is spent doing this, one might argue that there is a specialized system for carrying out this task. Of course, in dorsal premotor cortex there are many cells that fire in relation to different movements. So you may wish to argue instead that there is a movement vocabulary in premotor cortex as a whole.

Rizzolatti: Absolutely. It might be that F5 is a specialized system that evolved according to its own rules. It might be, however, that the dorsal premotor cortex has never been studied properly. By properly I mean using ethologically appropriate stimuli. It might be, therefore, that neurons in dorsal premotor cortex are not for reaching in general, as usually believed, but code reaching for climbing, reaching for fighting, and so on. This would imply, of course, that in the available studies on neural properties of the dorsal premotor cortex only unspecific elements of these hypothetical vocabularies had been selected.

Strick: Another feature of the PMv (F5) is that it is the only premotor area to receive substantial input from area 46 (Lu et al 1994). The prefrontal cortex gains its most direct access to the motor system at the cortical level via this premotor area. Thus, the PMv is a nodal point for inputs from three different cortical areas: area 46, portions of area 7 and SII. If the PMv is involved in the guidance of movement based on external cues, then one might speculate that input from area 7 could provide information about the location of objects in space, area 46 could provide information about where objects were in space and SII could provide important somatosensory information for guiding movement in the absence of vision.

References

Basso A, Faglioni P, Luzzatti C 1985 Methods in neuroanatomical research and an experimental study of limb apraxia. In: Roy EA (ed) Neurophysiological studies of apraxia and related disorders. North Holland, Amsterdam, p 179–202

Bell BD 1994 Pantomime recognition impairment in aphasia: an analysis of error types. Brain Lang 47:269–278

Carey DP, Perrett DI, Oram MW 1997 Recognizing, understanding and reproducing actions. In: Jeannerod M, Grafman J (eds) Handbook of neuropsychology, vol 11: Action and cognition. Elsevier Science, Amsterdam, p 111–130

Dum RP, Strick PL 1991 The origin of corticospinal projections from the premotor areas in the frontal lobe. J Neurosci 11:667–689

Fogassi L, Gallese V, Fadiga L, Luppino G, Matelli M, Rizzolatti G 1996 Coding of peripersonal space in inferior premotor cortex (area F4). J Neurophysiol 76:141–157

Gentilucci M, Fogassi L, Luppino G, Matelli M, Camarda R, Rizzolatti G 1988 Functional organization of inferior area 6 in the macaque monkey: I. Somatotopy and the control of proximal movements. Exp Brain Res 71:475–490

Godschalk G, Lemon RN, Nijs HJT, Kuypers HGJM 1981 Behaviour of neurons in monkey peri-arcuate and precentral cortex before and during visually guided arm and hand movements. Exp Brain Res 44:113–116

Godschalk G, Lemon RN, Kuypers HGJM, van der Steen J 1985 The involvement of monkey premotor cortex neurones in preparation of visually cued arm movements. Behav Brain Res 18:143–157

Grafton ST, Arbib MA, Fadiga L, Rizzolatti G 1996 Localization of grasp representations in humans by positron emission tomography: 2. Observation compared with imagination. Exp Brain Res 112:103–111

Graziano MS, Yap GS, Gross CG 1994 Coding of visual space by premotor neurons. Science 266:1054–1057

Graziano MS, Hu XT, Gross CG 1997 Visuospatial properties of ventral premotor cortex. J Neurophysiol 77:2268–2292

He SQ, Dum RP, Strick PL 1993 Topographic organization of corticospinal projections from the frontal lobe: motor areas on the lateral surface of the hemisphere. J Neurosci 13:952–980

Jeannerod M 1994 The representing brain: neural correlates of motor intention and imagery. Behav Brain Sci 17:187–245

Lu M-T, Preston JB, Strick PL 1994 Interconnections between the prefrontal cortex and the premotor areas in the frontal lobe. J Comp Neurol 341:375–392

Rizzolatti G, Gallese V 1997 From action to meaning: a neurophysiological perspective. In: Petit J-L (ed) Les neurosciences et la philosophie de l'action. Vrin, Paris, p 217–229

Rizzolatti G, Fadiga L, Matelli M et al 1996 Localization of grasp representations in humans by PET: 1. Observation versus execution. Exp Brain Res 111:246–252

General discussion II

Georgopoulos: I have two general questions relating to Peter Strick's talk. The first one deals with the premotor areas. I was impressed by the elegant and quantitative analysis, but there are still some discrepancies. I agree with you that the data are clear that the spatial distribution of the spinal projections is very similar, but the density of the projections differs for different areas; for example, it seems that motor cortical projections are more numerous in lamina IX than those of the premotor areas. I'm trying to reconcile this projection pattern with the fact that it is difficult to get post-spike facilitation responses from the medial wall (at least the SMA). Perhaps they are spatially confined to a small area, so that one misses them. However, the simplest explanatory factor would be the relatively small density of the projections onto lamina IX from these premotor areas, as compared with the motor cortex. Of course, there are many similarities in the projections from the motor and premotor areas, but there are differences as well, especially on the density of projections to specific spinal laminae. These differences can explain some physiological data.

I have a second point concerning the effects of lesions. You made a provocative statement: you said that you destroyed all the motor cortex and the reaching was fine. Now, you showed how to assess properly wrist movements following a motor cortical lesion. If I were visiting your lab, you could have shown me a seemingly normal monkey unless you said 'look at this oblique direction, that oblique direction, something is wrong with it' — otherwise I would have missed it. It is the same with reaching movements: it is important that you test them in the same quantitative way. The monkey may look normal but unless you test thoroughly the hand and/or joint movements, you can't really say that 'all is normal'.

Strick: In response to your first question, Wiesendanger has reported post-spike facilitation of EMGs from the SMA and Lemon and his colleagues have found physiological evidence for monosynaptic connections between SMA neurons and motoneurons innervating the distal limb. Thus, there is clear physiological evidence to support our conclusions that the SMA and several of the other premotor areas have direct access to motor output.

In response to your second comment about lesions of the primary motor cortex, let me say that I would definitely not want to be quoted as saying that reaching is entirely normal after removal of the primary motor cortex. However, I think one must recall that Lawrence & Kuypers (1968) found that bilateral section of the pyramidal tract (which interrupts corticospinal efferents from all the motor areas) resulted in major deficits in the generation of relatively independent movements of the fingers, but rather small deficits in the control of reaching movements. We didn't study reaching, instead we examined the control of wrist movements. We found that for 2 to 3 months after removal of the arm area of the primary motor cortex, monkeys are unable to move their wrist in any direction (Hoffman & Strick 1995). However, a remarkable recovery of motor function was seen in these animals when we worked with them for a 5 month to 2 year period. Ultimately, these animals could make wrist movements in all directions, albeit more slowly than normal animals. Several specific deficits remained. Some wrist movements in lesioned animals were misdirected. For example, most movements that required a combination of wrist flexion and radial deviation were made in two steps, instead of a single smooth trajectory. After the lesion, distinct bursts of muscle activity were no longer observed during step-tracking movements. In addition, suppression of antagonist activity at movement onset was abolished or reduced; and the relative timing of agonist and synergist muscle activity was markedly altered. On the basis of these and other observations, we concluded that M1 contributes to the precise spatiotemporal patterning of muscle activity during step-tracking movements of the wrist. Thus, one could look at the consequences of motor cortex lesions from two perspectives — the lesion initially causes some striking deficits in wrist movements. On the other hand, it does not lead to permanent paralysis and the recovery that can occur is remarkable.

Georgopoulos: Is that true for humans as well?

Strick: We've studied several patients with unilateral strokes. In fact, in the hand *ipsilateral* to the stroke, we observed deficits that were similar to those we observed in monkeys *contralateral* to the cortical ablation. Thus, in humans a lesion in one hemisphere results in bilateral deficits. Of course, the subjects we examined did not have lesions that were confined to the primary motor cortex.

Passingham: My memory is that you only removed the hand area as identified by microstimulation.

Strick: No, in one monkey we removed all the arm area of the primary motor cortex. In a second monkey our lesions also extended intentionally into part of the adjacent leg and face representations of area 4. In that monkey we may also have involved some of the PMd and PMv.

Marsden: Does this massive descending projection from the additional premotor areas travel in the pyramidal tract?

Strick: Yes.

Marsden: Then you are back into the problem of what really is the deficit after a pyramidal lesion in humans. Remarkably little is the general belief. A deficit in fractionating finger movements is the usual description.

Glickstein: Let me ask a simple question. What are the thalamic afferents to those two areas in the cingulate sulcus that you have studied?

Strick: The CMAd and the CMAv receive thalamic input from portions of VLc and VLo. It is likely that they're the target of cerebellar and basal ganglia output.

Glickstein: But they don't extend more ventrally to include any of the anterior thalamic nuclei?

Strick: No, they receive their inputs from traditional cerebellar and basal ganglia nuclei in the thalamus. They are quite different from the cingulate gyrus in that respect.

Fetz: Given the symmetrical organization of the pre-central and post-central gyrus, have you ever thought about an analogue of the cingulate regions in the post-central medial wall? Do these posterior midline regions show any retrograde labelling? And what do the cells in these regions do?

Strick: I would say that this has been explored but not quantitatively analysed.

Glickstein: I recognize that in your case we are talking about motor areas in the cingulate fissure, not the cingulate cortex, but that region has been a target for psychosurgeons. Do they include any of your motor areas in their lesions?

Strick: That is a good question. We have looked at this, but it's difficult to determine what they actually remove in these surgeries. I would say that, on the whole, the regions removed are rostral to the cingulate motor areas. In many cases, the removals undercut rostral cortical areas and thus, may interrupt some of the inputs and outputs of the cingulate motor areas. Perhaps the akinetic mutism associated with the anterior cerebral syndrome is more closely linked with the functions of the cingulate motor areas (e.g. Barris & Schuman 1953, Farris 1969). I have wondered whether there is any association between the motor symptoms of this syndrome and the akinesia of some basal ganglia disorders.

Marsden: You are exploring the uncertainty of clinicians to define the nature of the human motor syndrome following lesions of the supplementary motor area and, even more difficult, what is the motor syndrome of the lateral premotor cortex. (See Halsband et al 1993, Freund & Hummelsheim 1985 for discussion.)

Strick: We recently reviewed all of the PET studies that have been done on the medial wall (Picard & Strick 1996). For simple movements the story is very much like what we see in the monkey: that is, if you ignore the names that people call these structures and look at the coordinates of activation in the different studies, it's clear that even for simple movements the SMA is active in all tasks.

Marsden: I defer to you entirely, but when you knock out the SMA in humans not much happens after the initial recovery from such lesions.

Strick: And so this raises the question of what activity means.

Thach: I would like to hear David Marsden say more about Liepmann's ideas about kinetic apraxia from anterior lesions; I think Freund also supports those concepts. What do you see on these lesions? Is there a clumsiness or melo-kinetic apraxia?

Marsden: The whole business of limb-kinetic or melo-kinetic apraxia is beset with difficulties. Many have dismissed the deficits that are seen as merely a minor expression of a pyramidal lesion. I don't believe that's true. The problem in the human is that you very rarely get pure lesions, knocking out what Liepmann might have considered to have been the 'senso-motorium'. A contrast you can make in human beings is between the effect of a lesion of the cerebral cortex (including the premotor cortical areas and SMA) with mild pyramidal signs, compared with what you see in a patient with a spinal cord pyramidal lesion. People with cortical lesions may have an additional motor deficit that you don't see in spinal or indeed in capsular lesions. There appears to be a motor clumsiness and difficulty in manipulation of the hand with cerebral cortical lesions. I think there really is something in limb-kinetic apraxia, but this has been poorly studied and is not really defined.

Lemon: The best case in the literature of a complete section of the pyramidal tract in humans is the case documented by Bucy et al (1964). This was not only a surgically controlled lesion, but there was also histology after the death of the patient. Of course this is the famous patient that could produce fine, individual movements of the fingers fairly well with the affected hand which were only slightly less well executed than on the unaffected side. It's important to remember that the surgery was carried out after the patient had suffered for many years from a variety of motor disorders. Therefore it doesn't necessarily tell us very much about what the pyramidal tract does in ourselves or in monkeys, because this is a lesion that is applied to a system that is heavily disordered. That case is frequently cited as an example of the fact that there are a million fibres that don't know what they're doing. But what I think is much more striking is that in cases where you have a capsular infarct, which is one of the common causes of the motor problems that are seen in the clinic, that this still is referred to by physicians as pyramidal, even though the proportion of fibres in the internal capsule that the spinal cord is probably only a few per cent (see Porter & Lemon 1993, p 80).

Marsden: Bucy's patient wasn't a pianist and didn't play the violin, and neurosurgeons don't usually look for subtle motor deficits. In these human patients with cortical lesions of motor areas, when we say that nothing happens we probably haven't looked for the right thing.

References

Barris RW, Schuman HR 1953 Bilateral anterior cingulate lesions. Neurology 3:44–52
Bucy PC, Keplinger LE, Siqueira EB 1964 Destruction of the 'pyramidal tract' in man. J Neurosurg 21:3385–398
Farris AA 1969 Limbic system infarction. Neurology 19:91–96

Freund H, Hummelsheim H 1985 Lesion of the premotor cortex in man. Brain 108:697–733
Halsband U, Ito N, Tanji J, Freund H J 1993 The role of premotor cortex and the supplementary
    motor area in the temporal control of movement in man. Brain 116:243–266
Hoffman DS, Strick PL 1995 Effects of a primary motor cortex lesion on step-tracking
    movements of the wrist. J Neurophysiol 73:891–895
Lawrence DG, Kuypers HG JM 1968 The functional organization of the motor system in the
    monkey. I. The effects of bilateral pyramidal lesions. Brain 91:1–14
Picard N, Strick PL 1996 Motor areas of the medial wall: a review of location and functional
    activation. Cerebral Cortex 6:342–353
Porter R, Lemon RN 1993 Corticospinal function and voluntary movement. Physiological
    Society monograph. Oxford University Press, Oxford

Posterior parietal areas specialized for eye movements (LIP) and reach (PRR) using a common coordinate frame

R. A. Andersen, L. H. Snyder, A. P. Batista, C. A. Buneo and Y. E. Cohen

Division of Biology, California Institute of Technology, Mail Code 216-76, 1200 E California Boulevard, Pasadena, CA 91125, USA

Abstract. The posterior parietal cortex (PPC) has long been considered a sensory area specialized for spatial awareness and the directing of attention. However, a new, far reaching concept is now emerging that this area is involved in integrating sensory information for the purpose of planning action. Moreover, experiments by our group and others over the last two decades indicate that PPC is in fact anatomically organized with respect to action. PPC also is an 'association' cortex which must combine different sensory modalities which are coded in different coordinate frames. We have found, at least for two different cortical areas within PPC, that different sensory signals are brought into a common coordinate frame. This coordinate frame codes locations with respect to the eye, but also gain modulates the activity by eye and body position signals. An interesting feature of this coordinate representation at the population level is that it codes concurrently target locations in multiple coordinate frames (eye, head, body and world). Depending on how this population of neurons is sampled, different coordinate transformations can be accomplished by the same population of neurons.

1998 Sensory guidance of movement. Wiley, Chichester (Novartis Foundation Symposium 218) p 109–128

Historically, the posterior parietal cortex (PPC) has been considered a high-order sensory area important for the perception of space. The syndrome of neglect, in which patients with parietal lobe lesions have difficulty attending to stimuli or shifting their attention, first suggested that this area also plays an important role in attention (Critchley 1953, Andersen 1987 for review). Numerous physiological experiments in non-human primates demonstrated attention-related enhancements of activity in the PPC (see Colby et al 1995 for review). More recently, however, there have been a number of studies in humans and monkeys which suggest that the PPC is important in action and, more specifically, in transforming sensory signals into plans for action (Mountcastle et al 1975, Gnadt & Andersen 1988, Goodale & Milner 1992, Andersen 1995, Mazzoni et al 1996b, Snyder et al 1997).

In fact, over the last few years there has been an emerging view that parts of the PPC contain an anatomical specialization — or map — of intentions. As will be covered in this review, the lateral intraparietal area (LIP) appears to be specialized for making saccades. A medial and posterior area, which may include the medial intraparietal area (MIP) and the occipital parietal area (PO) appears to be specialized for reaching movements. We have referred to this area as the parietal reach region (PRR). A third area anterior to LIP, the anterior intraparietal area (AIP), appears to be specialized for grasping. We will also review studies of the reference frame in which space is represented in LIP and PRR. How are different modalities, that are originally represented in different coordinate frames, integrated in PPC? Also, how is communication achieved between these different areas, which are highly interconnected anatomically (Andersen et al 1990, Blatt et al 1990), and whose outputs are presumably closely orchestrated for coordinated movements? As we will see, there appears to be a common coordinate frame used by these two areas for several modalities. This coordinate frame has an extremely interesting feature of being distributed, and can be read out by other areas in several different coordinate frames, e.g. eye, head, body or even world-centred. Finally, we will see that the representations of space in both LIP and PRR are updated across eye movements for the remembered locations of targets for movement.

Coding of intention to saccade and reach

Although there has been considerable suggestion in the literature that the PPC may play a role in intention, it has been very difficult to approach this problem experimentally. This is because it is quite difficult to differentiate activities related to attention and intention. This difficulty is due to the obvious fact that animals attend to locations to which they plan movements. Recently we designed a task specifically to isolate activities related to these two cognitive functions. We reasoned that if PPC activity was simply related to attention, this activity should be indifferent to the type of movement an animal planned to make to a particular stimulus. On the other hand, if activity varied according to the animals' plans, given the same location and stimulus, then it is likely this activity reflects what the animal plans (intends) to do.

We trained monkeys to memorize the location of peripherally flashed lights and plan either an eye or an arm movement to that location (Snyder et al 1997). As demonstrated in Fig. 1, we found many cells that were active in the memory period only when an animal planned an eye movement and others that were only active when the animal planned an arm movement. In fact, about two-thirds of PPC neurons showed a significant response in the memory period for only one of

SACCADE TRIALS   REACH TRIALS

A. Saccade-specific cell

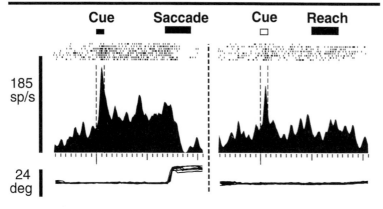

B. Reach-specific cell

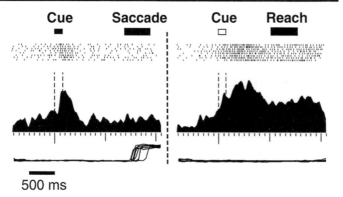

500 ms

FIG. 1.   Responses of two intention-specific neurons in the delayed-saccade (*left*) and delayed-reach (*right*) tasks. Each panel shows timing of peripheral flash ('Cue': red flashes indicated by filled bars, green flashes by open bars) and response ('Saccade' or 'Reach'); eight rows of rasters corresponding to every third action potential recorded during each of eight trials; a spike density histogram of neuronal activity, generated by convolution with a triangular kernel aligned on cue presentation, with cue onset and offset indicated by dashed lines; and eight overlaid traces showing vertical eye position. Neuronal responses in the cue interval (50 ms before to 150 ms after cue offset) were non-specific. However, during the delay interval (150–600 ms), firing depended specifically on motor intent. (A) A cell showing elevated delay period firing before a saccade (*left*) but not before a reach (*right*). For illustration purposes, data for this cell were collected using a fixed delay interval. (B) A second cell showing reach rather than saccade specificity during the delay interval. Reprinted from Snyder et al (1997).

the two plans. The remaining one-third of the cells responded to both plans. This activity in many cases is not merely attention/sensory memory activity, as the control experiment in Fig. 2 shows. This cell had activity for flashes in its receptive field regardless of whether the animal planned a reach or a saccade there. However, we also had the animal perform a two movement task in which he planned and made eye and reach movements simultaneously in opposite directions. As can be seen in the bottom panels of Fig. 2, when the animal planned an arm movement into the receptive field of this same cell, but an eye movement outside the receptive field, the cell was still active; however, when the eye movement was to be into the receptive field and the arm movement outside, the cell was not active. We interpret this result as the animal making a 'default' plan to make a reaching movement that was not executed. Half of the remaining 'sensory' cells demonstrated a covert preference for either saccades or reaches indicating that over 80% of the PPC cells tested had activity during the memory period that specified the intent of the animal.

An important feature of this intended movement activity is that it is anatomically localized. The eye movement planning activities were found predominantly for cells in LIP. This observation is consistent with previous research in LIP which has shown presaccadic bursts of activity (Barash et al 1991), saccade deficits after lesioning (Lynch & McLaren 1989, Li et al 1998), strong axonal projections to other saccade centres (Lynch et al 1985, Asanuma et al 1985, Blatt et al 1990, Andersen et al 1990) and evoked saccades due to electrical stimulation (Thier & Andersen 1996). The reach-selective responses were also found to be anatomically segregated within a continuous swath of cortex which appears to include areas MIP to PO. We referred to this region as the parietal reach region (PRR).

It could be argued that the selectivity in LIP is due to the fact that the animals attend to where they plan to saccade but not to where they plan to reach, and the differential activity reflects this difference in attention. If this were the case, however, then PRR neurons also should only be active when eye movements are planned in their receptive fields; instead we see the reverse phenomenon, with activity being present only when reaches are planned into the receptive fields. Moreover, in the experiments reviewed next, attention is maintained at the same location and the animal is asked to change movement plans. In this case, where attention is identical across trials, the activity of PPC neurons changes dramatically depending on the animals' plans.

Activity related to changing movement plans

A prediction of the above results is that activity should shift between areas LIP and PRR when monkeys change their movement plans. We decided to test this prediction directly with the paradigm shown in Fig. 3A (Snyder et al 1998). The experiment was similar to the one mentioned above, but once a target instructing a

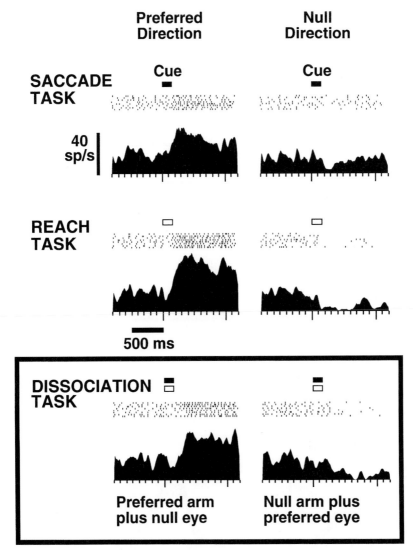

Preferred Direction **Null Direction**

SACCADE TASK — Cue / Cue

40 sp/s

REACH TASK

500 ms

DISSOCIATION TASK

Preferred arm plus null eye / Null arm plus preferred eye

FIG. 2. An intention-specific neuron whose motor specificity was revealed by the dissociation task. Delay activity was greater before movements towards the receptive field ('Preferred direction', left column) compared to away ('Null direction', right column) in both delayed saccade (top row) and reach (middle row) tasks. Thus in single-movement tasks, the neuron appears to code remembered target location independent of motor intent. However, motor specificity was revealed in the dissociation task (bottom row). Firing was vigorous before a preferred reach combined with a null saccade (bottom left), but nearly absent before a preferred saccade plus null reach (bottom right). Thus when both a reach and a saccade were planned, delay activity reflected the intended reach and not the intended saccade. Panel formats are similar to Fig. 1. Every other action potential is indicated by one raster mark. Reprinted from Snyder et al (1997).

Single flash trials:

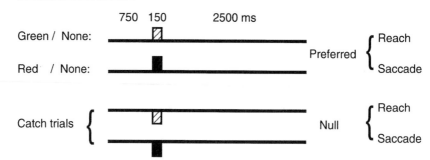

Double flash trials:

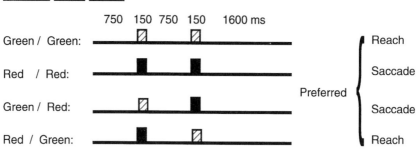

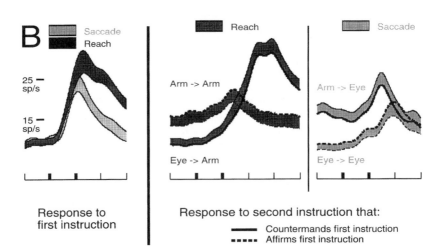

particular movement had been flashed in the receptive field of a cell, on some trials this plan would be changed by a second flash of a different colour, or reaffirmed by a flash of the same colour. Since the animal did not know what the subsequent flash would instruct, and since these flashes always appeared at the same location as the preceding flash, the monkeys' spatial attention was the same in these two conditions. However, the response to the flashes, and the subsequent activity in the memory period after the flash was strongly related to the animals' plans. An example of this plan dependency can be seen in Fig. 3B for the population response of reach neurons from PRR. The response to the first flash is always larger when it is green and thereby instructing a reach. This activity remains high during the first memory period when the monkey is still planning a reach. The middle part of the figure shows the responses to a second, green flash instructing a reach, segregated into two plots depending on whether this flash reaffirmed or changed the plan. It can be seen that the response to the identical flash, under identical attentional conditions, was much stronger if the animal changed his plan. This result indicates that a large component of activity to the flash reflects a shift in plans, suggesting that PPC may play a role in shifting plans. That this change-in-plan specific activity is not a result of the novelty of the stimulus is demonstrated in the plots on the right, which show the responses to the second flash when it is red and instructing an eye movement. The responses were small for the non-preferred plan, regardless of whether it was a change or reaffirmation of the previous plan. Thus the enhanced response to the flashes was only present when there was a change of plan to the preferred plan of the area. Essentially the same result was found for LIP neurons, but with saccades being the preferred plan.

Coding the next planned movement in LIP and PRR

Using a memory double-saccade paradigm we recently found that a majority of LIP neurons code the next planned eye movement (Mazzoni et al 1996b). For instance,

---

FIG. 3.   (A) Time course of eight single and double flash trials. The experiment was designed to force the animal to attend to the spatial location and colour of both flashes. Second flashes never required a shift in spatial attention. See text for details. (B) Population data from PRR (average of 17 cells). Responses to initial flashes instructing a saccade (light) or reach (dark) are shown on the left. Centre and right panels, respectively, show responses when a second flash, at the same location as the first, instructed either the preferred or non-preferred movement. Preferred responses were larger than non-preferred responses. Responses to the second flash were further subdivided by whether they countermanded (solid lines) or affirmed (dashed lines) the instruction of the first flash. Countermanding flashes elicited a greater response when a preferred movement was instructed. When non-preferred movement was instructed, responses were much more similar. Standard error was calculated across cells and mean ± 1 SEM is shown. From Snyder et al (1998).

if the second target in a double eye movement task fell within the receptive field of an LIP cell, but the animal was planning the first eye movement outside of the receptive field, then this cell would not be active in the memory period. However, if the same target fell within the receptive field of the cell and it was the target for the first eye movement, then the cell was active during the memory period. This result is consistent with a majority of the LIP neurons coding movement intention. There was also a minority of cells with activity for the second target during the memory phase, and we interpreted these cells as holding the memory of the location of the second target.

We have recently performed a similar experiment in PRR (Batista et al 1998). In this case we cue the monkey to a location for a reach. However, during the delay period we flash a second target which the animal uses to change his limb position. At the end of the delay the animal must make a second arm movement to the location of the first target. We find that, similar to LIP, the PRR cells typically will cease firing to the remembered location of the first reach target when the monkey is planning an arm movement to a location outside the receptive field of the cell. Thus PRR shares another similarity with LIP, i.e. PRR neurons code the next planned movement in double movement tasks. This result is consistent with the accumulating data that a large component of both PRR and LIP activity reflects the animals' plans or intentions for movement.

Coordinates for representing space within area LIP

Cells in LIP have receptive fields much like cells in other visual areas. These receptive fields are in the coordinates of the retina or eye, and the location in space that will activate these cells will move with the eyes. However, we also found that the activity of these cells is modulated by eye position and head position. Neural network simulations show that these 'gain field' effects can lead to a distributed coding in other coordinates besides eye-centred. Thus, for instance, neurons in another part of the brain which receive projections from LIP could construct receptive fields in head-centred coordinates by exploiting the eye position gain fields. Likewise the combination of eye and head position gains can be used to construct body-centred coordinates (see Figs 4 and 5).

Area LIP is a classic extrastriate visual area. In the hierarchy of visual areas based on feedforward and feedback patterns of cortico-cortical connections (Maunsell & van Essen 1983), it is at approximately the same level as area V4 (Andersen et al 1990, Blatt et al 1990). In other words, it is an area deeply embedded in visual extrastriate cortex, and it occupies a processing position relatively early in the visual pathway (i.e. close to area V1). This fact is reflected in the response properties of LIP neurons, which have brisk responses to visual stimuli, even

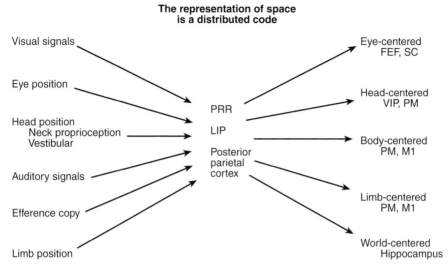

FIG. 4.   Schematic of the inputs and outputs of areas PRR and LIP. These areas receive a variety of sensory signals and body position signals. These signals are integrated in a very specific fashion and the population code can be read out in a variety of coordinate frames by other areas of the brain. SC, superior colliculus; FEF, frontal eye field; VIP, ventral intraparietal area; PM, premotor cortex; M1, primary motor cortex.

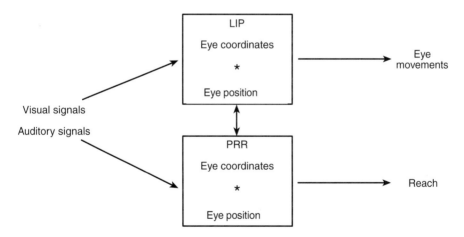

FIG. 5.   Schematic of the common coordinate representation within LIP and PRR. Visual and auditory signals are both inputted to these areas. These signals are to a large degree represented in eye coordinates, but the receptive fields are gain modulated by eye position signals. As indicated in Fig. 4, these gain modulations enable LIP and PRR activity to be read out in multiple coordinate frames by other cortical areas and thus act as a mechanism for coordinate transformations. The outputs of LIP are primarily for the purpose of saccades, and those of PRR for limb movements.

when the animal is ignoring the stimulus (Linden et al 1997) or is anaesthetized (Blatt et al 1990).

LIP cells do not respond to auditory stimuli if they are not meaningful to the animal. However, since LIP plays an important role in saccades, and since monkeys can obviously make eye movements to auditory stimuli, we hypothesized that LIP cells would be active when the monkey used auditory stimuli for the purpose of making saccades. We found this to be true (Mazzoni et al 1996a, Grunewald et al 1997). Moreover, we determined the coordinate frames of these auditory-triggered responses in a memory guided eye movement task. In early parts of the auditory pathway the auditory receptive fields are in head-centred coordinates, constructed from interaural time, intensity and spectral cues. In LIP, however, only 33% of the cells were in head-centred coordinates while a surprising 44% were in eye-centred coordinates (Stricanne et al 1996). Another 23% were intermediate between these two coordinate frames. One possibility is that LIP is responsible for converting head-centred auditory signals into eye-centred coordinates. The neurons with auditory responses typically also have eye position gain fields. These gain effects could provide the mechanism for this coordinate transformation.

The finding that many LIP neurons code auditory signals in eye-centred coordinates when the animals are considering these auditory stimuli as possible saccade targets, has interesting implications. This result suggests that vision provides the basic map for spatial location in LIP. It also suggests that the mapping of auditory space onto visual space occurs only when these auditory stimuli are significant to the animal (Fig. 5). This is a very different view of multimodal integration from that which is commonly held. As we will see, these ideas can also be extended to PRR, and may be a fairly general way of representing space and integrating different modalities within a particular spatial representation. This concept may explain why visual stimuli tend to dictate the perceived spatial location of auditory stimuli. For instance, if we see someone's lips moving, but the sound is coming from a distant location in space, we none the less perceive the sound as coming from the speaker's lips.

Coordinates for representing space in PRR

Recently we have examined the coordinates of the reach planning activity in PRR. One possibility is that the reach activity would be in the coordinates of the limb, as has been suggested for reach-related activity in the motor cortex. Alternatively, this activity could also be in the coordinates of the eye similar to LIP. We addressed this problem by having animals make the same reach, but with the eyes gazing in different directions, or alternatively to reach to the same location with respect to the eyes, but with the limbs starting from different initial positions. If the cells were coding in eye coordinates we would expect different activities for the former condition, since identical reaches would be made to different retinal locations. On the other hand, if the cells were coding in limb coordinates we would expect the activity to vary in the latter condition, since limb movements in different directions are being made to the same location on the retina. We found that most PRR cells code reaches in eye coordinates, although some do code in limb coordinates or intermediate between the two frames (Batista et al 1998). The eye-centred responses also often showed gain modulation by eye position. Thus these cells represent space in a similar distributed manner as LIP neurons, with eye-centred receptive fields modulated by gain fields for eye position.

On the basis of the results of a common coordinate frame for both LIP and PRR, we were led to make a rather non-intuitive prediction. This prediction is that reaches to the remembered locations of sounds in the dark should be coded in eye-centred coordinates. Of course there is, in principle, no need for such a result. Head-centred auditory signals could be converted directly to limb coordinates for these reaches; there is no need to have an intermediate representation of these reach signals in eye coordinates. However, if there is a common distributed coordinate frame in PRR and LIP, then the reach activity should code the target location in eye-centred coordinates and be modulated by eye and limb position signals. Moreover, the results for auditory saccades in LIP, outlined above, would also predict that the auditory signals would be transformed into eye-centred receptive fields. This prediction was substantiated in recent experiments from our lab (Y. E. Cohen & R. A. Andersen, unpublished results 1998). We find that the reach activity is often in eye coordinates for auditory targets, and that these eye-centred receptive fields are strongly gain modulated by eye and limb position. Thus, auditory and visual signals are brought into the same distributed representation in both LIP and PRR, with eye-centred receptive fields modulated by eye and body position signals (see Fig. 5). The advantage of such a representation is the ease of coordinating activity between these two areas, and the ability to read out multiple coordinate frames from this common representation (Fig. 4).

Updating the spatial representations within LIP and PRR across saccades

When a subject makes multiple saccades to different locations from memory, the remembered locations must be updated with each eye movement. This problem was first addressed in physiological experiments by Sparks & Mays (1980), who found that cells in the intermediate layers of the superior colliculus updated the location of the next planned eye movement in eye-centred coordinates across saccades. We later showed a similar phenomenon in area LIP (Gnadt & Andersen 1988). Duhamel et al (1992) extended these results to show that a second eye movement was not necessary for this updating to take place.

Although they interpreted this updated activity to be sensory, the results of Snyder et al (1997, 1998) and those outlined in a previous section ('Coding the next planned movement in LIP and PRR'), suggests that this activity may in fact represent default plans for eye movements to the flashed second targets.

Recently we asked if this same updating process might also occur in area PRR. To test this hypothesis we presented a visual target for a reach that the animal was required to remember. However, during the memory period we then had the animal make a saccade to fixate a new location in space. We found that the remembered location of the reach target was updated in eye coordinates to take into account the change in eye position (Batista et al 1998). For instance, if the monkey made a saccade that brought the remembered location of the target into the retinal receptive field of the PRR neuron, then the cell became active during the delay period prior to the reach. On the other hand, if the saccade brought the remembered location out of the receptive field of the PRR cell, then the cell fell silent. Again LIP and PRR were found to share an important similarity in updating remembered locations in eye coordinates across saccades (see Fig. 6).

This finding also has important implications for reading out the distributed representation of space accurately in non-retinal coordinates. For instance, if the eyes move, the eye position signals and gain modulations in LIP and PRR will change in accordance with the new eye position. If the remembered retinal location of a target remained the same after the eye movement it would be incorrectly coded in head or body centred coordinates. Thus the location in eye coordinates would by necessity need to be updated to read out the correct location with respect to the head or body.

Conclusions

The results reviewed above indicate that the PPC is specialized for transforming sensory signals into action. Two prominent areas within the PPC, areas LIP and PRR, are specialized for saccades and reaches. For both areas, the visual system appears to serve as an anchor for representing space. Thus, both visual and auditory receptive fields are in the coordinates of the eye. However, these signals

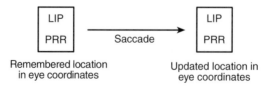

FIG. 6.   Schematic showing that in both area LIP and PRR the remembered locations of targets are updated, in eye coordinates, across saccades.

are also gain modulated by eye and head position signals, and this gain modulation allows multiple reference frames to be coded simultaneously within these areas. Thus LIP and PRR contain a common, distributed representation of space. This representation is updated each time the eye moves. Not only are the eye position signals changing across eye movements, but also the retinal locations of remembered sensory targets. Thus this distributed representation of space can faithfully code the location of remembered targets across eye movements in eye, head or body-centred coordinates. This updating is obviously useful for making accurate movements in spite of intervening saccades. However, we also perceive space as stable in spite of eye movements. It is not clear whether the spatial constancy of perception is also supported by activity in PPC. Alternatively, PPC may only operate for action and not conscious awareness and activity in the ventral visual pathway may support visual awareness (Goodale & Milner 1992). If this is the case, then receptive fields in the ventral pathway may also update across eye movements, and this may be the basis for the spatial stability of perception. Likewise, there have been several reports of gain field effects in ventral extrastriate areas not unlike those found in PPC which may also contribute to perceiving space as constant across eye and head movements. Future experiments will need to be done to determine whether the updating mechanisms that are found in the motor and dorsal extrastriate areas are also found in the ventral extrastriate cortex. It is possible that updating of signals in eye coordinates, and the gain modulation of eye-centred receptive fields, are a very general phenomenon for large parts of the mammalian brain.

References

Andersen RA 1987 The role of the inferior parietal lobule function in spatial perception and visuomotor integration. In: Plum F, Mountcastle VB, Geiger SR (eds) Handbook of physiology, section 1: The nervous system, vol V: Higher functions of the brain, part 2. American Physiology Association, Bethesda, MD, p 483–518

Andersen RA 1995 Encoding of intention and spatial location in the posterior parietal cortex. Cereb Cortex 5:457–469

Andersen RA, Asanuma C, Essick G, Siegel RM 1990 Cortico-cortical connections of anatomically and physiologically defined subdivisions within the inferior parietal lobule. J Comp Neurol 296:65–113

Asanuma C, Andersen RA, Cowan WM 1985 The thalamic relations of the caudal inferior parietal lobule and the lateral prefrontal cortex in monkeys: divergent cortical projections from cell clusters in the medial pulvinar nucleus. J Comp Neurol 241:357–381

Barash S, Andersen RA, Bracewell RM, Fogassi L, Gnadt J 1991 Saccade-related activity in the lateral intraparietal area. I: temporal properties. J Neurophysiol 66:1095–1108

Batista AP, Snyder LH, Buneo CA, Andersen RA 1998 A common reference frame for planning eye and hand movements in the posterior parietal cortex. Submitted

Blatt G, Andersen RA, Stoner G 1990 Visual receptive field organization and cortico-cortical connections of area LIP in the macaque. J Comp Neurol 299:421–445

Colby CL, Duhamel J-R, Goldberg ME 1995 Oculocentric spatial representation in parietal cortex. Cereb Cortex 5:470–481

Critchley M 1953 The parietal lobes. Hafner Press, New York

Duhamel JR, Colby CL, Goldberg ME 1992 The updating of the representation of visual space in parietal cortex by intended eye movements. Science 255:90–92

Gnadt JW, Andersen RA 1988 Memory related motor planning activity in posterior parietal cortex of macaque. Exp Brain Res 70:216–220

Goodale MA, Milner AD 1992 Separate visual pathways for perception and action. Trends Neurosci 15:20–25

Grunewald A, Linden JF, Andersen RA 1997 Auditory responses in LIP. II: behavioral gating. Soc Neurosci Abstr 23:16

Li C-SR, Mazzoni P, Andersen RA 1998 The effect of reversible inactivation of macaque lateral intraparietal area on oculomotor behaviors. I. Visual and memory saccades, submitted

Linden JF, Grunewald A, Andersen RA 1997 Auditory responses in LIP. I: training effects. Soc Neurosci Abstr 23:16

Lynch JC, McLaren JW 1989 Deficits of visual attention and saccadic eye movements after movements after lesions of parietooccipital cortex in monkeys. J Neurophysiol 61:74–90

Lynch JC, Graybiel AM, Lobeck LJ 1985 The differential projection of two cytoarchitectonic subregions of the inferior parietal lobule of macaque upon the deep layers of the superior colliculus. J Comp Neurol 235:241–254

Maunsell JH, van Essen DC 1983 The connections of the middle temporal visual area (MT) and their relationship to a cortical hierarchy in the macaque monkey. J Neurosci 3:2563–2586

Mazzoni P, Bracewell RM, Barash S, Andersen RA 1996a Spatially tuned auditory responses in area LIP of macaques performing delayed memory saccades to acoustic targets. J Neurophysiol 75:1233–1241

Mazzoni P, Bracewell RM, Barash S, Andersen RA 1996b Motor intention activity in the macaque's lateral intraparietal area. I. Dissociation of motor plan from sensory memory. J Neurophysiol 76:1439–1456

Mountcastle VB, Lynch JC, Georgopoulos A, Sakata H, Acuna C 1975 Posterior parietal association cortex of the monkey: command functions for operations within extrapersonal space. J Neurophysiol 38:871–908

Snyder LH, Batista AP, Andersen RA 1997 Coding of intention in the posterior parietal cortex. Nature 386:167–170

Snyder LH, Batista A, Andersen RA 1998 Change in plan activity without changing the focus of attention. J Neurophysiol, in press

Sparks D, Mays LE 1980 Movement fields of saccade-related burst neurons in the monkey superior coliculus. Brain Res 190:39–50

Stricanne B, Andersen RA, Mazzoni P 1996 Eye-centered, head-centered and intermediate coding of remembered sound locations in area LIP. J Neurophysiol 76:2071–2076

Thier P, Andersen RA 1996 Electrical microstimulation suggests two different kinds of representation of head-centered space in the intraparietal sulcus of rhesus monkeys. Proc Natl Acad Sci USA 93:4962–4967

DISCUSSION

Stein: I didn't quite understand your reconciliation with Micky Goldberg. Micky says that there is an updating of the retinal meaning, as it were, of a receptive field before an eye movement. Many of your experiments suggest a recalibration after the eye movement. I got the message from your paper that there is some reconciliation going on now, but I couldn't quite understand it.

Andersen: There is nothing much to reconcile, since we have both reported on updating of activity in LIP across saccades, that is in eye coordinates. Your question is about the timing of the update. When we look at memory responses, in that case the compensation usually occurs right at the time of the beginning of the eye movement or after, but not prior. Mickey looked at a different condition in which the stimulus was still visible and often saw the compensation occurring before the eye movement.

We have recently looked at the eye position signal itself. Interestingly, if a visual target is present, it begins to change prior to the eye movement. But if we look at a memory saccade, again it begins changing right about the time of the memory saccade. The idea is that the presence of the visual target somehow makes the compensation earlier in time.

Stein: But you never see it 100 ms before the eye movement?

Andersen: We haven't tried his experiment, but we do see the eye position signal updating sometimes even more than 100 ms prior to the eye movement. We think that the efference copy of the saccade command, possibly originating in the frontal lobe, is responsible, because the compensation is so early. This efference copy of eye displacement may be integrated by the parietal cortex to provide an eye position signal to then produce gain fields and maintain the spatial representation across eye movements.

Thier: You mentioned the early work by Mountcastle and co-workers on area 7a, in which they described the existence of saccade-related activity and reach-related activity in 7a (Mountcastle et al 1975). Now we have learnt, thanks to work from your lab and others, that there is a specific area involved in processing saccade-related information, area LIP, and another one, MST, processing pursuit-related information as well as signals related to optic flow. In addition, we now learn about another reach-related area in parts of the intraparietal sulcus, neighbouring area LIP. So what is left for area 7a to do?

Andersen: There are two answers. First, 7a does have reach activity. It also has eye movement activity but the responses are post-saccadic and not pre-saccadic; it's a very complicated area. As Dick Passingham was saying yesterday, it's all in the connections. If you look at 7a connections, it goes to the highest levels of the brain: the hippocampal gyrus, cingulate cortex and the anterior part of the superior temporal sulcus. It is not yet clear what area 7a does. Certainly, in the parietal reach region (PRR) the activity is incredibly robust; for saccades LIP is robust, and smooth pursuit seems to be found easily in area MST. No doubt in the early days when people were doing experiments in the posterior parietal region they were running electrode tracks deep through many of these regions. At that time 7a was defined as a much bigger area, which included areas LIP and

MST. Today, we define 7a as a much smaller area located on the surface of the inferior parietal lobule.

Thier: Does it also hold for the reach-related activity in 7a that it comes later than reach-related activity in the intraparietal sulcus?

Andersen: We haven't looked at that in detail. With this parietal reach area you can see in the rasters that the reach activity precedes the reach movement. In 7a their activity can also precede the reach, but we haven't analysed quantitatively whether 7a tends to have a higher proportion of post-reach responses.

Miller: I have trouble in understanding your interpretation of the last part of your extinction series of experiments. Wouldn't a fairly simple description be that as the eyes approach the edge of the oculomotor range, the monkey didn't care to look further in that direction and looked back?

Andersen: In the normal condition, when gaze is straight ahead the animal will choose with about equal frequency to look to the left and right targets. When the eyes are deviated to one side (say left), the monkey will generally choose to look in the direction that will centre the eye in the orbit (right). After LIP inactivation the monkey will generally not look into the unhealthy field even when the eye is deviated in the opposite direction. Thus the 'equilibrium' point for gaze direction at which the animal will choose the left and right targets equally shifts far into the ipsilesional field after inactivation. This result demonstrates an eye position (head-centred) deficit after LIP inactivation.

Savaki: Have you found any cells in area LIP which encode target position in head-centred coordinates?

Andersen: No it has always been in eye coordinates, but modulated by eye and head position.

Savaki: The discharge of cells which encode target position in head-centred coordinates (target *re* head position) should be completely unaffected by changes of eye position and affected only by changes of head position. As far as I know, you have not found any cells in area LIP coding target position in head-centred space. Moreover, a signal coding target *re* head position (even if it existed in area LIP) should be transformed back into a signal coding eye displacement *re* retina position to be used by the superior colliculi. Thus, cells in area LIP which send information out to the superior colliculi cannot be the LIP gain field neurons. Actually, the LIP output neurons have not been described yet. My impression is that the neurons which you have described to encode 'intention' or 'planning of movement' or 'memory of the intended eye-position' in area LIP have similar properties to the quasivisual (Qv) cells described in the deep layer of the superior colliculi by Mays & Sparks (1980). Moreover, it has been demonstrated by Moschovakis et al (1988) that these cells receive (a) visual retinotopic input from the superficial layer of SC (retinal error signal from L neurons) and (b) feedback input concerning the degree of eye displacement from RTLLB cells (cells which discharge in proportion to eye displacement). Thus, retinal error minus eye displacement computation in Qv cells provides information about 'eye-position error' or 'memory of the desired eye displacement'. As far as I know, there is no anatomical support in any area of the brain, of eye position information subtracted from target *re* head position signal. Thus, LIP neurons may encode 'memory of the desired eye displacement' rather than 'memory of the intended eye-position'. The spatial hypothesis (which implies eye-position signal) is neither anatomically nor functionally substantiated, neither in area LIP nor in any other eye movement-related area. In contrast, the vector subtraction hypothesis (which implies eye displacement signal) has been substantiated in the superior colliculi both anatomically and functionally (Moschovakis et al 1996).

Andersen: That is the beauty of this distributed representation. I could think about looking to a remembered place in space, or a location with respect to some part of my body, through reading out that representation. In this distributed framework, the retinal location of a target is also retained, and a plan to move the eyes in eye-centred coordinates can also be read out from the population of LIP cells and used by the superior colliculus. Whenever you convert from a retinal receptive field to a receptive field in another coordinate frame, you lose information, whereas with this distributed representation you simultaneously have several coordinate frames that can be read out and you don't lose any information.

Savaki: But we haven't found the output cells of area LIP yet.

Andersen: I think cells that receive output from LIP that have other reference frames would be like VIP, which contains many cells which code the visual targets in head-centric coordinates. Dr Rizzolatti's experiments in F4 show coding with respect to body parts, and Graziano, Gross and colleagues have reproduced that result. Thus there are places in the brain which do combine information, and in a sense lose information when they make these conversions. An interesting question concerns why you would ever want to do that. In other words, the brain could stay within this distributed coordinate framework until motor cortex (M1) or the oculomotor nuclei.

Ebner: I'm interested in the general properties of the PRR cells. How is their amplitude tuning? Do these cells encode other parameters such as speed or velocity?

Andersen: That's a fascinating question, but we haven't looked at amplitude or speed tuning yet. We plan to look at this. My guess from what we know so far is that it will look like a receptive field, such as a retinal receptive field. Thus it would be amplitude tuned, but not velocity tuned.

Ebner: But your sense is that they're going to be spatially tuned; they're going to be tuned along an amplitude axis, as opposed to simply linear.

Andersen: Yes, but I'm guessing.

Kalaska: I want to follow up on the issue of directional tuning of these cells. When I looked at your results, I got the impression that the reach-related cells seemed to have more of a preferred spatial target location in retinal coordinates for reaching movements. They would discharge whenever the monkey moves into that target area but they're not actually tuned *per se* in terms of the metrics of the movement the monkey makes into that area — for instance, in which direction they must move the arm to get into the target location. Putting this another way, when you move into that field from many different directions, the cell seems to be active. It is non-directional in that sense. This clearly is quite different from motor cortical cells.

Andersen: That's the basis of my guess that it is going to be spatial because, as you say, the animal can move in two different directions but to the same location on the retina, and they're tuned with respect to the retina.

Kalaska: To continue along this line, you were recording a very medial location in the medial bank of the parietal sulcus. Donald Crammond and I recorded in an area that was slightly lateral to that, although still probably in MIP (Kalaska & Crammond 1995). The behaviour of the cells there didn't leave us with the impression or a suspicion that they had a retinotopic or eye-coordinate framework. I'm not upset about that: again, we're not in the same part of the brain, and also in our tasks we didn't fixate the eyes. The monkey is constantly saccading around and fixating at random throughout the performance of the task. When we turned on a target in a particular spatial location relative to where the hand was, in a delayed task, a cell would commonly emit a stable tonic discharge during the delay period before movement that was a function of the direction in which the monkey had to move to get to the target. In the meantime, during this delay period, the monkey is saccading all over. If the cells had retinotopic movement-target fields, the image of the spatial location of the movement-location signal we gave should fall on different locations on the retina relative to its movement-target field, and you should hear changes in the tonic discharge as the eye is saccading about during the delay period. However, we didn't see that property in those cells that we recorded in a part of area 5 only a few millimetres lateral to where you were recording. Instead, the tonic activity usually remained very stable. Thus there may be a very rapid shift in the nature of the coordinate frameworks, within a few millimetres along the bank of the intraparietal sulcus, from one that is retinotopic or at least strongly influenced by eye position, to one that appears to be more egocentric or even limb centred.

Andersen: Sure. This distinction of MIP from the convexity of area 5 is somewhat arbitrary. We have begun examining whether area 5 proper, up on the surface, was going to show a similar activity (C. A. Bueno, A. P. Batista & R. A. Andersen, unpublished observations). In this task the activity appears to be very different. We don't see the memory activity, by and large. Also, it appears to be

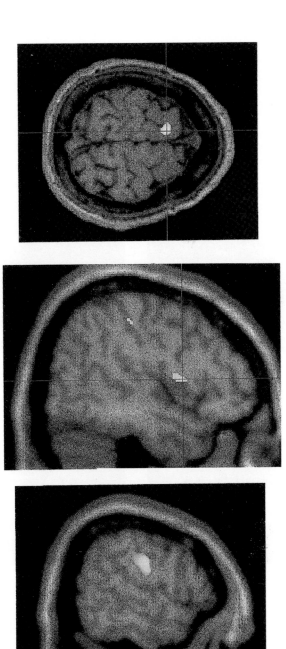

PLATE 1   Comparison of visuomotor associative task (VMA) and reach and grasp (RG). (*Top*)
Dorsal premotor cortex (VMA–RG). (*Middle*) Ventral opercular premotor cortex (RG–VMA).
(*Bottom*) Anterior parietal cortex (RG–VMA).

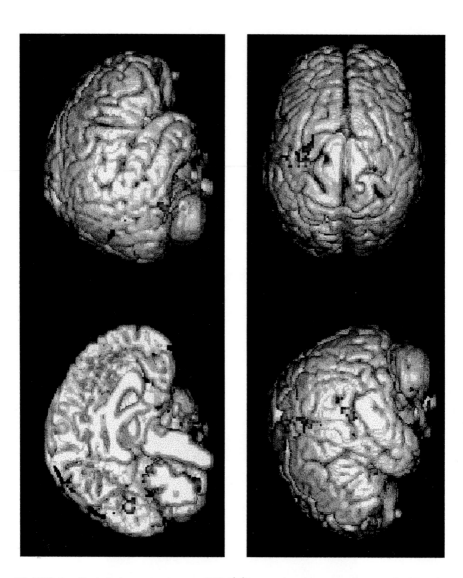

PLATE 2   Statistical parametric map (SPM{F}) map showing areas that are significantly activated on a visuomotor associative task in which there was a variable delay between the visual instruction cues and the auditory trigger cues. The areas are shown for one subject scanned with event-related fMRI (Schluter et al 1997). The activations are superimposed on a standard brain. (*Top*) Areas in which the evoked haemodynamic response was statistically significant when aligned to the visual instruction cues. (*Bottom*) Areas in which the evoked haemodynamic response was statistically significant when aligned to the auditory trigger cue (time of response).

more limb related, but in some very complex way. Just as you discuss intrinsic coordinates, it is as if we're sampling a lot of the position signals from the limb from area 5; it is very different.

Kalaska: Donald Crammond and I saw exactly the same gradient: as we proceeded further laterally along the intraparietal sulcus and then onto the exposed surface of what most would still consider to be area 5, or the 2/5 transition area, the delay period discharge becomes much less prominent and cell activity becomes more coupled in time to the movements of the arm itself.

Andersen: We think this shared coordinate frame for PRR and LIP may help in hand–eye coordination, for instance. It would be nice and much simpler to plan arm movements under visual guidance in eye coordinates, and thus share a common coordinate frame with area LIP for that task.

Goodale: Would you like to comment on differences in the topology of what we know about the activation patterns that occur with reaching as opposed to those that occur with saccadic eye movements in neuroimaging studies of human brain? I'm thinking primarily of the recent work by Kawashima et al (1996), in which they showed that an area was activated in the intraparietal sulcus when subjects reached towards a visual target that was slightly more rostral and medial to the area that was activated when subjects made saccades towards the same targets. Is this a difference in the topological arrangement of the same areas that are seen in the monkey or are they different areas that have emerged in the human brain?

Andersen: I meant to mention at the end of the talk that Mel Goodale and his colleagues and I have been doing an fMRI experiment that shows the separation of saccade and reach in the parietal lobe of humans. The reach activation is located medial to the saccade area (similar to the monkey) but more anteriorly than we found in the monkey parietal lobe. There could be some difference in topography between the monkey and human.

Yesterday we touched briefly on some of the differences between monkeys and humans in terms of the superior and inferior parietal lobules. Also, in extrastriate cortex, the story is somewhat different between the two species: it is as if in human the monkey map has been dragged down and back. For instance, MT is located much more ventrally and posterially than we would have expected from monkeys. Although there are some small differences in topography between the species, it is important to emphasize that we can see the segregation for reach and saccade in the human and monkey parietal cortex.

References

Kalaska JF, Crammond DJ 1995 Deciding not to go: neuronal correlates of response selection in a GO/NOGO task in primate premotor and parietal cortex. Cerebral Cortex 5:4110–428

Kawashima R, Naitoh E, Matsumura M et al 1996 Topographic representation in human intraparietal sulcus of reaching and saccade. Neuroreport 7:1253–1256

Mays LE, Sparks DL 1980 Dissociation of visual and saccade-related responses in superior colliculus neurons. J Neurophysiol 43:207–232

Moschovakis AK, Karabelas AB, Highstein SM 1988 Structure–function relationships in the primate superior colliculus. II. Morphological identity of presaccadic neurons. J Neurophysiol 60:263–302

Moschovakis AK, Scudder CA, Highstein SM 1996 The microscopic anatomy and physiology of the mammalian saccadic system. Progr Neurobiol 50:133–254

Mountcastle VB, Lynch JC, Georgopoulos A, Sakata H, Acuna C 1975 Posterior parietal association cortex of the monkey: command functions for operations within extrapersonal space. J Neurophysiol 38:871–908

How do visual instructions influence the motor system?

R. E. Passingham*†, I. Toni†, N. Schluter*, M. F. S. Rushworth*

*Department of Experimental Psychology, University of Oxford, South Parks Road, Oxford OX1 3UD and †Wellcome Department of Cognitive Neurology, Institute of Neurology, 12 Queen Square, London WC1N 3BG, UK

Abstract. The paper distinguishes the use of visual cues to guide reaching and grasping, and the ability to learn to associate arbitrary sensory cues with movements. Using positron emission tomography (PET), we have shown that the arbitrary association of visual cues and movements involves the ventral visual system (prestriate, inferotemporal and ventral prefrontal cortex), the basal ganglia and the dorsal premotor cortex. Using functional magnetic resonance imaging (fMRI), we have shown that the evoked haemodynamic responses in the ventral visual system are time-locked to the presentation of the visual cues, that the response in the motor cortex is locked to the time of response, and that the response in the dorsal premotor cortex shows cue-related, movement-related and set-related components. Using PET we have shown that there are learning-related changes in activation in both the ventral prestriate cortex and the basal ganglia (globus pallidus) when subjects learn a visuomotor associative task. We argue that the basal ganglia may act as a flexible system for learning the association of sensory cues and movements.

1998 Sensory guidance of movement. Wiley, Chichester (Novartis Foundation Symposium 218) p 129–146

People can associate any stimulus with any response. Depending on the instructions, they can move one finger given one stimulus and a different finger given another. The stimuli could be different colours, different tones or even different tastes, and the responses could be made with the hand, eyes or toes. This is not a trivial ability. Human subjects can obey the written instruction to 'pull', even though the association between the shape of the word and the movement is arbitrary.

One's first thought is that there must be cortico-cortical paths from each sense modality to the motor system. And this thought is encouraged by the observation that there are visual pathways from parietal cortex to the premotor cortex (Matelli et al 1986, Tanné et al 1995, Johnson et al 1996), and that there are projections from the premotor cortex to the motor cortex (Strick 1985). In the macaque brain, cells in parietal area AIP code information about the shape of objects to be grasped (Sakata et al 1996), and this area sends projections to ventral premotor cortex (PMv) (Matelli et al 1986). Cells in this premotor region (area F5) become active when the animal prepares to grasp an object (Murata et al 1997). Inactivation of cells in both areas (AIP, PMv) severely impairs the pre-shaping of hand and wrist in preparation for grasping (Gallese et al 1997).

Arbitrary cues

It would, however, be naïve to suppose that all sensory cues influence the premotor cortex via cortico-cortical projections of this sort. Both animals and human subjects can learn to associate *arbitrary* sensory cues with movements. In the laboratory this situation can be modelled by teaching a 'visuomotor associative task'. For example, monkeys can be taught to make movement A given one colour (or pattern), and movement B given another colour (or pattern) (Passingham 1993). Here the response is conditional on the stimulus, and thus the design is sometimes referred to as a 'visual conditional task' (Passingham 1993).

Where visual information is used to *guide* the hand, 3D visual information is used to specify the reach and the shape of the grasp. There is a *spatial correspondence* between the location in space of the object and the termination of the reach, and also between the 3D shape of the object and the size and shape of the appropriate grasping movement. Both the object information and the movement can be described in a spatial coordinate system, and there can be a direct interaction between the dorsal visual system (parietal cortex) and premotor cortex. There *is no such spatial correspondence* between 2D colours or tones and movements. Wise et al (1996) draw the distinction by comparing 'standard' with 'non-standard' mapping.

In the case of 2D colours or patterns, there is no common coordinate system in which both cues and movements can be described. It is not clear how the premotor cortex could directly interpret such information. The visual cues must first be identified, and information about colour and pattern is processed in the ventral visual system, including the inferotemporal cortex (Heywood et al 1995). Whereas there are direct projections to premotor cortex from parietal cortex, there are no direct projections from the inferotemporal cortex to the premotor cortex.

There is a further point. Monkeys do not have to learn to reach for and grasp objects. They spend most of their day picking fruit and leaves, and the brain has dedicated pathways to make this possible. But monkeys have to *learn* what response to make to arbitrary cues. Like human subjects, monkeys can learn associations for any modality: for example they can learn to press one pedal given a light and another pedal given a sound (Delacour et al 1972). It is implausible that this ability depends on simple cortico-cortical connections between each modality and the premotor system. Instead, a flexible system is needed that has inputs from all modalities and that also has motor outputs — a system that can reinforce associations via learning.

Imaging visual guidance and visuomotor association

It is now possible to use functional brain imaging to delineate, and thus contrast, the systems involved in visual guidance and in visuomotor associative learning. In a recent experiment using PET, two conditions were compared (Toni et al 1998a): in one ('reach and grasp') the subjects saw an object, waited, and then reached for it and grasped it. In the other condition ('visuomotor associative task') the subjects saw an object, waited and then made a manual gesture. In both cases there were four objects. In the second condition the gestures that were appropriate for each object were taught before scanning.

When performance of the visuomotor associative task (VMA) was contrasted with those for reaching and grasping (RG) (comparison VMA–RG), there was an activation in the dorsal premotor cortex (Plate 1, top). For the opposite contrast (RG–VMA) there was an activation ventrally in premotor cortex; the peak lay in the opercular cortex (Plate 1, middle). Kurata & Hoffman (1994) have compared the effects of inactivating either the dorsal premotor cortex (PMd) or the ventral premotor cortex (PMv) in monkeys. They report that inactivation of the dorsal, but not the ventral premotor cortex, caused the animals to make the wrong movements on a visuomotor association task.

When comparing visuomotor associative learning with visual guidance (VMA–RG), there was also an activation in the ventral prefrontal cortex. The peak lay in the ventral bank of the inferior frontal sulcus, probably within the region identified by Petrides & Pandya (1995) as area 45A. This area receives an input from the inferotemporal cortex (Webster et al 1994). If performance of a visual conditional task is compared with a baseline condition in which no visual stimuli are presented, activation can also be measured in the ventral visual system including the inferotemporal cortex (area 37) (Toni et al 1998b) (Plate 2, top).

By contrast, when reaching and grasping was compared with performance of the visuomotor associative task (RG–VMA), there was an activation anteriorly in parietal cortex (area 40). It lay in the region where the intraparietal sulcus touches on the somatosensory strip (Plate 1, bottom). This area appears to be similar to the region identified as AIP in a related positron emission tomography (PET) study by Faillenot et al (1997).

Visual versus motor activations

PET can be used to map the visual and motor areas that are involved in visuomotor mapping where there is an arbitrary association between cues and movements. However, to understand the visuomotor transformation, it is also necessary to characterize the contribution that is made by the different areas. We have devised a novel method for event-related functional magnetic resonance imaging (fMRI), which allows one statistically to associate the activations on a visuomotor associative task with either the presentation of the cues or the motor response (Schluter et al 1997, Toni et al 1998b).

The subjects were required to move their forefinger given one shape and their second finger given another shape. The visual instruction cue was briefly presented, there was a variable delay, and the subject then responded to an auditory trigger cue. The areas activated can be seen in Plate 2. Because the delay was varied, it was possible to analyse the data by aligning the data either to the presentation of the visual instruction cue or to the auditory trigger cue (Schluter et al 1997). When the data were aligned to the visual instruction cue, there were significant activations in the striate, prestriate and inferotemporal cortex (Plate 2, top), but when the data were aligned to the time of response (auditory trigger cue) there were significant activations in the dorsal premotor cortex and motor cortex (Plate 2, bottom).

The evoked haemodynamic responses for striate cortex and motor cortex are shown in Fig. 1. For each area, the evoked haemodynamic response is shown as averaged either to the visual instruction cue or to the auditory trigger cue. For striate cortex there was a significant haemodynamic response when the data were aligned to the visual cue but not when they were aligned to the auditory trigger cue (Fig. 1, top). In the inferotemporal cortex (area 37) the haemodynamic response was also statistically associated with the visual instruction cue; the response appears to be slightly delayed (Fig. 1, middle). For motor cortex there was a significant haemodynamic response when the data were aligned to the trigger cue but not when they were aligned to the visual instruction cue (Fig. 1, bottom).

Figure 2 shows the activity in the dorsal premotor cortex for trials with a delay of 12.8 s, and compares it with the activity for motor cortex. It can be seen that in the premotor cortex there is a response to the visual cue, followed by a sustained response, followed by a further response to the trigger cue. The evoked haemodynamic response for the population of cells, as demonstrated by fMRI,

---

FIG. 1. Evoked haemodynamic responses in three cortical areas while three subjects performed a visuomotor associative task in which there was a variable delay between the visual instruction cues and the auditory trigger cues. Data from study by Schluter et al (1997) and Toni et al (1998b). (*Top*) Striate cortex: continuous line (circles) gives the response when the data are aligned to the visual instruction cues; dotted line (crosses) gives the response when the data are aligned to the auditory trigger cue (time of response). (*Middle*) Inferotemporal cortex (area 37): continuous line (circles) gives the response when the data are aligned to the visual instruction cues; dotted line (crosses) gives the response when the data are aligned to the auditory trigger cue (time of response). (*Bottom*) Motor cortex: continuous line (circles) gives the response when the data are aligned to the auditory trigger cue (time of response); dotted line (crosses) gives the response when the data are aligned to the visual instruction cues.

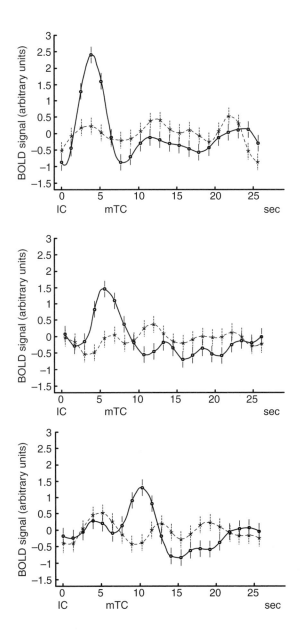

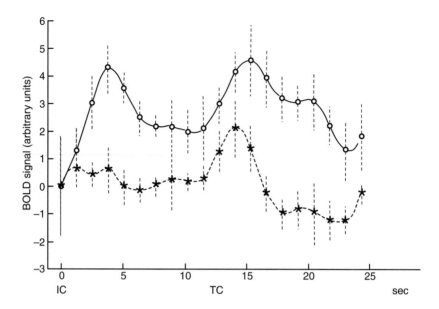

FIG. 2.   Evoked haemodynamic responses in premotor and motor cortex while three subjects performed a visuomotor associative task in which there was a delay between the visual instruction cues and the auditory trigger cues. The responses are shown for a delay of 12.8 s. The response for the dorsal premotor cortex is shown by the continuous line (circles), and the response for motor cortex by the dotted line (crosses). Data from study by Schluter et al (1997) and Toni et al (1998b).

can be compared with that expected on the basis of recording the activity of single neurons in this area while monkeys perform a visuomotor associative task. Weinrich et al (1984) reported that in PMd 47% of the cells had activity that was cue related, 34% set related and 65% movement related (any neuron could belong to more than one class). The profile for the population of cells shown in Fig. 2 appears to have cue-related, set-related and movement-related components.

Learning movements

In the imaging studies described above, the subjects had learned the association between cues and responses before scanning, and they were scanned later while they *performed* the task. However, in a further study (Toni & Passingham 1998) the subjects were scanned while they *learned* which finger movement to make for each of the nonsense shapes presented (visuomotor associative task). The task was taught by trial and error in the same way that we had previously taught motor sequence tasks (Jueptner et al 1997), with tones for feedback cues.

Between the four scans, the subjects were given further training so that the task was overtrained by the time of the last two scans. Four baseline scans were also taken in which the subjects were presented with irrelevant nonsense shapes but made no movements. In the learning condition the nonsense shapes served as pacing cues as well as instructing which movement to make.

An analysis was performed to see whether there were brain areas in which there were changes in activity that were related to learning over the four scans. There were two areas in which there was an increase in activation as learning progressed. The first peak lay in ventral prestriate cortex (lingual gyrus). The change in activation here is shown in Fig. 3 (top). It may reflect changes in attention to the distinguishing features of the nonsense shapes as the subjects learned to identify them.

The second peak lay in the globus pallidus, near to the border with the putamen. In the previous study comparing non-standard with standard mapping (VMA–RG), we also found an activation in the globus pallidus (Toni & Passingham 1998). Figure 3 (bottom) shows the increase in activation in this region as the subjects learned the visuomotor associative task. This change in the basal ganglia suggests that the anatomical connections with the basal ganglia from the temporal cortex may be important for the process by which associations are learned between visual stimuli and motor outputs. Saint-Cyr et al (1990) have shown that the ventral prestriate and temporal cortex sends projections to the posterior striatum, and that there are projections from there to the globus pallidus (Fig. 4).

There is other evidence that the basal ganglia are involved in motor learning. In the study of visuomotor associative learning, we also taught a motor sequence (Toni & Passingham 1998). Again the sequence was taught by trial and error as in Jueptner et al (1997), with tones for feedback cues. For the sequence, as for the visuomotor associative task, there was an increase in activation in the globus pallidus across the four learning scans (Toni & Passingham 1998).

Several authors (e.g. Passingham 1987, 1993, Hikosaka 1993, Houk & Wise 1995, Dominey et al 1995) have proposed that the basal ganglia may play an essential role in motor learning, and in particular in the process by which movements are reinforced. They cite as supporting evidence the fact that the dopaminergic projections from the substantia nigra to the striatal medium spiny neurons could modulate cortico-striatal inputs (Houk & Wise 1995); that there are cells that are responsive to reward in the ventral third of the striatum (Apicella et al 1991); and that there are cells that change their activity during learning (Schultz et al 1993, Aosaki et al 1994). It is of particular interest that in monkeys there are changes in cell activity in the striatum that are associated with the learning of a visual conditional motor task (Tremblay et al 1994).

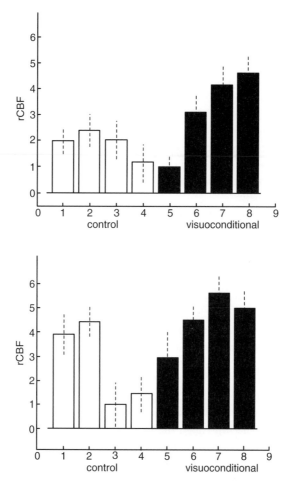

FIG. 3.   Changes in activation for two brain areas over four scans of learning a visuomotor
associative task. White, baseline; black, visuomotor associative learning. The ordinate gives
the relative regional cerebral blood flow (rCBF). The baseline (0) is arbitrarily set at 1% below
the smallest activation. Data from Toni et al (1998b). (*Top*) Ventral prestriate cortex (lingual
gyrus) (coordinates in standard space for Montreal Neurological Institute [MNI] = 16, −60,
−10). (*Bottom*) Globus pallidus (MNI coordinates = −26, −8, −6).

The effects of interference

It is one thing to show which areas are *active* during the learning of visuomotor
association tasks; it is another to show which areas are *essential* for the learning
and performance of these tasks. For example, it has been shown using PET that
the dorsal premotor cortex is active when subjects perform a visuomotor

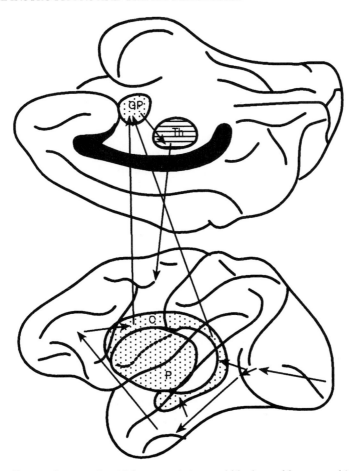

FIG. 4.   Proposed routes via which an association could be learned between arbitrary visual cues and movements. GP, globus pallidus; Th, ventral thalamus; C, caudate; P, putamen. For references see text and reviews by Passingham (1993) and Wise (1996). Figure loosely based on Wise (1996).

associative task (Plate 1); but to demonstrate that this region is essential for response selection, one needs to interfere. We have used transcranial magnetic brain stimulation (TMS), and have stimulated over the dorsal premotor cortex while subjects perform a visuomotor associative task (Schluter et al 1998). As in the imaging experiments described above (Schluter et al 1997), the subjects were required to move their forefinger given one shape and their second finger given another shape. The difference was that the subjects were required to respond as soon after presentation of the shape as possible (choice reaction time). TMS over the dorsal premotor cortex 140 ms after presentation of the cue delayed the movement on the choice reaction time task, but not on a simple reaction time task (Schluter et al 1998).

To find out via which routes the visual cues influence premotor cortex it is necessary to interfere in the various candidate pathways. The effects of lesions at different stages has been reviewed by Passingham (1987, 1993) and Wise et al (1996). We have trained monkeys on a visuomotor associative task and have compared the effects of placing lesions in either the dorsal or ventral visual stream. Rushworth et al (1997a) found no effect on retention when the lesion included the upper bank of the intraparietal sulcus (including some of MIP) and the lower bank of the anterior part of the intraparietal suclus (including AIP). Similarly there was no effect when a lesion was placed in the posterior part of the inferior parietal cortex (including area 7a). However, further experiments are needed to check these negative findings, because recent anatomical studies have suggested that there are other visually receiving areas of parietal cortex that project to the dorsal premotor cortex (Tanné et al 1995, Johnson et al 1996).

It has been suggested above that where an arbitrary association is learned between movements and colours or shapes, it is more likely that the analysis of the identity of the cues depends on the ventral visual stream. The inferotemporal cortex sends projections to the ventral prefrontal cortex (Webster et al 1994), and Murray & Wise (1997) have shown that lesions in the ventral prefrontal cortex interfere with the learning of visuomotor associative tasks. We have also shown that ventral prefrontal lesions severely impair the retention of a visuomotor associative task on which the monkeys had to select between colour shapes on the basis of a visual cue (visual matching) (Rushworth et al 1997b).

The crucial question is whether the basal ganglia are necessarily involved in the process by which the visuomotor associations are learned. The striatum receives inputs from all cortical areas, including the ventral prestriate and inferotemporal cortex (Saint-Cyr et al 1990), the ventral prefrontal cortex and the dorsal premotor cortex (Selemon & Goldman-Rakic 1985) (Fig. 4). In an early study (Canavan et al 1989) we showed that monkeys were very severely impaired indeed at re-learning a visuomotor associative task after large bilateral lesions in the basal ganglia territory of the ventral thalamus. The lesion included the ventral nuclei (VAmc, VApc and VLo) that receive an input from the global pallidus pars interna (GPi) (Ilinsky & Kultas-Ilinsky 1987) and that project to the premotor areas (Strick et al 1995, Matelli & Luppino 1996). Because the lesion might also have invaded the cerebellar territory of the ventral thalamus (nucleus X), in a later study Passingham & Nixon (1996) placed total excitotoxic lesions in the dentate and interpositus nuclei of the cerebellum in monkeys. The monkeys showed normal retention and normal new learning of visuomotor associative tasks. We are now comparing the effects of placing different excitotoxic lesions in the globus pallidus. That the globus pallidus is essential for motor learning in general is shown by the experiments of Hikosaka et al (1996) in which injections of muscimol in the globus pallidus impaired the learning and retention of motor sequences.

Conclusions

This paper has distinguished two problems. The first is how visuospatial cues serve to guide and orient movements; the second is how arbitrary visual instructions influence which movement it is appropriate to perform. The first problem is the more commonly studied, and it is clear from this meeting that much progress has been made.

The second problem is the more intractable. Any sensory stimulus can be associated with any motor response. It has been argued that the dorsal premotor cortex forms a critical stage in the circuit, but it is less clear how this area receives the relevant inputs. No projections to the dorsal premotor cortex have been described from either the inferotemporal cortex or the ventral prefrontal cortex (Fig. 4), though the latter does send a projection to the ventral prefrontal cortex. Furthermore, even if such projections were to exist it is not clear that they would allow the *learning* of an association between stimulus and response. One possibility is that the learning of this association makes demands on a general learning mechanism with sensory inputs from all modalities and outputs to the cortical motor system. The basal ganglia serve as a candidate for such a mechanism.

It is not clear whether the fine details of anatomical wiring in the basal ganglia permit such sensory–motor integration. The relevant literature has been reviewed by Passingham (1993) and Wise (1996). It has been controversial whether there is overlap in the basal ganglia between the loops connecting with the different cortical regions (Strick et al 1995, Sidibe et al 1997). One possibility is that the visual and motor representations are associated in the ventral prefrontal cortex, and this association is reinforced through the operation of prefrontal–basal ganglia loops.

Acknowledgement

Dr I. Toni was supported by a European BIOMED grant.

References

Aosaki TA, Graybiel M, Kimura M 1994 Effect of the nigrostriatal dopamine system on acquired neural responses in the striatum of behaving monkeys. Science 265:412–415

Apicella P, Ljungberg T, Scarnati E, Schultz W 1991 Responses to reward in monkey dorsal and ventral striatum. Exp Brain Res 85:491–500

Canavan AG, Nixon PD, Passingham RE 1989 Motor learning in monkeys (*Macaca fascicularis*) with lesions in motor thalamus. Exp Brain Res 77:113–126

Delacour J, Libouban S, McNeil M 1972 Premotor cortex and instrumental behavior in monkeys. Physiol Behav 8:299–305

Dominey P, Arbib M, Joseph J-P 1995 A model of corticostriatal plasticity for learning oculomotor associations and sequences. J Cogn Neurosci 7:311–336

Faillenot I, Toni I, Decety J, Gregoire M-C, Jeannerod M 1997 Visual pathways for object-oriented action and object recognition: functional anatomy with PET. Cereb Cortex 7:77–85

Gallese V, Fadiga L, Fogassi L, Luppino G, Murata A 1997 A parietal-frontal circuit for hand grasping movements in the monkey: evidence from reversible inactivation experiments. In: Thier P, Karnath HO (eds) Parietal lobe contributions to orientation in 3D space. Springer-Verlag, Heidelberg, p 255–269

Heywood CA, Gaffan D, Cowey A 1995 Cerebral achromatopsia in monkeys. Eur J Neurosci 7:1064–1073

Hikosaka O 1993 Role of the basal ganglia in motor learning: a hypothesis. In: Ono T, Squire LR, Raichle ME, Perrett DI, Fukuda M (eds) Brain mechanisms of perception and memory: from neuron to behavior. Oxford University Press, Oxford, p 497–513

Hikosaka O, Miyachi S, Miyashita K, Rand MK 1996 Learning of sequential procedures in monkeys. In: Bloedel JR, Ebner TJ, Wise SP (eds) The acquisition of motor behavior in vertebrates. MIT Press, Cambridge, MA, p 303–318

Houk JC, Wise SP 1995 Distributed modular architectures linking basal ganglia, cerebellum and cerebral cortex: their role in planning and controlling action. Cereb Cortex 5:95–110

Ilinsky IA, Kultas-Ilinsky K 1987 Sagittal cytoarchitectonic maps of the *Macaca mulatta* thalamus with a revised nomenclature of the motor-related nuclei validated by observations of their connectivity. J Comp Neurol 262:331–364

Johnson PB, Ferraina S, Bianchi L, Caminiti R 1996 Cortical networks for visual reaching: physiological and anatomical organization of frontal and parietal lobe arm regions. Cereb Cortex 6:102–119

Jueptner M, Stephan KM, Frith CD, Brooks DJ, Frackowiak RSJ, Passingham RE 1997 Anatomy of motor learning. I. Frontal cortex and attention to action. J Neurophysiol 77:1313–1324

Kurata K, Hoffman DS 1994 Differential effects of muscimol microinjection into dorsal and ventral aspects of the premotor cortex of monkeys. J Neurophysiol 64:1151–1164

Matelli M, Luppino G 1996 Thalamic input to mesial and superior area 6 in the macaque monkey. J Comp Neurol 372:59–87

Matelli M, Camarda M, Glickstein M, Rizzolatti G 1986 Afferent and efferent projections of the inferior area 6 in the macaque monkey. J Comp Neurol 251:281–298

Murata A, Fadiga L, Fogassi L, Gallese V, Raos V, Rizzolatti G 1997 Object representation in the ventral premotor cortex (area F5) of the monkey. J Neurophysiol 78:2226–2230

Murray EA, Wise SP 1997 Role of orbitoventral prefrontal cortex in conditional motor learning. Soc Neurosci Abstr 23:12.1

Passingham RE 1987 From where does motor cortex get its instructions? In: Wise S (ed) Neural and behavioral approaches to higher brain function. Wiley, New York, p 67–97

Passingham RE 1993 The frontal lobes and voluntary action. Oxford University Press, Oxford

Passingham RE, Nixon PD 1996 Lesions of the cerebellar nuclei do not impair the acquisition of a visual-motor conditional learning task. Soc Neurosci Abstr 22:116.1

Petrides M, Pandya DN 1995 Comparative architectonic analysis of the human and macaque frontal cortex. In: Grafman J, Boller F (eds) Handbook of neuropsychology. Elsevier Science BV, Amsterdam

Rushworth M, Nixon PD, Eacott MJ, Passingham RE 1997a Ventral prefrontal cortex is not essential for working memory. J Neurosci 117:4829–4838

Rushworth M, Nixon PD, Passingham RE 1997b Parietal cortex and movement. I. Movement selection and reaching. Exp Brain Res 117:292–310

Saint-Cyr J, Ungerleider LG, Desimone R 1990 Organization of visual cortical inputs to the striatum and subsequent outputs to the pallido-nigral complex in the monkey. J Comp Neurol 298:129–156

Sakata A, Gallese V, Kaseda M, Sakata H 1996 Parietal neurons related to memory-guided hand manipulation. J Neurophysiol 75:2180–2186

Schluter ND, Josephs O, Toni I, Friston K, Passingham RE 1997 Testing the association of haemodynamic responses with different task events using fMRI. Neuroimage 5:S359

Schluter ND, Rushworth MFS, Passingham RE, Mills KR 1998 Temporary inactivation of human lateral premotor cortex suggests dominance for the selection of movements: a study using transcranial magnetic stimulation. Brain 121:785–799

Schultz W, Apicella P, Ljungberg T 1993 Responses of monkey dopamine neurons to reward and conditioned stimuli during successive steps of learning a delayed response task. J Neurosci 13:900–913

Selemon LD, Goldman-Rakic PS 1985 Longitudinal topography and interdigitation of corticostriatal projections in the rhesus monkey. J Neurosci 5:776–794

Sidibe M, Bevan MD, Bolam JP, Smith Y 1997 Efferent connections of the internal globus pallidus in the squirrel monkey: I. Topography and synaptic organization of the pallidothalamic projection. J Comp Neurol 382:323–347

Strick PL 1985 How do the basal ganglia and cerebellum gain access to the cortical motor areas? Behav Brain Res 18:107–124

Strick PL, Dum RP, Picard N 1995 Macro-organization of the circuits connecting the basal ganglia with the cortical motor areas. In: Houk JC, Davis JL, Beiser DG (eds) Models of information processing in the basal ganglia. MIT Press, Cambridge, MA, p 117–130

Tanné J, Boussaoud D, Boyer-Zeller N, Roullier E 1995 Parietal inputs to physiologically defined regions of dorsal premotor cortex in macaque monkey. Neuroreport 7:267–272

Toni I, Passingham RE 1998 Learning movements according to visual instructions. Soc Neurosci Abstr 24:254.14

Toni I, Rushworth MFS, Ramnani, Passingham RE 1998a Visually instructed and visually guided movements. Neuroimage 7:5980 (abstr)

Toni I, Schluter ND, Josephs O, Friston K, Passingham RE 1998b Signal, set and movement-related activity in the human brain: an event-related fMRI study. Submitted

Tremblay L, Hollerman J, Schultz W 1994 Neuronal activity in primate striatum neurons during learning. Soc Neurosci Abstr 20:780

Webster MJ, Bachevalier J, Ungerleider LG 1994 Connections of inferior temporal areas TEO and TE with parietal and frontal cortex in macaque monkeys. Cereb Cortex 4:471–483

Weinrich M, Wise SP, Mauritz SP 1984 A neurophysiological study of the premotor cortex in the rhesus monkey. Brain 107:385–414

Wise SP 1996 Evolution of neuronal activity during conditional motor learning. In: Bloedel JR, Ebner TJ, Wise SP (eds) The acquisition of motor behavior in vertebrates. MIT Press, Cambridge, MA, p 261–286

Wise SP, di Pellegrino D, Boussaoud D 1996 The premotor cortex and nonstandard sensorimotor mapping. Can J Physiol Pharmacol 74:469–482

DISCUSSION

Strick: We injected area TE with a retrograde strain of our herpes virus to look at one aspect of this issue of integration. We reported that the pars reticulata of the nigra projects to a thalamic nucleus which in turn projects to TE (Middleton & Strick 1996). This was the same part of the pars reticulata that ultimately receives input from the caudate and ventral putamen regions that are the target of TE projections. Your animals obviously do the task, but I don't think that it is based on any kind of TE/TEO inferotemporal input into a region of the striatum that ultimately gets into the motor system.

Passingham: I still wonder whether that might not be a possible route. We find learning-related increases in the globus pallidus, and if we make a ventral thalamic lesion the animals are unable to relearn the task. We have not checked with pallidal lesions, but will do so. Of course, it could be that even if a pallidal lesion were to impair performance on the task, the integration between sensory input and motor output happens elsewhere than in the basal ganglia — for instance in the prefrontal cortex. All such a result would show is that the basal ganglia are necessary for learning the task.

If the integration does not occur in the basal ganglia, one other possibility is that the ventral visual system has access to the dorsal visual system in parietal cortex and that the sensory–motor integration depends on the projections from parietal to premotor cortex. Baizer et al (1991) showed that there are connections from inferotemporal area TEO to parietal areas VIP and LIP. But we have not found that monkeys with lesions in parietal areas 5 or 7b or in area 7a are impaired on retention of a visuomotor associative task (Rushworth et al 1997).

Strick: Neurosurgeons are currently making pallidal lesions in human subjects to ameliorate some of the symptoms of Parkinson's disease. I wonder whether such lesions influence the patients ability to perform conditional motor tasks?

Passingham: Two groups are already looking at that. The problem is that the patients have very severe Parkinson's disease, and we have already shown that patients with Parkinson's disease can be impaired on a visuomotor associative task (Canavan et al 1989). Thus they will be impaired before the pallidal surgery, and it may be difficult to detect an increase in the impairment.

Stein: Can I offer another suggestion about the integration in the globus pallidus? I am going to be controversial, to try to expose the question of whether or not these circuits going through the basal ganglia are truly separate. There are radial dendrites in the internal globus pallidus that actually cross over many of these circuits. It is possible that this is where the integration is occurring.

Passingham: Those who argue that there is no sensory–motor integration in the basal ganglia argue that the integration that occurs from striatum to pallidum occurs within cortico–basal ganglia loops and not between them. There has been no demonstration that integration occurs between these loops.

Stein: But the dendrites extend many millimetres, across more than one circuit.

Passingham: The dendrites can collect from a wide distance, but this does not prove that they are collecting between loops. The question remains open.

Marsden: Can we go to the fine detail of that second point? According to Percheron's view, with the size of the dendritic tree in the internal globus pallidus, it must span different circuits.

Strick: No.

Marsden: Percheron disagrees?

Strick: I guess when we get in the same room together he doesn't. The bottom line is that we have done experiments in which we have put virus into different cortical areas and examined whether the neurons and the processes that we can see are segregated. We have looked at primary motor cortex, SMA, ventral premotor area, area 46, area 12 and medial and lateral area 9. What is clear from these experiments is that the centres of pallidal projections to each of these cortical areas are quite separate. However, the real way to address this issue is with double-labelling procedures with two viruses that travel transneuronally in the retrograde direction. We are currently developing this technique for future experiments.

Passingham: The problem with the experiments using viruses is that you may see the peak labelling, and it may not be easy to judge the degree of overlap.

Strick: We do see dendritic fields. Essentially, the virus transport labels some of these cells as if they were stained by the Golgi technique. In general, the dendritic fields of the labelled neurons fall within the same territory as labelled cell bodies.

Goodale: I want to return to this visual association versus visual grasp as a behavioural concept. When you reach for objects, for example a hammer, it's true that you institute a reach and grasp, but you also presumably bring in some visual associations. You have associated the hammer in the past with particular kinds of tasks. So there's got to be some integration between the metrical properties of reaching and grasping and the functional properties presumably called up by visual association. Is the prediction, therefore, that if you were to make homologous lesions in humans of these areas that produce deficits in monkeys, you would lose the functional aspects of grasp and preserve the metrical scaling?

Passingham: Clinicians have claimed that it is parietal lesions that produce an inability to perform movements to command or to copy movements. The problem that we have been studying is how you get from the word 'pull' to the appropriate movement, and at the moment our research does not point to a route via parietal cortex. I have two comments on apraxia. First, many patients have kinematic impairments, and we have shown that removal of parietal areas 5 and 7b causes kinematic impairments (Rushworth et al 1998). Second, it is possible that the ability to copy movements depends on the operation of 'mirror' neurons, and there may be mirror neurons in parietal cortex.

Marsden: You have got two problems as I see it. First, how do you learn your visual association task, which does appear to involve globus pallidus (lentiform nucleus)? Second, having learnt it, how do you execute it?

Passingham: It is, of course, possible that once you have learned a visuomotor associative task, it comes to depend on visual inputs to the parietal cortex. It is just that, at the moment, this is not what our lesion experiments show. The monkeys in the experiment by Rushworth et al (1997) were tested on retention of such a task, and the parietal lesions still had no effect.

Rizzolatti: To clarify better the anatomical issue, which is the motor region crucial for associative motor learning? My impression is that in your monkey experiments the lesion producing associative learning deficits was rostral. The area you showed today in humans is, on the contrary, rather caudal.

Passingham: In our monkey experiments we removed PMd and F7. The area that is activated during performance of the visuomotor task but not during performance of reaching and grasping lies at the back of the superior frontal sulcus, but we think within area 6.

Rizzolatti: Does it correspond to monkey area F7?

Passingham: I think that we should be very careful about identifying areas such as F7 in the human brain until Karl Zilles has mapped the whole of the premotor cortex in the human brain.

Rizzolatti: If I remember correctly, in some monkeys operated by Michael Petrides (1985), the lesion was essentially in F7.

Passingham: Mike Petrides' lesions look as if they extend back into part of PMd (Petrides 1987).

Lemon: This random time interval between the instruction and the performance is a good design feature. But what do human subjects do when they have to wait 12 seconds between receiving information and acting upon it? There must be other things going on.

Passingham: I agree. But one thing that we know is going on is preparation for the response, and we can detect preparatory activity in the evoked heamodynamic responses in dorsal premotor cortex.

Lemon: The point I was making is that there are lots of other things going on that have nothing to do at all with the task that you're doing. Could the blood flow changes be related to other brain events ('wandering mind') during the long delay period?

Passingham: Our subjects were trained to concentrate on the task. If they were thinking in the way you suggest, one might have expected activation in the dorsal prefrontal cortex.

Thach: I appreciate that lesions of the dentate nucleus don't interfere with 'set'.

Passingham: Nor were there learning-related increases in the cerebellum during our PET study in which subjects learned a visuomotor associative task.

Thach: That is what I was going to ask. In the cerebellum, have you looked at motor learning tasks or learning tasks?

Passingham: What we have done is to compare four scans of visuomotor associative learning with four scans in which the subjects learned a motor sequence. There was a learning-related increase in activation in the cerebellum for the sequence but not for visuomotor associative learning. The reason, we think, is that as you learn the sequence task you come to prepare the next response, whereas on the visuomotor association task you do not know what response to make until the visual stimulus is presented. On the sequence task, but not the visuomotor associative task, one can coordinate a series of movements.

Thach: But your results might question the generality some of the eye-blink conditioning.

Passingham: Yes.

Lemon: This relates to the point Helen Savaki made yesterday, about how much you infer from the lesion situation. The problem that you have is marrying up the lesion data in monkeys with fMRI data in humans. Take the situation with your monkey lesions where you're making strategic lesions in the posterior parietal lobe and the monkeys are still not impaired on the association task. Can it not be that in those situations that you can revert, for instance to the learning circuit, to start using this as the execution circuit?

Passingham: I agree that this is possible.

Marsden: You say that patients with Parkinson's disease are impaired on your visual association task, from which it is deduced that the basal ganglia must be involved. However, have you done the same experiment in drug-induced Parkinsonism? The crucial control for all Parkinson's disease work is to compare the results in patients with drug-induced Parkinson's in whom there is pharmacologically induced basal ganglia dysfunction. For example, some patients with Parkinson's disease exhibit ideomotor apraxia, but those with drug-induced Parkinsonism do not. Such apraxia is unlikely to be due to basal ganglia dysfunction; more likely it is due to cortical changes in Parkinson's disease. Your visual association task is showing a figure and asking the human subject to adopt a hand posture in response to a visually perceived figure. Is that any different from a bedside clinical test in which the patient is asked to copy the examiner's hand posture?

Passingham: I think it is, because copying may depend on the operation of mirror neurons.

Marsden: The reason I raised this is because with people with Parkinson's disease have no problems in copying hand postures.

Strick: But do they have problems saluting to command or waving goodbye?

Marsden: Some patients with Parkinson's disease do fail on gesture production of the nature you mentioned. None with drug-induced Parkinson's fail on gesture reproduction. In this small proportion of people with Parkinson's disease who do fail on gesture production, it's not the basal ganglia but something else that is responsible.

Passingham: The problem with Parkinson's disease is a loss of cells in the substantia nigra. The critical test is still going to be a global pallidus lesion.

Lemon: Are we forcing ourselves into a corner, because conceptually we want to have a dorsal and a ventral stream? Mel Goodale, in your paper showing that the visual lesion doesn't transfer to the motor performance, wouldn't you accept that there is some transfer, i.e. that the separation is not absolute?

Goodale: Yes. Pictorial illusions can sometimes have an effect on grip aperture. But compared with the effect they have on perceptual judgements, that effect is extremely small. In fact, in a recent extension of the original study by Aglioti et al (1995), we did not find any effect of the Ebbinghaus Illusion on grasp aperture (Haffenden & Goodale 1998). Thus, although the effect of illusion on grasp is sometimes there, it is not particularly reliable.

Passingham: We have deliberately tried to make the problem as hard as possible. We have taught monkeys with plain colours as cues. Colours are not known to drive parietal cells.

References

Aglioti S, DeSouza J, Goodale MA 1995 Size-contrast illusions deceive the eyes but not the hand. Curr Biol 5:679–685

Baizer JS, Ungerleider LG, Desimone R 1991 Organization of visual inputs to the inferior temporal and posterior parietal cortex in macaques. J Neurosci 11:168–190

Canavan AGM, Passingham RE, Marsden CD, Quinn N, Wyke M, Polkey CE 1989 The performance on learning tasks of patients in the early stages of Parkinson's disease. Neuropsychologia 27:141–156

Haffenden A, Goodale MA 1998 The effect of pictorial illusion on prehension and perception. J Cognit Neurosci 10:122–136

Middleton FA, Strick PL 1996 The temporal lobe is a target of output from the basal ganglia. Proc Natl Acad Sci USA 93:8683–8687

Petrides M 1985 Deficits in non-spatial conditional associative learning after periarcuate lesions in the monkey. Behav Brain Res 16:95–101

Petrides M 1987 Conditional learning and primate frontal cortex. In: Perecman E (ed) The frontal lobes revisited. IRBN Press, New York, p 91–108

Rushworth MFS, Nixon PD, Passingham RE 1997 Parietal cortex and movement. I. Movement selection and reaching. Exp Brain Res 117:292–310

Rushworth MFS, Johansen-Berg H, Young SA 1998 Parietal cortex and spatial-postural transformation during arm movements. J Neurophysiol 79:478–482

Online visual control of the arm

Apostolos P. Georgopoulos

Brain Sciences Center (11B), Veterans Affairs Medical Center, Minneapolis, MN 55417, and Departments of Physiology, Neurology and Psychiatry, University of Minnesota Medical School, Minneapolis, MN 55455, USA

Abstract. The psychophysical and cerebrocortical mechanisms in visually guided reaching movements and isometric force pulses are discussed. The results of psychophysical studies of pointing movements have demonstrated a tight coupling between the visual information and the direction of the movement, and those of studies of directed isometric force pulses have documented the sensitive dependence of the motor system on the continuous availability of visual information for the ongoing correction of directional deviations from the instructed direction. Recordings of the activity of single cells in the motor cortex and parietal areas 2 and 5 have revealed the same tight, online coupling between visual information and cell discharge, and have partially elucidated the neural mechanisms underlying this function at the cortical level.

1998 Sensory guidance of movement. Wiley, Chichester (Novartis Foundation Symposium 218) p 147–170

Vision plays a major role in the motor repertoire of primates. Commonly, purposeful arm and hand movements are directed towards, and adapted for the use of, objects of interest within the visual field. The visual aspects of this problem are dealt with in other chapters of this symposium (e.g. this volume: Goodale 1998, Jeannerod et al 1998). In this chapter I review the results of psychophysical and neural studies pertaining to arm movements and isometric forces that are instructed, controlled and/or guided by visual information. Altogether, these results show that the arm motor output is tightly coupled to, and sensitive to changes of, ongoing visual information. This results in an efficient and effective visuomotor control function which apparently involves the cooperation of several brain areas and which is reflected in the neural activity of motor cortical and parietal cells.

Visual control of arm movements

Discrete movements to stationary visual targets

Reaching movements to stationary visual targets have been studied extensively (for a review see Georgopoulos 1986). Typically, such movements are learned

147

during infancy, and their trajectories are fairly stereotyped and show invariant properties (Soechting & Lacquaniti 1981). With respect to the neural mechanisms involved, many studies have been performed by recording the impulse activity of single cells in several brain areas of behaving monkeys trained to reach towards visual targets (for a review see Georgopoulos 1990a).

Basically, two kinds of analyses have been carried out. In one, the average firing rate during reaching has been analysed with respect to motor variables; this provides a robust estimate of the intensity of activation and of its relation to movement but destroys the fine time-course of cell activity. Those studies have revealed that the activity of single cells in several brain areas, including cerebrocortical and cerebellar areas (see Georgopoulos 1990a), varies in an orderly fashion with the direction of reaching so that cells are directionally tuned: cell discharge is highest for reaching in a particular direction (the cell's 'preferred direction') and decreases progressively with reaching in directions farther and farther away from the preferred one. The directional tuning is generally broad and can be expressed as a cosine function (Georgopoulos et al 1982, Schwartz et al 1988). Preferred directions differ for different cells and are distributed throughout the directional continuum in 3D space (Schwartz et al 1988). A neuronal population vector code provides accurate information concerning the direction of movement under various experimental conditions (see Georgopoulos et al 1993 for a review).

Finally, cell discharge also varies with the amplitude of the movement but the preferred direction remains the same for movements of different amplitudes (Fu et al 1993). Directional tuning is observed during both the reaction and movement time whereas the variation with movement amplitude is observed during the movement time (Fu et al 1995).

In a different study (Ashe & Georgopoulos 1994) the fine time-course of single-cell activity (e.g. every 20 ms) was analysed with respect to the direction of the visual target as well as with respect to time-varying motor parameters, including position, velocity and acceleration. It was found that cell activity was related to all of these parameters, but that target direction and movement velocity were the most important determinants of the time-varying cell activity. The importance of the ongoing movement velocity signal was also indicated by neural studies of tracing movements (Schwartz 1993) and of simultaneous recordings from several cells (Humphrey et al 1970). It is reasonable to suppose that these effects reflect motor control signals as well as the effects of peripheral inputs. A contribution of feedback is supported by the known inputs to the motor cortex from the somatic periphery. A feedforward signal could relate to the length-tension state of the muscles (Fromm 1983), in which case this signal could be tailored to the current states of the muscles to be controlled. This combination of afferent and efferent signals could be quite complex, given the appreciable divergence of corticospinal axons at the spinal level, the wide distribution of motor cortical output signals to various cortical and subcortical structures, and the convergence of peripheral inputs to cortical areas (e.g. areas 2 and 5) which provide major inputs to the motor cortex. If one adds the known inputs from subcortical structures (basal ganglia, cerebellum) and considers the large divergence (Shinoda & Kakei 1989) and convergence (Darian-Smith et al 1990) of the thalamic projections to the motor cortex, then a picture emerges in which the motor cortex occupies a nodal point at the cross-section of many interacting sensorimotor circuits.

Reaching in a target shift task

Many times the object of interest towards which the hand is directed changes location, and therefore it is interesting to know whether the motor system can follow the target and change the movement in mid-flight. We studied this problem in monkeys (Georgopoulos et al 1981) and human subjects (Massey et al 1986) who moved an articulated manipulandum on a planar working surface. Two peripheral lights in opposite locations were used (e.g. at 12 and 6 o'clock). The subject held the handle in the centre for a variable period of time after which one of the two peripheral targets was turned on; it remained on for 50, 100, 150, 200, 250, 300 or 400 ms and then was turned off and the other target was turned on. The animal was rewarded after holding at the second light for 0.5 s. Trials in which the first light stayed on without changing location were interspersed among those in which the target location changed so that the subject could not predict whether the target would change location in a certain trial; moreover, the subject could not predict for how long the first target would stay on in the trials in which it changed location. The effect of the change in target location on the movement trajectory is shown in Fig. 1A. The first target was at 12 o'clock and the second target at 6 o'clock. Single trajectories of arm movements are shown in the lower trace. It can be seen that the arm moved initially towards the first target, then changed direction and moved towards the second target. Therefore, the arm movement could change online depending on the target instructed.

There are several aspects of these experiments that are noteworthy. First of all, how consistently is a movement made towards the first target? This question was examined by varying systematically the duration of the first target and observing the arm movement towards it. It was found that the occurrence of a movement towards the first target depends on how long the first light stays on. This is illustrated in Fig. 1B which plots the probability of occurrence of a movement towards the first target versus the duration of presentation of the first target. It can be seen that this probability increases steeply and becomes one when the first light stays on for at least 100 ms.

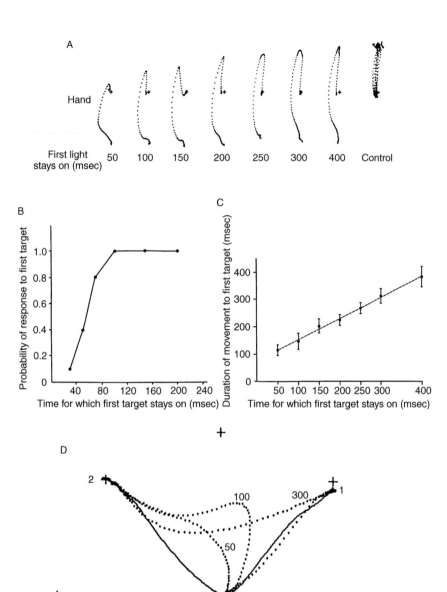

The second question concerns the temporal relations between the direction of the target and the duration of the movement. Figure 1C illustrates the finding that the duration of the arm movement towards the first target is a linear function of the time for which the first target stayed on.

The third question concerns the spatial characteristics of the trajectory of the first movement. In most cases tested, the two target lights were located along the same line, so that the first and second movements were in opposite directions. However, when the two target lights were arranged in such a way that the corresponding movements were not in opposite directions, a modification of the direction of the trajectory of the first movement was observed in some trials. An example is shown in Fig. 1D. The first light (#1) was at approximately 2 o'clock, and the second light (#2) was at 90° angle from it. The two continuous lines in Fig. 1D show examples of trajectories made directly to each of the lights in control trials. The dotted lines plot trajectories obtained at the interstimulus interval indicated in the plot (50, 100 and 300 ms). It can be seen that the trajectory deviated towards the direction of the second target, the more so the shorter the interstimulus interval was. These results indicate that the motor command for the direction of movement generated after the appearance of the first target can be modified by the second target when the targets shift early in time.

The fourth question concerns the velocity characteristics of the trajectories of the movements towards the second target, after their reversal. It can be seen in Fig. 1A that these movements were faster than those made towards the first target. In fact, the peak velocity of the movements towards the second target was approximately three times that of the movement towards the first target. This was true even for the interstimulus interval of 50 ms, in which case the movement towards the first light was small and, therefore, the amplitude of the second movement was very similar to that of the movement made directly to the second target in control trials. These results can be explained by the strategy that monkeys and human subjects used to solve the problems posed by this target-shift task. This

FIG. 1. (A) Modification of hand movement trajectories in the target shift task. The first target light was at 12 o'clock; it stayed on for the time indicated and then changed location to 6 o'clock. Single trajectories are shown (X–Y data points were recorded every 10 ms). At the far right (control), seven trajectories to the target at 12 o'clock are superimposed. (B) Probability of response to first of two targets presented in quick succession. (C) Duration of movement towards the first of two targets (ordinate) presented in succession at specified interstimulus intervals (abscissa). Data from one monkey. (D) Modification of the direction of movement elicited by the first target (#1) when the second target (#2) was at an angle of 90°. Solid lines indicate control trajectories of movements made directly to targets A and B. Dotted lines are trajectories of movements made at the stated interstimulus interval (X–Y data points were sampled every 10 ms). (Adapted from Georgopoulos et al 1981 and Georgopoulos 1990b.)

strategy was revealed by an analysis of the forces exerted on the manipulandum during performance of the task (Massey et al 1986).

The problem is that if the trajectory is to be interrupted at different points along its extent, the dynamics of the hand and the manipulandum will differ in these points reflecting different velocities and accelerations; therefore, the braking forces will have to be precalculated in accordance with the anticipated kinematic and dynamic conditions. However, the subjects ignored the differences between the mechanical conditions associated with different interruption points and, instead, produced a large braking force in the opposite direction in response to the second target that stopped the limb and moved it to the second target. These braking forces were excessive for the short movements towards the first target but were effective for all cases and did not require individual adjustments for particular trials. Therefore, the computational load was reduced at the expense of increased spending of mechanical energy; in other words, a simple and mechanically effective but energy-inefficient strategy underlay the efficient eye–hand coordination in this task.

A correlate of this increased efficiency in information processing might lie in the observation by Soechting & Lacquaniti (1983) that under similar conditions of rapid response to a target change there is a reduction in the degrees of freedom of the movement; this is achieved by imposing constraints on the kinematic variables (angular deceleration at the shoulder and elbow joints), and by generating more stereotyped patterns of activity in the muscles acting on these two joints.

Neural mechanisms of visuomotor coupling

When the location of visual stimuli is changed in quick succession, the patterns of cell activity in motor (Georgopoulos et al 1983) and parietal (Kalaska et al 1981) cortex follow these changes with remarkable temporal fidelity and attest to the efficient engagement of those areas during eye–hand coordination. An example is shown in Fig. 2A. The location of the first and second target, and the required movement direction, are shown in the top of the figure. The pattern of cell activity associated with movements directly to these targets consisted of an increase in cell activity when moving to target A and of a decrease in activity when moving to target B. When the first target was target A, the pattern of cell activity was that associated with movement to that target; this pattern lasted for a time proportional to the time for which the first target stayed on, and then became like the pattern of activity associated with movement to target B. These results indicate that when a sequence of hand movements is generated towards targets that change location, the motor cortical activity follows the changes in visual information well and generates the appropriate motor commands without temporal smearing. This apparently underlies, at least in part, the efficient eye–hand coordination observed at the behavioural level.

Visual control of isometric force pulses: an information-theoretical analysis

In these experiments we investigated the effects of an external constant force bias and of various manipulations of the visual information on the information transmitted (T_i) by the direction of isometric force exerted in a two-dimensional space by human subjects. For that purpose we used an isometric manipulandum and random dot stereograms generated in a colour display (Massey et al 1991a,b). Human subjects viewed the display through appropriate colour filters and perceived the image of a disk rotated about a horizontal axis on the frontal plane; the top of the disk was rotated around that axis by 45° away from the subject. Subjects were instructed to exert force pulses of >200 g force intensity in the direction of a visual target ($n = 20$ targets) presented on the disk in a reaction time task. The instantaneous force exerted by the subjects on the manipulandum was shown on the disk in the form of a feedback cursor. The T_i was calculated as described previously (Georgopoulos & Massey 1988). The time course of force development and the gain of directional information transmitted (i.e. the rate of increase of T_i) during force development were studied under three experimental conditions; namely, (a) in the absence and presence of a constant force bias, (b) when the force feedback cursor was frozen or (c) turned off when the force developed exceeded 100 g force. Each one of these experimental manipulations probed different aspects of the specification and generation of net force in a visually specified direction.

Online gain of directional information

In order to determine the gain of directional information during force development, we calculated the T_i at various levels of force intensity, ranging from ~ 50 g force to >200 g force. There was a gain of information (i.e. the T_i increased) with force intensity for all experimental conditions studied (i.e. stereoscopic depth, absence of visual force feedback and presence of force bias). This suggests that the specification of the direction of force improves as the force intensity increases, which could be due to a continuous comparison and correction of the force produced so that it is in the visually defined direction, as was suggested by the results of other studies (Cordo 1987, Gordon & Ghez 1987).

Quantitatively, the curves of T_i vs. force intensity, F, were negatively accelerating. The relation between T_i and F was a power function of the form:

$$T_i = kF^m \tag{1}$$

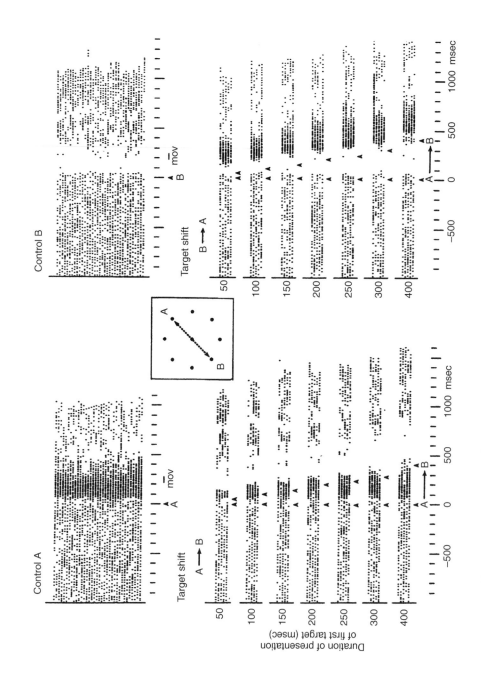

where k and m are constants. Equation (1) is linear in a log–log scale:

$$\ln T_i = A + m\ln F \qquad (2)$$

where $A = \ln k$ ('ln' refers to the natural logarithms, that is to base e).

Effects of force bias

Subjects exerted force pulses so that the force feedback cursor moved in the display past the target cursor. In the absence of force bias, the force exerted by the subject (Fig. 3A) increased from near zero to >200 g force at the end of a trial and was close to the visually defined direction. When a constant bias force of 110 g force was applied in various directions in blocks of trials, the force exerted by the subject increased in time, as above; however, its direction also changed in time (Fig. 3B) so that the instantaneous vector sum of the bias force and the force exerted by the subject pointed close to the visually defined direction. The T_i calculated at 200 g force and the reaction time did not differ significantly in the two experimental conditions (Massey et al 1991b). Figure 3C is a log–log plot of the T_i against force in the absence (open circles, interrupted line) and presence (filled circles, solid line) of force bias. (The lines are fitted regression lines.) It can be seen that the lines are very similar; the slopes did not differ statistically at the 5% level of significance. (The values of the constants k and m are given in Table 2 in Massey et al 1991b.) Altogether, these results demonstrated that presence of a constant force bias did not degrade performance: subjects were able to specify accurately (i.e. at a high T_i) the net force output of the manipulandum to be in the visually defined direction by changing continuously the direction and magnitude of the

---

FIG. 2.   Changes in discharge of a motor cortical cell in the target shift task. Beneath each control raster are seven rasters of trials during which the target changed location after 50–400 ms, as indicated; the first target to appear in each trial was the same as that for the control trials plotted above it. The initial change of activity seen in the target shift trials was of the same sign as that during the corresponding control trials, i.e. an increase in cell activity on the left and a decrease on the right. The initial pattern of activity did not continue as long as in control trials, however, for a short while after the target changed it was replaced by a pattern of activity similar to that recorded during movement to the other target. Thus, the initial increase in activity during movements to target A was truncated by a complete suppression of activity similar to that seen in control trials during movements to target B, while the decrease in activity on the right side was terminated by a brisk increase in activity like that seen for movements to target A. This was true for all interstimulus intervals tested. The time at which the switch in the pattern of activity occurred was related to the time of the target shift (second arrows). The horizontal bar labelled MOV indicates the range of the times of movement onset. The first and second arrows indicate the time of presentation of the first target and of the target shift, respectively. (From Georgopoulos et al 1983; reproduced with permission.)

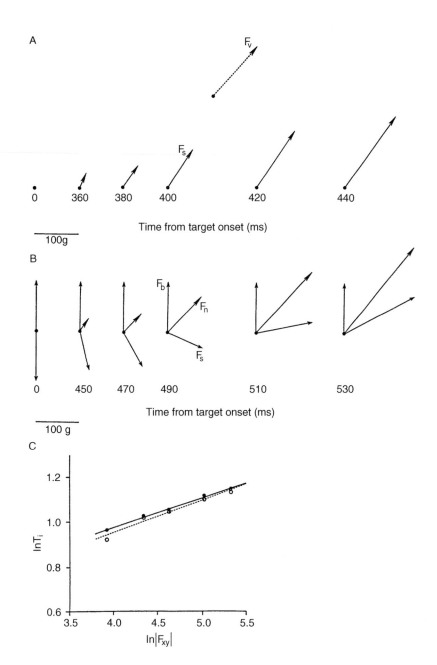

active force they exerted at no extra time (i.e. without a longer reaction time). Thus external loads are processed very efficiently even under dynamic conditions.

Effects of manipulations of visual information

Figure 4 A–D illustrates individual trials of force development and angular deviations of the force from the stimulus direction in the presence (Fig. 4A) and absence (Fig. 4 B–D) of force-feedback cursor. It can appreciated qualitatively from the plots in Fig. 4 A–D and quantitatively from the plots in Fig. 4E that manipulation of the visual force-feedback had a significant effect on the gain of information. The plots of the gain of information for the three conditions used (force feedback cursor intact, frozen or absent) are shown in Fig. 4E. It can be seen that the absence of the force feedback cursor resulted in lowering of the line (Fig. 4E, line labelled A), whereas freezing the cursor at the centre of the disk resulted in an intermediate positioning of the line (line labelled F), between those obtained in the presence (line P) and absence (line A) of the force feedback cursor. The gradients m did not differ statistically at the 5% level of significance.

Discussion

In the present experiments, subjects exerted forces on an immobile manipulandum so that a cursor reflecting the net X–Y forces exerted on the manipulandum moved in a direction defined by a target in the display. Enough force had to be exerted to exceed a 200 g force threshold but an upper limit was not defined. Indeed, subjects performed accordingly and generated force pulses; the intensity of force kept increasing even after the 200 g force threshold was exceeded. Therefore, the data can be regarded as reflecting specification and/or control of force direction but not its termination.

Inspection of individual trials indicated that the direction of force was not specified accurately from the beginning of force change; instead, there was a period of gain of directional information as the force intensity increased (Fig. 4).

FIG. 3. (A) Force vectors (F_s) generated in the absence of force bias. Data are from a single trial. The visually defined direction (F_p) is indicated at the top of the figure. Numbers indicate the time (in ms) from the target onset. (B) Force vectors generated in the presence of force bias (F_b) for the same visually defined direction (F_p) as in A. The force bias vector was towards 12 o'clock. The subject's force vector (F_s) was initially equal and opposite (towards 6 o'clock) to the force bias vector. With the development of more force, the force exerted by the subject changes in direction and magnitude so that the net force (F_n), that is the resultant of F_b and F_s, is in the visually defined direction (F_p). Numbers indicate the time (in ms) from the target onset. (C) T_i is plotted against force intensity in a log–log scale. Open and filled circles correspond to absence and presence of force bias (at 90°), respectively. Interrupted and solid lines are fitted regression lines for absence and presence of force bias data, respectively. (Adapted from Massey et al 1991b.)

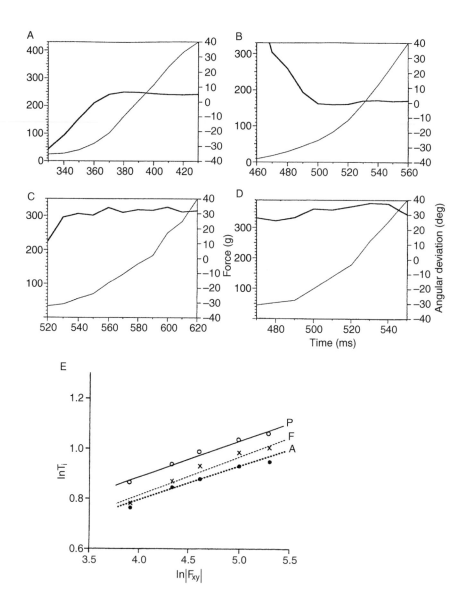

The gain of directional information during increasing force intensity was observed under all experimental conditions. This suggests that there may be a process by which the direction of force is continuously corrected with respect to the visually specified direction. A continuous effect of visual information on the direction of an upcoming movement was shown previously (Georgopoulos et al 1981, van Sonderen et al 1988). It is remarkable that the rate of gain of information was very similar for the different conditions but the whole curve was transposed to lower levels in the cases in which the visual definition of direction was degraded. These findings suggest that the process of gain of directional information is fundamentally the same for a variety of conditions but that it operates at various levels depending on the actual information available. This information was reduced when the force-feedback cursor was absent or fixed in the centre.

It is noteworthy that, in contrast to the effect of visual manipulations, the presence of a constant force bias had no adverse effect on information gain. This indicates that the motor system is very efficient in controlling the direction of force. It is possible that when a constant force bias is present, this is offset actively by an opposite force vector, and then the required force is exerted in the visually specified direction. The results of neurophysiological studies in the motor cortex of behaving monkeys (Georgopoulos et al 1992) supported this hypothesis as discussed below.

Neural mechanisms of visually instructed isometric force pulses

The exertion of an isometric force pulse involves the production of a rapid change in force in the absence of limb motion. When such a force pulse is instructed by a

FIG. 4. *A–D* are plots of force development (thin line, left Y-axis) and angular deviations of that force from the stimulus direction (thick line, right Y-axis) at the time from stimulus onset indicated in the abscissa. All four plots are from single trials. For the angular deviations, positive and negative values are counterclockwise (CCW) and clockwise (CW), respectively, from the stimulus direction (0 value). (A) A trial in which the force-feedback cursor was present throughout the trial. When a direction of force was attained close to the stimulus direction (approximately 5° CCW) at approximately 370 ms after stimulus onset, it was maintained for the rest of the trial. Stimulus direction was at 113°. Plots B–D are all from trials in which the force-feedback cursor was eliminated at the onset of the RT. In (B) the subject attained and maintained the correct direction of force. Stimulus direction was at 353°. In (C) the subject attained and maintained a force that was approximately 32° CCW from the stimulus direction. Stimulus direction was at 137°. Finally, in (D) the subject maintained from the beginning a force that was more than 30° CCW from the stimulus direction. Stimulus direction was at 99°. (E) log–log plots and regression lines of T_i vs. force intensity for three conditions in which the visual force-feedback was manipulated. Visual force-feedback cursor was present throughout the trial (P), was absent from the beginning of the reaction time (A), or was frozen at the centre of the disk from the beginning of the reaction time (F). Data points are means of 12 subjects. (Adapted from Massey et al 1991b.)

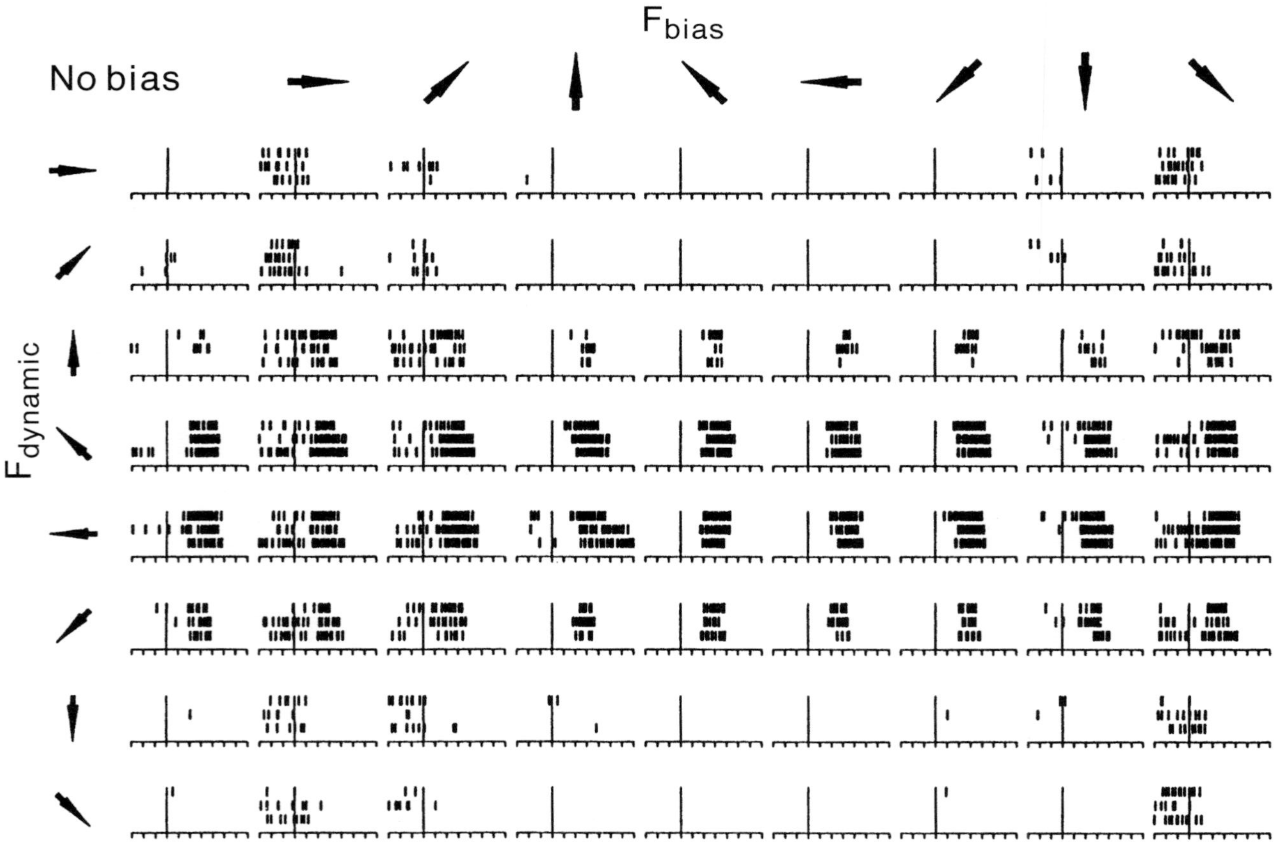
F_bias
No bias
F_dynamic

visual signal, it allows the study of the relations of neural activity to visuomotor parameters at the isometric force domain, as was done in recent studies (Georgopoulos et al 1992). The following experimental arrangement allowed the dissociation between dynamic and static components of the force exerted. Monkeys produced pure force pulses on an isometric handle in the presence of a constant force bias so that the net force (i.e. the vector sum of the monkey's force and the bias force) was in a visually specified direction. The net force developed over time had to stay in the specified direction and to increase in magnitude in order to exceed a required intensity threshold. Now consider the case in which the directions of the net and bias forces differ, by being, for example, orthogonal. In order for the task to be performed successfully under these conditions, the animal's force has to change continuously in direction and magnitude, so that, at any moment during force development, the vector sum of this force and the bias force is in the visually specified direction. Thus this experimental arrangement effectively dissociated the animal's force vector, the direction of which changed continuously in a trial, from the net force vector, the direction of which remained invariant. Eight net force directions and eight bias force directions were employed. Recordings of neuronal activity in the motor cortex revealed that the activity of single cells was directionally tuned in the absence of bias force, and that this tuning remained invariant when the same net forces were produced in the presence of different directions of bias force (Fig. 5). These results show that, during the generation of the force pulse, cell activity does not relate to the direction of the animal's force *per se* but to its dynamic component. In fact, in this experimental design, three vectors possess the same direction but different time-varying magnitudes, namely the dynamic component of the force, the first time-derivative of the force, and the visually instructed target direction. The magnitude of the first two vectors varies over time but in different ways, whereas the magnitude of the last one remains constant. The potentially different relations between these parameters and the time-varying cell activity was investigated recently using a pulse-and-step isometric force task (Ashe & Boline 1997). A time-course analysis (as described in Ashe & Georgopoulos 1994) revealed that the visual target direction and the first time-derivative of force had the most substantial effects on the time-varying cell activity (J. Boline & J. Ashe, personal communication 1998). This finding is formally similar to the result obtained for

---

FIG. 5.   Force directional tuning and its invariance across force biases are illustrated for the impulse activity (three repetitions) of one motor cortical cell. The directions of $F_{dynamic}$ and F_{bias} are shown in the rows and columns, respectively, including the case of no force bias (first column). Rasters are aligned to the onset of the peripheral stimulus (0 time); the time scale is 100 ms per division. (From Georgopoulos et al 1992; reproduced with permission. Copyright AAAS 1992.)

movement, in which the direction of the target and movement velocity (i.e. the first time derivative of position) had the strongest effects on cell activity (Ashe & Georgopoulos 1994). These findings underscore the importance of the visual information and the change in the motor output for the ongoing cell discharge.

Concluding remarks

The results of the studies reviewed above attest to the remarkably efficient and effective eye–hand coordination in primates. They also document the involvement of the motor cortex in this function, obviously as part of a dynamically interconnected, widespread brain network. Recent studies of the neural mechanisms underlying manual interception of moving targets (e.g. Port et al 1994, 1996, Lee et al 1997) have provided additional support for the involvement of the motor cortex in processing visual information for the initiation and online control of arm movements aimed at catching accurately moving visual targets. A major challenge for future research is the elucidation of the interplay of the various areas participating in online control of arm movements.

Acknowledgements

This work was supported by United States Public Health Service grants NS17413 and MH48185, the Department of Veterans Affairs and the American Legion Chair in Brain Sciences.

References

Ashe J, Boline J 1997 Neural activity in motor cortex and the direction and magnitude of isometric force. Soc Neurosci Abstr 23:1399
Ashe J, Georgopoulos AP 1994 Movement parameters and neuronal activity in motor cortex and area 5. Cereb Cortex 6:590–600
Cordo PJ 1987 Mechanisms controlling accurate changes in elbow torque in humans. J Neurosci 7:432–442
Darian-Smith C, Darian-Smith I, Cheema SS 1990 Thalamic projections to sensorimotor cortex in the macaque monkey: use of multiple retrograde fluorescent tracers. J Comp Neurol 299:17–46
Fromm C 1983 Changes of steady state activity in motor cortex consistent with the length-tension relation of muscle. Pflügers Archiv 398:318–323
Fu Q-G, Suarez JL, Ebner TJ 1993 Neuronal specification of direction and distance during reaching movements in the superior precentral premotor area and primary motor cortex of monkeys. J Neurophysiol 70:2097–2116
Fu Q-G, Flament D, Coltz JD, Ebner TJ 1995 Temporal coding of movement kinematics in the discharge of primary motor and premotor neurons. J Neurophysiol 73:836–854
Georgopoulos AP 1986 On reaching. Ann Rev Neurosci 9:147–170
Georgopoulos AP 1990a Neurophysiology of reaching. In: Jeannerod M (ed) Attention and performance, vol XIII. Lawrence Erlbaum, Hillsdale, NJ, p 227–263

Georgopoulos AP 1990b Eye–hand coordination and visual control of reaching: studies in behaving animals. In: Berkley MA, Stebbins WC (eds) Comparative perception, vol I: Basic mechanisms. Wiley, New York, p 375–403

Georgopoulos AP, Massey JT 1988 Cognitive spatial-motor processes. 2. Information transmitted by the direction of two-dimensional arm movements and by neuronal populations in primate motor cortex and area 5. Exp Brain Res 69:315–326

Georgopoulos AP, Kalaska JF, Massey JT 1981 Spatial trajectories and reaction times of aimed movements: effects of practice, uncertainty and change in target location. J Neurophysiol 46:725–743

Georgopoulos AP, Kalaska JF, Caminiti R, Massey JT 1982 On the relations between the direction of two-dimensional arm movements and cell discharge in primate motor cortex. J Neurosci 2:1527–1537

Georgopoulos AP, Kalaska JF, Caminiti R, Massey JT 1983 Interruption of motor cortical discharge subserving aimed arm movements. Exp Brain Res 49:327–340

Georgopoulos AP, Ashe J, Smyrnis N, Taira M 1992 Motor cortex and the coding of force. Science 256:1692–1695

Goodale MA 1998 Vision for perception and vision for action in the primate brain. In: Sensory guidance of movement. Wiley, Chichester (Novartis Found Symp 218) p 21–44

Gordon J, Ghez C 1987 Trajectory control in targeted force impulses. III. Compensatory adjustments for initial errors. Exp Brain Res 67:253–269

Humphrey DR, Schmidt EM, Thompson WD 1970 Predicting measures of motor performance from multiple cortical spike trains. Science 170:758–762

Jeannerod M, Paulignan Y, Weiss P 1998 Grasping an object: one movement, several components. In: Sensory guidance of movement. Wiley, Chichester (Novartis Found Symp 218) p 5–20

Kalaska JF, Caminiti R, Georgopoulos AP 1981 Cortical mechanisms of two-dimensional aimed arm movements. III. Relations of parietal (areas 5 and 2) neuronal activity to direction of movement and change in target location. Soc Neurosci Abstr 7:563

Lee D, Port NL, Kruse W, Georgopoulos AP 1997 Neuronal clusters in the primate motor cortex during interception of moving targets. Soc Neurosci Abstr 23:1400

Massey JT, Schwartz AB, Georgopoulos AP 1986 On information processing and performing a movement sequence. Exp Brain Res Suppl 15:242–251

Massey JT, Drake RA, Lurito JT, Georgopoulos AP 1991a Cognitive spatial-motor processes. 4. Specification of the direction of visually guided isometric forces in two-dimensional space: information transmitted and effects of visual force-feedback. Exp Brain Res 83:439–445

Massey JT, Drake RA, Georgopoulos AP 1991b Cognitive spatial-motor processes. 5. Specification of the direction of visually guided isometric forces in two-dimensional space: time course of information transmitted and effect of constant force bias. Exp Brain Res 83:446–452

Port NL, Kruse W, Dassonville P, Georgopoulos AP 1994 Motor cortex and interception of moving targets: single cell analysis. Soc Neurosci Abstr 20:982

Port NL, Lee, D, Kruse W, Georgopoulos AP 1996 Motor cortical activity during target motion in the presence and absence of manual target interception. Soc Neurosci Abstr 22:12

Schwartz AB 1993 Motor cortical activity during drawing movements: population representation during sinusoid tracing. J Neurophysiol 70:28–36

Schwartz AB, Kettner RE, Georgopoulos AP 1988 Primate motor cortex and free arm movements to visual targets in three-dimensional space. I. Relations between single cell discharge and direction of movement. J Neurosci 8:2913–2927

Shinoda Y, Kakei S 1989 Distribution of terminals of thalamocortical fibers originating from the ventrolateral nucleus of the cat thalamus. Neurosci Lett 96:163–167

Soechting JF, Lacquaniti F 1981 Invariant characteristics of a pointing movement in man. J Neurosci 1:710–720

Soechting JF, Lacquaniti F 1983 Modification of trajectory of a pointing movement in response to a change in target location. J Neurophysiol 49:548–564

van Sonderen JF, van der Gon JJD, Gielen CCAM 1988 Conditions determining early modification of motor programmes in response to changes in target location. Exp Brain Res 71:320–328

DISCUSSION

Jeannerod: We have done similar experiments in humans, by changing the position of the target at movement onset and looking at the movement. We found very similar results including this very strong braking of the movement before the change in direction.

Georgopoulos: Were they in opposite directions in your case?

Jeannerod: No, they were at 90°.

Georgopoulos: That may make a difference.

Jeannerod: Another difference would be the accuracy requirement. In our case, because the target had to be grasped, the movement had to be more accurate.

Georgopoulos: Absolutely. There was a positional window within which the movement should end. However, these were reaching movements and did not involve grasping.

Jeannerod: There was no accuracy requirement in distance, because the monkey could hit the target.

Georgopoulos: No, in our case the movements were in two dimensions: they had to stop within a positional window, so they were pretty accurate. Our human subjects did as well as they could: in about 7% of trials they overshot, so they were just at the limit of performing 'as quickly and as accurately as possible'.

Fetz: It might be worth discussing what is actually being coded in motor cortex populations. You have data consistent with a variety of things being coded. Your initial studies showed that various kinematic variables (displacement, velocity and so forth) could all be represented. In those experiments force wasn't measured, but force is another important variable.

Georgopoulos: Acceleration was as close as we could get to force.

Fetz: But you also published an experiment in which you measured isometric forces in different directions (Taira et al 1996). So the question is whether the displacement or the force is the more primary variable. Force is generated by muscle activity and muscle activity is generated by motor neurons, and motor neurons are driven by neural activity. This would argue that perhaps force is the primary variable and the displacement is a secondary variable.

Georgopoulos: The key point is not the change in just *any* force, but the change in the *net* force. This a crucial point. The data show that during the generation of an isometric force pulse, it is the net force that is the important variable both for cell and population activity; this 'net force' is defined as the vector sum of the force bias and the force exerted by the subject. Alternatively, the vector of the force exerted by the subject can be decomposed to a 'static' and a 'dynamic' component: the static component is equal in magnitude and opposite in direction to the force bias vector, whereas the dynamic component is in the visually instructed direction. This dynamic force vector is the same as the net force vector above. (These vectors are illustrated in Massey et al 1991, Georgopoulos et al 1992.) Changes in motor cortical activity relate to this dynamic (or net) force but not to the total force exerted by the monkey. There is a major difference between this 'total' force and its 'dynamic' component: we claim that, under conditions of changing force, motor cortical activity reflects the dynamic component of the total force exerted.

Fetz: The net force would be the resultant of many individual muscle forces.

Georgopoulos: Exactly, but only a component of them: The resultant of *all* the muscle forces is the *total* force exerted, but only the *dynamic component* of this total force (and, therefore, of all the muscle forces) would be under motor cortical control under conditions of force change.

Miller: I'm interested in both the force that you talk about, but also the position, velocity and acceleration regression you mentioned at the beginning. You mentioned that acceleration seems to contribute such a small component, and implied the equivalence to inertial force. But there are other sources of force, for example, gravity and segmental coupling forces, as well as elastic forces. Isn't it difficult to estimate these forces, unless you can go in and measure them directly?

Georgopoulos: Apparently the best way to do it is to concentrate on the isometric force case where there is no limb mass to be moved. And in that case, the second time derivative of force did not have a significant effect on cell activity in a time-varying multiple regression analysis (J. Boline, J. Ashe & A. P. Georgopoulos, unpublished results).

Miller: What is the significance of the second derivative of force?

Georgopoulos: I am referring to the isometric force case (J. Boline, J. Ashe, A.P. Georgopoulos, unpublished observations). In that experiment the monkey exerted an isometric force pulse in various visually instructed directions and single cell activity was recorded in the contralateral motor cortex. The time-varying variables available for analysis included the following: the spike train as the dependent variable; the isometric force, its first and second time derivatives, and the visually instructed direction as the independent variables. A multiple linear regression analysis (as formally described in Ashe & Georgopoulos 1994) showed major effects of the first time derivative of force and of the visually instructed direction (J. Boline, J. Ashe & A. P. Georgopoulos, unpublished results).

Miller: The force in this case is the isometric force.

Georgopoulos: Yes.

Miller: Speaking of target direction, I'd like to go back to the discharge measured during movement, rather than the isometric case. In your earlier work, you've shown the nice relation between movement direction and neuronal discharge. Now more recently you've also attempted to account for the time-course of discharge during movement. It seems to me that the main conclusion you need to draw from those regression studies is that the truly dynamic signals (position, velocity, acceleration) accounted for a relatively small proportion of the firing rate. For most of your cells, the static target direction variable accounted for most of the discharge. Doesn't this suggest that the dynamics of the hand movement-related signals don't really match those of the cells terribly well?

Georgopoulos: No, this is not correct. The time-varying velocity and position of the hand were major explanatory factors for the time-varying cell activity.

Miller: Although your direction reversal task would suggest that there's a big torque component that you haven't considered directly in that first regression case.

Georgopoulos: The time-varying regression analysis was not carried out in the reversal task. The analyses published (Ashe & Georgopoulos 1994) came from the centre-out task.

Miller: You said there was a large deceleration force.

Georgopoulos: The large deceleration force was observed in the reversal task (Massey et al 1986). As I mentioned above, we did not perform the temporal analysis on those data.

Miller: But you had a large increase in discharge in neurons at the time of that reversal: is that correct?

Georgopoulos: Actually, no. The cell activity switched abruptly from the pattern of activity appropriate for the first direction, to that appropriate for the second direction, as predicted by the control task of moving directly towards the first or the second target without any reversal. This is nicely illustrated in the published records in Georgopoulos et al (1993). This was surprising: in spite of the huge reversing braking forces, the changes in cell activity seemed to reflect just pure kinematics. We didn't see anything reflecting that huge force which was quite evident in the EMG records.

Miller: What was the signal with the large peak at the time of discharge?

Georgopoulos: That was the peak velocity of the second movement.

Gibson: During testing, when did you change the bias force?

Georgopoulos: It was constant.

Gibson: The bias force was constant for an entire block of trials? When you stepped the bias force to a new direction, did the cells discharge as if the monkeys were generating a force equivalent to and in a direction opposing the new bias force?

Georgopoulos: You mean during the static phase. During the static phase, cell activity was tuned to the direction of the static force. Interestingly, when the animal started generating the dynamic pulse, it seemed that this pattern related to the pre-existing static force was replaced promptly by the proper one for the dynamic case.

Lemon: So do you have a situation where you put the bias force on, the cell shows a relationship to the direction of that bias force, and then once you instruct the monkey to make the pulses, it drops out?

Georgopoulos: Yes. The relation to the dynamic pulse takes over.

Lemon: What is doing the compensation?

Georgopoulos: Reticular formation cells, of course! I don't want to sound like an evolutionary biologist, but we live under the constant effect of gravity. Beyond these laboratory situations animals have been exposed continuously to gravitational fields. It is a reasonable idea that components of the antigravity system could be involved in this compensation for static loads. In fact, I would reverse the question, and ask why would the motor cortex have anything to do with this compensation in the first place? It is possible that the motor cortical signal is not important for compensating for the static load but that it may be providing an internal calibration signal, and the true compensation comes from the antigravity system.

Wolpert: There seems to be controversy in the literature about the coordinate systems which motor cortex operates in. At the single cell level do you believe neurons are coding for Cartesian- or joint-based parameters, and at the population level are they coding for joint- or Cartesian-based parameters?

Georgopoulos: Lacquaniti et al (1995) have recently examined this question with respect to area 5. The various parameters are quite interrelated. The activity of a good number of cells can be accounted for by analysing the data with respect to a Cartesian system; then if you re-express everything in terms of joint angles you find some relationship there as well. It is a problem that needs to be re-examined.

Wolpert: Is the transformation of Cartesian- to muscle-based coordinates upstream or downstream of the motor cortex?

Kalaska: We've been publishing data on this issue. I'll show in my presentation that when you start to try to dissociate these Cartesian spatial coordinate systems from what we call intrinsic (others might call them joint-centred) coordinate systems by changing task conditions, many cells in primary motor cortex show modulations of discharge that are systematic with both conditions: the extrinsic kinematics (the direction of movement) and also the changes in the arm geometry and the intrinsic details of how to perform a task. But that doesn't mean that any evidence of a covariation in cell activity with arm geometry is proof that the cell is representing movement exclusively in terms of intrinsic or 'joint-centred' parameters. It only shows that the cell's activity is not totally *independent* of arm geometry and so must be receiving information about it. Beyond that, it is very difficult to define more exactly the parameter space in which a given cell is representing movement, and that is only partly due to the biomechanical complexity of multiarticular arm movements and the inextricable coupling of many movement parameters through the laws of motion. I'm becoming increasingly discouraged that we won't ever be able to resolve this issue in the motor cortex. Perhaps it is a silly question to ask in a biological system, whereas in an engineering system it's a perfectly valid question.

Wolpert: Are you suggesting that single cells can show attributes of both?

Kalaska: Yes. You find some cells you swear are absolutely irrefutable proof that cells in the motor cortex are coding Cartesian spatial coordinates. They seem to be insensitive to anything we do in a particular task to dissociate spatial coordinates from other possible parameter spaces. And then there are other cells that look exactly like the posterior deltoid muscle. But then you get everything else in between.

Jeannerod: When the same pointing movement is performed in different conditions (a free movement constrained by a lever, for example), the set of coordinates used to plan the movement may change completely. In the first case, the movement kinematics will fit a model using coordinates of the endpoint of the limb as a reference; in the other case, it will fit a model using joint coordinates.

Georgopoulos: The endpoint is a different story: I wouldn't put it together with joint coordinate issue. For example, John Kalaska, Roberto Caminiti and myself did experiments in which monkeys moved a handle from the centre of a plane to peripheral targets, and vice versa. We found that the activity of cells in both the motor cortex and area 5 varied with the direction of movement (Georgopoulos et al 1985). In fact, we did not find any cell with endpoint-related activity.

Miall: I want to go back to the question of which other circuits might be filling in this gap between directional coding and what you see in the movements. You mentioned in terms of the bias force experiments that the reticular formation might compensate for those static forces. In the reversal experiments, you showed that the second movement was very fast and yet the motor cortex wasn't coding for that. Do you see the same thing with the reticular formation, or might it be switching in very quickly there?

Georgopoulos: It is possible. For example, visually guided trajectory reversal has been studied in the cat (Petersson et al 1997). It was found that cortical (i.e. the corticospinal system) as well as subcortical systems, including the tecto-reticulo-spinal and rubrospinal system, were important for this function. I don't know whether such subcortical systems (e.g. the tectospinal system) in the monkey may contribute to this function but I wouldn't be surprised if that were to be the case.

Miall: Could we just take one more extreme step? If you had an animal without a motor cortex, could it still do these tasks perfectly well?

Georgopoulos: I don't believe that this would be the case in the monkey, but it may quite different in the cat. I'm afraid it would be more like what we talked about yesterday: namely, that when you remove the motor cortex, the animal may somehow recover function, but it may take a lot of retraining and there may still remain a behavioural deficit.

Johansson: What you suggest is that initially after imposing the static force field in your experiments, there is some engagement of motor cortex, but after some time it's not a cortical business anymore. If you were to do slow changes or continuous changes in the background force during the task, will it become a motor cortical affair again?

Georgopoulos: This is an interesting question. In fact, this experiment has been done by Humphrey & Reed (1983). They recorded the activity of cells in the wrist area of the motor cortex while the force exerted by monkeys varied continuously in time to compensate for a time-varying load applied to the hand in the flexion–extension direction at various frequencies. At low frequencies ($<0.6\,\mathrm{Hz}$) the animals opposed the changing load by exerting appropriate, alternating flexion–extension forces at the wrist. However, at higher frequencies the animals adopted a strategy of co-contraction of flexor and extensor muscles of the hand; thus the mechanical stiffness at the wrist joint was increased and the handle was kept in a steady position. These behavioural events were reflected in the activity of cells recorded in the motor cortex. Thus, at frequencies of load modulation below $0.6\,\mathrm{Hz}$, the cell activity in the wrist area varied with the direction of the load in a reciprocal fashion. Moreover, microstimulation applied in that region elicited distinct EMG activation of wrist flexor or extensor muscles. However, at higher frequencies of load modulation a new class of cells became engaged. The tonic background level of discharge of these cells shifted progressively to higher or lower rates, in different cells, as the frequency of force perturbation was increased. These cells were located slightly more anteriorly than the 'reciprocal' cells; microstimulation at that locus elicited co-contraction of wrist flexors and extensors, and of other more proximal muscles. These findings suggest that separate motor cortical populations are concerned with the control of joint stiffness.

Johansson: Were they predictable?

Georgopoulos: This is a little controversial, because the experiment hasn't been repeated. They found that at low frequency the cell activity was nicely modulated, but at higher frequencies, they claim they discovered a new class of cells that became active with the co-contraction.

Fetz: We have rarely encountered cotricomotoneuronal cells that produce post-spike facilitation in both flexors and extensors.

Georgopoulos: The cells they described may not have had monosynaptic connections with motoneurons. In any case, that finding needs to be confirmed.

Fetz: These cells that could be recruited with contraction were never tested with respect to corticospinal projections or effects on muscles, so they could be intracortical. With microstimulation they evoked effects in flexors and extensors, but this again could be understood in terms of simultaneously stimulating separate flexor and extensor projections.

References

Ashe J, Georgopoulos AP 1994 Movement parameters and neuronal activity in motor cortex and area 5. Cereb Cortex 6:590–600

Georgopoulos AP, Kalaska JF, Caminiti R 1985 Relations between two-dimensional arm movements and single cell discharge in motor cortex and area 5: Movement direction versus movement endpoint. Exp Brain Res Suppl 10:176–183

Georgopoulos AP, Ashe J, Smyrnis N, Taira M 1992 Motor cortex and the coding of force. Science 256:1692–1695

Georgopoulos AP, Kalaska JF, Caminiti R, Massey JT 1993 Interruption of motor cortical discharge subserving aimed arm movements. Exp Brain Res 49:327–340

Humphrey DR, Reed DJ 1983 Separate cortical systems for control of joint movement and joint stiffness: reciprocal activation and coactivation of antagonist muscles. Adv Neurol 39:347–372

Lacquaniti F, Guigon E, Bianchi L, Ferraina S, Caminiti R 1995 Representing spatial information for limb movement: role of area 5 in the monkey. Cereb Cortex 5:391–409

Massey JT, Schwartz AB, Georgopoulos AP 1986 On information processing and performing a movement sequence. Exp Brain Res Suppl 15:242–251

Massey JT, Drake RA, Georgopoulos AP 1991 Cognitive spatial-motor processes. 5. Specification of the direction of visually guided isometric forces in two-dimensional space: Time course of information transmitted and effect of constant force bias. Exp Brain Res 83:446–452

Petersson L-G, Lundberg A, Alstermark B, Isa T, Tantisira B 1997 Effect of spinal cord lesions on forelimb target-reaching and on visually guided switching of target-reaching in the cat. Neurosci Res 29:241–256

Taira M, Boline J, Smyrnis N, Georgopoulos A, Ashe J 1996 On the relation between single cell activity in the motor cortex and the direction and magnitude of three-dimensional static isometric force. Exp Brain Res 109:367–376

General discussion III

Hoffmann: The superior colliculus has superficial and deep layers, and the general view is that there is a precise retinotopic map in the superficial layers and a precise motor map in the deeper layers which is an oculomotor map. We have a wealth of information on how the colliculus is involved in eliciting and governing saccades. Anatomical studies have shown the cortico–collicular connections involved in this task. In addition, there are several anatomical reports of projections from skeletomotor areas of the frontal cortex to the deep layers of the colliculus. This finding prompted us several years ago to look for other motor aspects in the deep layers of the colliculus, such as arm movements. Surprisingly, we found that many cells in these deep layers are involved in arm movements (Werner et al 1997a,b, Kutz et al 1997). After what we've heard this morning, I would like to describe the type of responses we have found. In particular, I want to show that very similar response types, be they motor, intentional or sensory, exist in the colliculus. We had to repeat many of the experiments which were done on the various cortical motor areas, because we wanted to know whether the colliculus receives and transforms information from these motor areas. So, the monkeys were trained to perform the centre–out/centre–in test. In the colliculus of these monkeys we find the same spectrum of response types as was found in the motor cortex, premotor cortex and parietal cortex. One type of neuron displays arm movement-related activity which only occurs when the contralateral arm is being moved. There is no activity when the eyes move, nor is there activity when the stimulus is presented. The activity can be seen as early as several hundred milliseconds before movement onset, and analysis of the directions of hand movements shows that these neurons display a pattern which is very much like that in the motor cortex for neurons coding the direction of hand movement.

A second type of neuron in the colliculus seemed to code the actual position and maybe the desired final position of the hand. In these neurons, irrespective of where the movement starts from, the strongest response is seen when the hand goes to a particular target in space. The third type of neuron may be the most interesting in the context of the paper we heard earlier by Richard Andersen. These neurons respond strongest to an arm movement to a target with a fixed vector to the fovea in a gaze-centred coordinate system. If gaze is shifted to a new position the preferred target shifts by the same amount as gaze did. This behaviour is irrespective of whether the contra- or ipsilateral arm with respect to the recorded colliculus is being used. Again the responses are very tightly locked to the arm movement and we don't see this activity with stimulus onset or during the waiting phase. Thus, in contrast to what Richard Andersen showed, these neurons seemed to be much closer to the motor aspect of the response. In addition we could also show that the response of this type of collicular neuron is modulated by eye position. Similar gain fields as they have been reported for neurons in the parietal cortex could be demonstrated.

Neurons in the colliculus seem to be the target of many cortical projections. For instance, in the premotor and parietal cortex we can find neurons with very similar types as their subcortical possible target which could be the superior colliculus. In the future we should do experiments with antidromic identification of neurons in the cortex projecting to the colliculus to find out whether cortical areas provide a specific type of information for the skeletomotor function of the superior colliculus. In summary we have found an additional structure in the skeletomotor system within deep layers of the superior colliculus and the underlying reticular formation. Anatomically, the border between deep colliculus and reticular formation is not clearly defined. Functionally, we find the distribution of the neurons in different depths as it is depicted in Fig. 1 (*Hoffmann*). The gaze-related reach neurons are distributed in about the same layers as the saccade neurons. The gaze-independent neurons are distributed even deeper and stretch out into the reticular formation. We could, however, not find a difference between the gaze-independent neurons in the deep layers of the colliculus and in the reticular formation. So far we have no information about the target of these neurons in the brain stem which makes speculations about their functions premature.

Thier: Do you find a distinct population of cells that is related to arm movements not discharging in relation to eye movements, whereas cells related to eye movements ignore arm movements, or are there also cells related to both eye and arm movements?

Hoffmann: We find very little overlap, but then the neurons have different properties if they are contributing to saccades or arm movements. This can be reconciled if a single neuron can be a member of different ensembles, one population coding eye movements in a specific direction and another population arm movements in another direction.

Thier: Are the oculomotor and the hand motor cells located in different places?

Hoffmann: One neuron can be involved in both aspects but can have different spatial properties. The gaze-related reach neurons are the most superficial and they overlap totally with the band of saccade cells. The more arm-related and muscle-related cells are deeper.

Thier: Have you tried to stimulate electrically the superior colliculus in an attempt to evoke hand or arm movements?

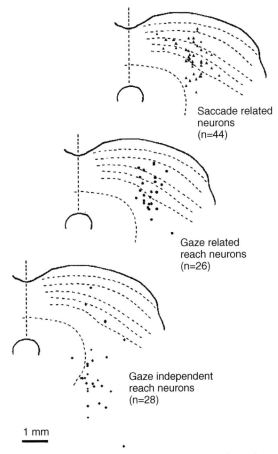

Saccade related
neurons
(n=44)

Gaze related
reach neurons
(n=26)

Gaze independent
reach neurons
(n=28)

1 mm

FIG. 1. (*Hoffmann*) The distribution of gaze-related, gaze-independent and saccade-related neurons in different depths of the colliculus and reticular formation.

Hoffmann: Yes. But we did not get goal-directed movements; electrical stimulation would only lead to twitches of the shoulder.

Ebner: Investigators who work behind the central sulcus have been more generous than those who work ahead of it. Richard Andersen showed very nicely that posterior parietal neurons encode several sensory and motor parameters. I think that we need to start thinking about similar multi-parameter processing ahead of the central sulcus, and not become so dogmatic about whether only kinematics or dynamics are processed. In the primary motor cortex and dorsal premotor cortex we have shown that direction, amplitude, velocity and speed are all represented. I'm certain that dynamic signals, and probably multiple coordinate systems are also represented. As Richard Andersen suggests, perhaps different structures will make use of these different classes of information. I also suspect that in different tasks, different information may be processed. Kinematics may be the dominating factor in some tasks and the processing will reflect that need. Similarly, in a purely dynamic task, dynamic information will be processed.

Lemon: That is all very well, except that there's one part of the motor system that will have problems with that — the motoneuron. The motoneuron is unable to interpret all those different frames of reference: it has to respond to the commands it receives.

Kalaska: I agree that it's possible that within the primary motor cortex and across the whole precentral gyrus including the premotor cortex, there is a strong temporal progression in the nature of the information that these cells might be processing, especially in the time interval between the presentation of a target and the initiation of movement towards that target. I am thinking in particular of the recent work by Shen & Alexander (1997a,b) and of Zheng et al (1997) suggesting that if you analyse the activity of these cells in time, you find initially that the earliest activity in premotor and primary motor cortex appears to be best correlated with the visuospatial attributes of the stimulus. Progressively in time you get more and more representation of the response the monkey must perform by the learned stimulus response associations. Thus within these structures we see a progressive shift in the nature of the information that a given cell may be coding or processing. Steve Scott and I also found evidence of a similar process (unpublished results). Again, when we trained monkeys to make movements with similar hand paths but using different arm geometries, we found that if you just take the activity over an extended period of time and average, you see a variety of changes, amongst other things, in the directional tuning of the cells. But if you now take a 50 ms sliding window and look at the directional tuning of these cells only within the window, the very earliest activity in the primary motor cortex, about 150 ms before movement onset, shows a relatively small directional tuning difference when the monkey is making reaching movements using two arm orientations. Then, very rapidly over about 100 ms, as one advances the window in time but still well before the onset of movement, you see a rapid increase in the size of the typical directional difference of the cells between the two arm orientations. Again, this is consistent with the idea from Shen & Alexander and Zhang et al that the very earliest activity in this area might reflect more visuospatial attributes of the input and less the nature of the motor output the monkey must perform to respond to the visual stimulus.

Marsden: Is what you are saying that firing of motor cortical units changes during the stimulus response from the sensory driven attribute to a motor execution attribute?

Kalaska: That seems to be the implication of the analysis that Shen & Alexander (1997a,b) and Zhang et al (1997) have done. You can see a temporal evolution of the nature of correlation of cells to the motor instructional attributes versus the nature of the response the monkey must make.

Marsden: Does that apply to both single units and populations?

Kalaska: Yes, at both levels.

Miller: To go back to the force bias business in relation to motor cortex static forces and dynamic forces and so forth. Another observation of Eb Fetz from a number of years back which I've never been able to quite put together is that during the ramp and hold task, he found lots of motor neurons with decreasing patterns of activity (Palmer & Fetz 1985). How does this relate to this observation of Apostolos Georgopoulos of initial discharge during statically applied force?

Fetz: Those decrementing patterns in the motor units probably reflect an adaptation of motor neurons to sustained input (Palmer & Fetz 1985). This is the simplest interpretation.

Miller: But could this be part of the effect that Apostolos describes, in which this initial tonic force-related discharge in motor cortex disappears?

Fetz: During the torque ramp, which is the dynamic component, many motor units and most motor cortex cells showed phasic discharge (Cheney & Fetz 1980). But the CM cells never showed decrementing discharge.

References

Cheney PD, Fetz EE 1980 Functional classes of primate corticomotoneuronal cells and their relation to active force. J Neurophysiol 44:773–791

Kutz D, Dannenberg S, Werner W, Hoffmann K-P 1997 Population coding of arm movement-related neurons in and below the superior colliculus of macaca mulatta. Biol Cybernetics 76:331–337

Palmer SS, Fetz EE 1985 Discharge properties of primate forearm motor units during isometric muscle activity. J Neurophysiol 54:1178–1193

Shen L, Alexander GE 1997a Neural correlates of a spatial sensory-to-motor transformation in primary motor cortex. J Neurophysiol 77:1171–1194

Shen L, Alexander GE 1997b Preferential representation of instructed target location versus limb trajectory in dorsal premotor area. J Neurophysiol 77:1195–1212

Werner W, Hoffmann K-P, Dannenberg S 1997a Arm movement-related neurons in the primate superior colliculus and underlying reticular formation: comparison of neuronal activity with EMGs of muscles of the shoulder, arm and trunk during reaching. Exp Brain Res 115:191–205

Werner W, Hoffmann K-P, Dannenberg S 1997b Population coding of arm movement-related neurons in the primate superior colliculus and underlying reticular formation in comparison to visual or saccadic cells. Exp Brain Res 115:206–216

Zhang J, Riehle A, Requin J, Kornblum S 1997 Dynamics of single neuron activity in monkey primary motor cortex related to sensorimotor transformation. J Neurosci 17:2227–2246

Cortical control of whole-arm motor tasks

John F. Kalaska, Lauren E. Sergio and Paul Cisek

Centre de Recherche en Sciences Neurologiques, Département de Physiologie, Faculté de Médecine, Université de Montréal, C.P. 6128, Succursale Centre-ville, Montréal, Québec, Canada H3C 3J7

Abstract. Making an arbitrary motor response to a sensory signal would appear to require at least two sequential steps — planning the appropriate response and generating a motor command to implement it. However, neuronal correlates of these two putative steps do not occur in strict serial order, nor are they subserved by separate cortical regions. Instead, they are distributed in a continuous, overlapping and non-uniform manner across the cerebral cortex, including primary motor, premotor and parietal regions. These processes take the form of temporal and spatial gradients of cell activity that are distributed within and across cortical regions. Instead of two serial steps, these neuronal events may be better described in terms of two parallel functions — action specification and action selection. These processes occur continuously, both before and during movement. Recent studies show that the activity of single cells in the caudal part of the primary motor cortex is strongly modulated by arm geometry and by task dynamics during whole-arm isometric and reaching tasks. This indicates that these cells contribute to the transformation between neural representations of the global attributes of motor actions and of the mechanical details of their implementation.

1998 Sensory guidance of movement. Wiley, Chichester (Novartis Foundation Symposium 218) p 176–201

In keeping with the theme of this meeting, this chapter begins with some speculations on the general role of sensory input in motor control, and their implications for the functional architecture of the motor system. Many of these ideas are not original to the authors of this chapter, but are derived from the work of others, including several of the participants in this conference. Some neurophysiological data relevant to this discussion will then be surveyed.

Action specification versus action selection: a useful dichotomy for motor control?

A distinction is traditionally made in motor control theory between 'planning' and 'execution' of movements (Fig. 1A). This makes sense from an engineering

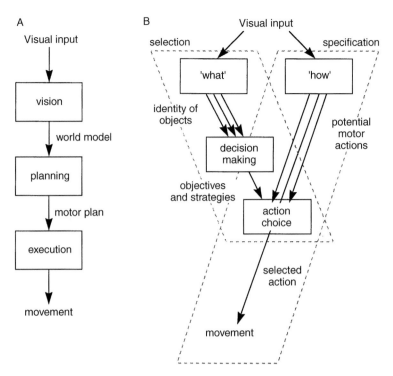

FIG. 1.(A)   The planning versus execution dichotomy within a traditional hierarchical model of the processing stages between vision and action. Note how planning is preceded by perceptual/cognitive processes that generate a world model from visual input. (B) Schematic representation of the specification versus selection dichotomy for visually guided behaviour. Action selection encompasses the ventral 'what' visual pathway and other decision-making mechanisms. Action specification begins in the dorsal 'how' visual pathway. It progressively transforms visual information into the parameters of potential motor actions, and includes all processes that dynamically generate and shape the outgoing motor command during movement, including specification via feedback from the unfolding movement. A striking feature of this architecture is the absence of an a priori central model of the visual world. In this perspective, visual input processing is pragmatic, biased toward analysis of visual input in terms of potential motor actions.

perspective because the task is decomposed into two sequential steps with different computational demands solved by separate systems. A 'planner' generates a spatiotemporal description of a desired movement, ideally in a form that is independent of the details of its implementation. A 'controller' subsequently converts that description into an overt movement. A serial relationship between planning and execution is obligatory in some optimization models (Flash & Hogan 1985, Uno et al 1989). In those models, a complete temporal profile of the intended response from its start to its end is planned and optimized for some cost function, before the controller can generate the motor commands that implement the optimized plan.

However, it is useful to consider whether the distinction between planning and execution is fundamental from an evolutionary perspective. One could argue that primitive creatures did a lot of *acting* or *reacting*, but very little *planning* per se. Instead of formulating a prior central description of an intended movement, including all desired intermediate states, these primitive creatures possessed neural circuits that directly generated motor commands in real time. Virtually all of their motor control processes would fall under the rubric of execution.

Nevertheless, their motor system undoubtedly did not function in purely open-loop mode. Their actions could be guided by sensory inputs about the environment and the organism's own moving body, signalled by primitive exteroceptors and proprioceptors. Some of these inputs projected onto motor circuits to shape the motor commands as the movement unfolded. Others elicited simple responses such as scratch and wipe reflexes, and righting, orienting and escape responses. These behaviours were stereotypical but not invariant. Instead, they were tailored by the sensory input that elicited them to accomplish a behavioural goal. This suggests that one ancient role for sensory input was the *specification* of the parameters of motor actions (Fig. 1B).

Action *selection* is a second important role for sensory input (Fig. 1B). An animal is continually bombarded by sensory inputs, but compulsive responsiveness to every input has low survival value. Often, the barrage of sensory inputs calls simultaneously for different responses that cannot be executed concurrently without interfering with each other. Furthermore, as the behavioural repertoire becomes more sophisticated and diverse, even a single environmental event may specify several possible alternative courses of action. Mechanisms for selecting from among the impinging sensory inputs those that warrant a response and the action most appropriate at that moment were essential early in evolution. In more advanced nervous systems, action selection encompasses a broad range of perceptual and cognitive processes, as well as mechanisms that permit the acquisition of arbitrary stimulus–response associations.

Action specification and selection are not necessarily independent processes (Fig. 1B), but their differing roles likely impose different demands on the nature of processing of sensory inputs that would require at least partially independent neuronal systems. Action specification requires information about the topography of sensory input systems, the spatial locations of stimulus sources and the spatial structure of the environment with which the organism is interacting. In contrast, properties of stimuli that are location- and orientation-invariant, such as the nature and identity of visual objects, are more critical for selecting what actions to take.

These demands appear to correspond well to the differing properties of the dorsal and ventral visual streams (Goodale & Milner 1992, Goodale 1996, 1998 this volume). Different parietal cortical cell populations in the dorsal ('how') stream contribute to visuospatial representations and visuomotor trans- formations that specify parameters of motor responses (Colby & Duhamel 1996, Johnson et al 1996, Andersen et al 1997, Sakata et al 1997, Wise et al 1997, this volume: Andersen et al 1998, Jeannerod et al 1998). Even in medial and caudal areas of the parietal lobe traditionally considered to have strictly visual functions, visual responses are shaped by movement-related processes (Ferraina et al 1997a,b), suggesting that visual inputs may be interpreted very quickly in terms of potential actions that they specify. In contrast, the evidence implicating the ventral stream in object identification ('what') and related perceptual and cognitive operations (Tanaka 1996) supports a role for it in early stages of action selection. The implicit bias in this interpretation of dorsal and ventral stream function is that sensory systems evolved initially to serve the needs of the motor system, not to generate an internal model of the world (Fig. 1). This is reminiscent of Koffka's notion of 'demand character' whereby objects are linked with associated actions ('. . . a fruit says "eat me", water says "drink me" . . .'; Koffka [1935], p 7). It is also consistent with Gibson's theory of 'affordances' (Gibson 1979), which proposes that perception of objects is fundamentally concerned with determining the actions that they permit.

Separating action specification and selection into partially independent neuronal systems permits aspects of both to be performed in parallel, rather than in strict serial order like many formal motor control models. Furthermore, several potential motor responses may begin to be specified by the available sensory information, and such specification may in turn influence which action is finally selected (Fig. 1B). These features of motor system organization are implicit in recent cognitive psychological models of motor planning (Kornblum et al 1990). According to these models, the motor system is predisposed to efficiently and rapidly map a behaviourally relevant sensory input into a motor response of high stimulus–response compatibility. In parallel, other cognitive processes evaluate the sensory input and the behavioural context, to identify alternative response strategies. If an action of lower compatibility is more appropriate, the motor system suppresses the ongoing preparation of the response to which it is predisposed and replaces it with the alternative.

One might argue that action specification and action selection are sub- processes of planning, and so are not incompatible with a strict serial dichotomy between planning and execution. However, specification encompasses all processes that define attributes of the movement, from the most global properties of its form to the details of muscle activity patterns. As a result, action specification is distributed across all levels of the motor system, from the 'highest-order' cortical structures to spinal interneuronal networks and α-motoneuron pools.

Specification is distributed not only across neural space, but across time, occurring both before and *during* movement. Using the inherent dynamical properties of neuronal circuitry and sensory signals about the evolving act, the motor system specifies each intermediate state of the act in real time. This obviates the need for complete specification of the desired movement in the form of a continuous sequence of pre-planned intermediate states prior to its generation. It may only be necessary to specify in advance certain critical features of the potential movements, such as the target location, direction and amplitude of linear arm movements, or the general form of more complex motions such as via-points for curved figures. The remaining details would be specified in real time during movement generation. Some recent formal motor control models possess this dynamic architecture (Jordan 1990, Bullock et al 1998). This suggests that neuronal correlates of much of what might otherwise be considered aspects of motor planning may in fact be expressed only as the movement is unfolding and might therefore be confounded temporally with presumed neuronal mechanisms of movement execution.

Cortical mechanisms of reaching movements

The simplest neuronal implementation of the planning versus execution dichotomy would entail one cell population that formulates a plan and a separate population that subsequently executes it. This organization should be most evident in instructed-delay tasks, in which subjects receive an instructional cue about the nature of a desired response but must withhold that response for a delay period before producing it. In theory, the subject could completely plan all aspects of the movement signalled by the cue during the delay period, as if mentally rehearsing the intended response. To initiate the movement, the neuronal circuits that execute the plan would be activated. Neurophysiological evidence shows that such a rigid separation of function at either the single-cell or population levels is untenable.

For instance, neurophysiological evidence that a representation of the complete spatiotemporal profile of a movement or movement sequence exists during the delay period of instructed-delay tasks is not compelling to date (Hocherman & Wise 1991, Mushiake et al 1991, Ashe et al 1993, Kettner et al 1996). Instead, the delay period activity appears to contain only enough information to specify a general outline of the intended motor response. The neuronal correlates of all the instantaneous intermediate states along the movement must therefore be generated dynamically as the movement is initiated. How the complete spatiotemporal form of a movement could be mentally rehearsed during the brief behavioural reaction time before movement onset in reaction-time tasks is even less obvious.

The idea that a movement is not completely pre-specified prior to initiation is further supported by psychophysical evidence that the pattern of initial activation of muscles (Karst & Hasan 1991) and the initial direction of displacement of the hand toward targets (Gordon et al 1994) is not always appropriate for the desired direction of movement. This indicates that at the moment of movement initiation, the motor response is not yet 'optimized'. Specification continues and the initial errors are corrected as the movement is performed.

Furthermore, changes in activity during both instructed-delay periods and movement execution have been observed in virtually all cortical regions implicated in motor control. Similarly, motor-imagery studies have shown that many of the same cortical areas are activated when one performs a movement, or simply imagines that one is performing it (Crammond 1997, Jeannerod & Decety 1995).

Finally, while some cells in a given area may be uniquely activated during only the delay period or the subsequent movement itself, many cells show activity changes during both phases of the task, as if contributing to both planning and execution. Two recent studies using tasks that dissociated the direction of instructional signals from the direction of signalled motor responses shed important new light on this property of cell activity in primary motor (M1) and dorsal premotor cortex (PMd) (Zhang et al 1997, Shen & Alexander 1997a,b). Both studies found that the discharge of a single cell could be better correlated at different times throughout a trial to spatial attributes of the instructional signal, to the associative rules coupling instruction to response, or to parameters of the instructed movement. Even during the movement itself, activity did not represent only details of the overt motor output. Instead, neuronal correlates of visuospatial and sensory-motor associative aspects of the task could also be observed in the activity of cells as the movement progressed. This is consistent with the idea that the generation of central representations of global features of a motor response ('planning') and of the details of its implementation ('execution') are not strictly serially ordered. Instead, they are dynamically generated in real time as the movement unfolds.

This does not mean that there was no temporal order to these processes. Both studies reported a strong serial progression in the nature of cell activity. The earliest activity was best correlated with visuospatial aspects of the instructional signals, followed by an increased representation of the associative rules. Finally, neuronal correlates of the signalled movements themselves became most prominent, either just before or during the movement. This temporal sequence is gradual, not abrupt, and at any given time neuronal correlates of all three stages coexist, but with relatively different prominence.

These temporally overlapping and progressively changing neuronal correlates do not fit readily into a serial planning/execution scheme. Instead, the role of these cell populations can be unified if it is proposed that they are continually involved in specification and selection of the motor response without an abrupt transition from one serial stage to another. At any given moment, the precise contribution of the cell would be determined by the dynamical flow of information within the distributed cortical network. The changing correlations in cell discharge suggest that the earliest activity within the network is dominated by information about visuospatial constraints of the task (specification) and cognitive processes related to the nature of stimulus–response associations (selection). Later activity becomes dominated by specification of the details of implementation of the selected motor response.

Along with a temporal gradient of activity, there is also a spatial gradient. Cell activity in PMd shows more prominent relations to visuospatial and context-dependent aspects of a motor task than do cells in M1. They also show more prominent activity than M1 cells during the delay period of instructed-delay tasks. Activity in M1 is more tightly coupled temporally to the actual performance of movement than is activity in PMd. These differences in the nature of activity change gradually over the rostrocaudal axis of the precentral gyrus. A corresponding and oppositely oriented gradient of cell properties has been demonstrated in the parietal cortex (Johnson et al 1996). Moreover, cells at different parts of the rostrocaudal gradient in precentral cortex tend to be reciprocally connected via cortico-cortical projections to cells with matching response properties along the rostrocaudal gradient in the parietal cortex.

The distinction between action specification and action selection within this distributed network was strikingly demonstrated in a study of parietal area 5 and PMd cell activity in a visually guided reaching task, in which visual cues in different spatial locations signalled the direction of movement (Kalaska & Crammond 1995). The colour of the signal indicated whether the monkey should move to the signal's location after a delay (GO trials), or remain at the initial position for a period of time to receive a reward (NO-GO). Cells in both area 5 and PMd were strongly directionally tuned during the delay period of GO trials prior to movements in different directions (Fig. 2). Many PMd cells also responded to the NO-GO cues, indicating that their presentation provided behaviourally relevant information that the cells processed. However, their activity was typically much less directionally tuned throughout most of the delay period compared to their activity in GO trials. These differences in response patterns between GO and NO-GO trials in PMd are presumed neuronal correlates of processes involved either in selecting whether to move or not on the basis of the colour of the cue, or in specification of the selected response. In contrast, many cells in area 5 continued to discharge in the same directional manner in NO-GO trials as in GO trials (Fig. 2). This suggests that the area 5 cells continued to specify attributes of the potential arm movements to the cue locations even after the monkey had

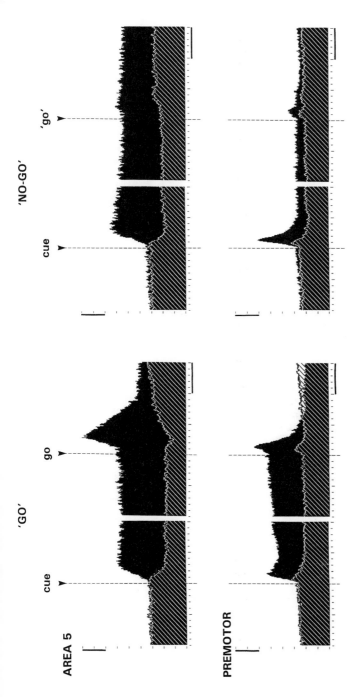

FIG. 2. Mean histograms of the discharge of 51 cells in parietal area 5 and 97 cells in PMd in an instructed-delay task. Visual cues in different spatial locations instructed the monkeys either to move to the cue after a delay ('GO', left) or not to move ('NO-GO', right), when a second 'go' cue was presented. Activity is from trials in which cues appeared at the preferred movement direction of each cell (solid histograms) or in the opposite direction (hatched histograms). Activity is oriented to the appearance of the cue (left vertical line) and to the go signal (right vertical line) in each histogram. During the delay period in GO trials, cells in both areas generated strong directional activity. Activity was much less directional in PMd within 300 ms after the cue in NO-GO trials than in GO trials. This is a presumed neuronal correlate of the monkey's decision not to move. In contrast, area 5 activity continued to be strongly directional after the NO-GO cues, as if continuing to specify attributes of the potential movements toward the cues that the monkeys were not authorized to make after the 'go' signal. Horizontal calibration bars = 500 ms; vertical calibration bars = 10 spikes/s. (Figure reproduced with permission from Kalaska et al 1997.)

A) Central location

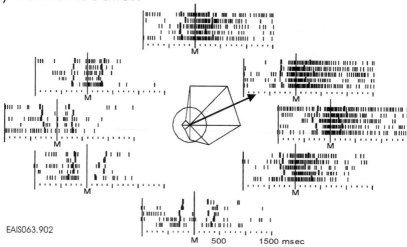

EAISO63.902

M   500   1500 msec

B) Nine locations

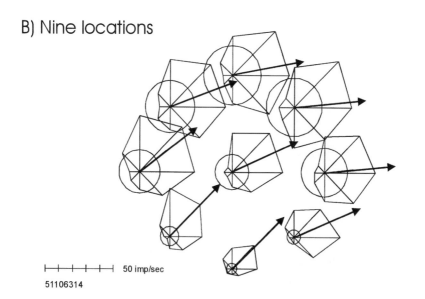

├─┼─┼─┼─┼─┤ 50 imp/sec

51106314

recognized, as indicated by the PMd activity, that the NO-GO cue did not authorize a movement. While both areas may contribute to action specification, area 5 did not appear to be as implicated as PMd in the selection of whether to move or not. This study also demonstrated that neuronal correlates of more than one motor response can coexist within the distributed cortical motor system. During NO-GO trials, area 5 activity covaried with the parameters of a potential but unauthorized motor response, whereas PMd activity reflected the monkey's final selection of what to do.

Coexisting neuronal correlates of multiple potential motor responses have also been observed within the parietal cortex itself in a task in which a monkey made either arm or eye movements to targets in different spatial locations (Snyder et al 1997). Even after the monkey was instructed to move only the eyes or the arm, neuronal correlates of both potential responses continued to be generated in the parietal cortex.

Neuronal correlates of these early decision-making processes are also found in M1, but with diminishing prominence as one proceeds caudally across the precentral gyrus. In contrast, M1 receives a major input from primary somatosensory cortex and parietal area 5, and from other sources of proprioceptive inputs that transmit information about the posture and motion of the limb and about the contractile state of the muscles (Prud'Homme & Kalaska 1994). This input would allow M1 to contribute to processes that convert a representation about the desired spatiotemporal form of a movement into motor signals that reflect the mechanical details of its implementation. These motor signals would have to covary with the geometry of the arm by which the

---

FIG. 3.   (A) Discharge pattern of a primary motor cortex cell during isometric force generation in eight directions in a horizontal plane while the hand is in a central location in the workspace, and (B) changes in that discharge pattern when generating the same forces while the hand is in different locations on a horizontal plane. Each of the eight rasters in the top figure show cell activity during five trials in one force direction; the position of each raster corresponds to force direction away from a starting force value. Data from each trial are oriented to the time of the first significant change in force measured by the force transducer (vertical line 'M') after the appearance of the force target in a trial (heavy tick marks to the left of the vertical line). Heavy ticks to the right of the line show time when the final target static force level was attained within the peripheral force target. At the centre of the raster plots is a polar plot depiction of the cell activity. Radius of the circle in the polar plot indicates mean cell discharge rate before peripheral force target appearance. Length of each axis of the polar plot indicates mean activity level during static force generation at each peripheral target. Heavy arrow indicates the preferred direction of the cell during static force generation in the eight directions. This polar plot is duplicated in the centre of the bottom figure. The other eight polar plots illustrate how the activity of the cell changes in intensity and directionality when the monkey generates the same forces against a force transducer while holding the hand in eight different locations arranged in a circle of 8 cm radius about the central location. (Sergio & Kalaska 1997, unpublished cell.)

movements are performed, and with the concomitant changes in causal forces and muscle activity patterns. This hypothesis is being tested in a series of studies using whole-arm reaching and isometric-force tasks.

The first study recorded the activity of M1 and PMd cells while monkeys made reaching movements along similar handpaths in eight directions in a horizontal plane at shoulder level, with the arm held in either the natural parasagittal plane or abducted into the horizontal plane at the shoulder (Scott & Kalaska 1997, Scott et al 1997). The contractile activity of most prime-mover muscles of the arm showed changes in their overall level and directional tuning between the two arm orientations. These changes reflected the arm posture-dependent changes in muscular forces required to produce the movements along similar handpaths. Many cells in the most caudal part of M1 in the bank of the central sulcus also showed changes in the level and directional tuning of their activity both during movement and while holding the arm over the same spatial target locations but with the arm in two different orientations. This showed that the activity of many single M1 cells covaried not only with the spatial attributes of the endpoint trajectory, but also with the arm-posture dependent changes in the intrinsic mechanical details of how to produce the arm movements using different arm geometries. The effects of arm orientation were not as strong in PMd as in M1 (Scott et al 1997). This is consistent with the hypothesis that PMd is more concerned with specification of global attributes of a movement, and less about the mechanical details of its implementation.

The complex dynamics of movement, however, complicate the interpretation of these changes. Therefore, a second study sought evidence of arm-posture dependent changes in M1 activity by training a monkey to use its whole arm to generate static forces in constant spatial directions in a horizontal plane against a force transducer held in its hand, when the transducer was located in different parts of space (Sergio & Kalaska 1997). Because arm geometry changes with hand spatial location, the muscle activity required to produce output forces in constant spatial directions varies systematically in level and in directional tuning as a function of hand spatial location. The activity of many M1 cells in the bank of the central sulcus likewise changes its directionality and level systematically with hand location (Fig. 3). As with the arm-movement study (Scott & Kalaska 1997), this result indicates that single-cell discharge in caudal M1 does not only signal global features of the motor task, such as the directionality of net static output forces at the hand. Instead, single-cell activity often covaries systematically with both the direction of desired net output forces and with hand spatial location and arm geometry while generating the forces, in a manner qualitatively similar to prime-mover muscles. This supports the hypothesis that M1 contributes to the neuronal processes specifying how to alter muscle activity to achieve the desired output.

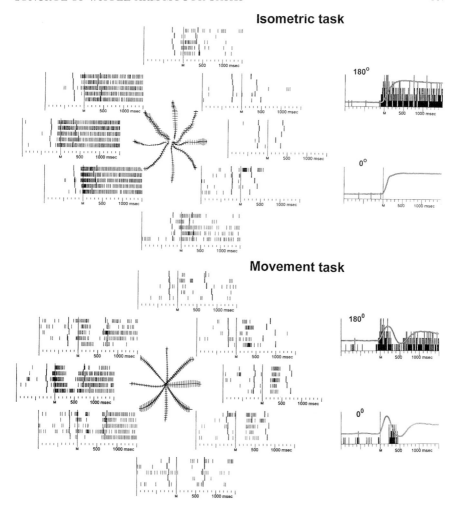

FIG. 4. Discharge pattern of a primary motor cortex cell during isometric force production in eight directions in a horizontal plane (*top*) and during arm movements in the same plane (*bottom*). For each task, the eight rasters to the left show the cell activity during five trials in each direction, and the location of each raster corresponds to the direction of force or movement away from the starting central target. Data are oriented to the first significant force change detected by a force transducer (vertical line 'M'). The mean force or movement trajectories are shown at the centre of the raster displays (crosses show standard deviations of five trajectories at 20 equidistant points). Panels to the right display cell activity in histogram format for the motor output aimed to the left (180°) and the right (0°), overlaid with the average temporal force profile for those responses. (Sergio & Kalaska 1998, unpublished cell.)

In a third study, a monkey either generated isometric forces at the hand in eight directions in a horizontal plane, or moved a handle in the same eight directions to targets in specific spatial locations (Sergio & Kalaska 1998). In the isometric task, the controlled variable was the net output force vector at the hand, and the force temporal profile was a simple ramp directed towards the target force value (Fig. 4). In contrast, the behaviourally controlled variable in the movement task was hand spatial location, and the handpath of each movement was a simple ramp displacement towards the target. Because of the combined mass and inertia of the monkey's limb and the handle, however, the forces generated at the hand were more complex in the movement task, including a transient reversal of the direction of forces to decelerate the limb and handle as they approached the target (Fig. 4). In the isometric task, muscles showed simple directionally tuned ramp-and-hold response patterns, whereas in the movement task their activity changed to a more complex triphasic burst–pause–step pattern in their preferred direction and a reciprocal pattern in the opposite direction. The activity of many caudal M1 cells showed corresponding differences between the two tasks (Fig. 4). Therefore, the temporal profile of activity of many caudal M1 cells was strongly modified by the change in task dynamics between the isometric and movement tasks.

These three studies demonstrate that the representation of limb motor behaviour in the caudal motor cortex reflects not just global task constraints, but also incorporates information about arm geometry, the mechanical properties of the arm and the causal forces necessary to produce the desired motor output. This does not imply that these cells generate explicit muscle control signals. The specification of muscle activity patterns implicates several neural structures, culminating only at level of the spinal motor apparatus itself. The primary motor cortex is one part of an interconnected parietal and precentral cortical network within which spatially and temporally distributed dynamic processes of action specification and action selection effect a gradual transformation of visuospatial inputs and cognitive constraints into a representation of the desired response. These processes occur continuously, both before and during movement.

References

Andersen RA, Snyder LH, Bradley DC, Xing J 1997 Multimodal representation of space in the posterior parietal cortex and its use in planning movements. Annu Rev Neurosci 20:303–330
Andersen RA, Snyder LH, Batista AP, Buneo CA, Cohen YE 1998 Posterior parietal areas specialized for eye movements (LIP) and reach (PRR) using a common coordinate frame. In: Sensory guidance of movement. Wiley, Chichester (Novartis Found Symp 218) p 109–120
Ashe J, Taira M, Smyrnis N et al 1993 Motor cortical activity preceding a memorized movement trajectory with an orthogonal bend. Exp Brain Res 95:118–130

Bullock D, Cisek PE, Grossberg S 1998 Cortical networks for control of voluntary arm movements under variable force conditions. Cereb Cortex 8:48–62

Colby CL, Duhamel J-R 1996 Spatial representations for action in parietal cortex. Cereb Cortex 5:105–115

Crammond DJ 1997 Motor imagery: never in your wildest dream. Trends Neurosci 20:54–57

Ferraina S, Johnson PB, Garasto MR et al 1997a Combination of hand and gaze signals during reaching: activity in parietal area 7m of the monkey. J Neurophysiol 77:1034–1038

Ferraina S, Garasto MR, Battaglia-Mayer A et al 1997b Visual control of hand-reaching movement: activity in parietal area 7m. Eur J Neurosci 9:1090–1095

Flash T, Hogan N 1985 The coordination of arm movements: an experimentally confirmed mathematical model. J Neurosci 5:1688–1703

Gibson JJ 1979 The ecological approach to visual perception. Houghton Mifflin Press, Boston, MA

Goodale MA 1996 Visuomotor modules in the vertebrate brain. Can J Physiol Pharmacol 74:390–400

Goodale MA 1998 Vision for perception and vision for action in the primate brain. In: Sensory guidance of movement. Wiley, Chichester (Novartis Found Symp 218) p 21–44

Goodale MA, Milner AD 1992 Separate visual pathways for perception and action. Trends Neurosci 15:20–25

Gordon J, Ghilardi MF, Cooper SE, Ghez C 1994 Accuracy of planar reaching movements. II. Systematic extent errors resulting from inertial anisotropy. Exp Brain Res 99:112–130

Hocherman S, Wise SP 1991 Effects of hand movement path on motor cortical activity in awake behaving rhesus monkeys. Exp Brain Res 83:285–302

Jeannerod M, Decety J 1995 Mental motor imagery: a window into the representational stages of action. Curr Opin Neurobiol 5:727–732

Jeannerod M, Paulignan Y, Weiss P 1998 Grasping an object: one movement, several components. In: Sensory guidance of movement. Wiley, Chichester (Novartis Found Symp 218) p 5–20

Johnson PB, Ferraina S, Bianchi L, Caminiti R 1996 Cortical networks for visual reaching: physiological and anatomical organization of frontal and parietal lobe arm regions. Cereb Cortex 6:102–119

Jordan MI 1990 Motor learning and the degrees of freedom problem. In: Jeannerod M (ed) Attention and performance XIII: motor representation and control. Lawrence Erlbaum Associates Inc, Hillsdale, NJ, p 796–836

Kalaska JF, Crammond DJ 1995 Deciding not to go: neuronal correlates of response selection in a go/no-go task in primate premotor and parietal cortex. Cereb Cortex 5:410–428

Kalaska JF, Scott SH, Cisek P, Sergio LE 1997 Cortical control of reaching movements. Curr Opin Neurobiol 7:849–859

Karst GM, Hasan Z 1991 Initiation rules for planar, two-joint arm movements: agonist selection for movements throughout the workspace. J Neurophysiol 66:1579–1593

Kettner RE, Marcario JK, Port NL 1996 Control of remembered reaching sequences in monkey, II. Storage and preparation before movement in motor and premotor cortex. Exp Brain Res 112:347–358

Koffka K 1935 Principles of Gestalt psychology. Harcourt Brace, New York

Kornblum S, Hasbroucq T, Osman A 1990 Dimensional overlap: cognitive basis for stimulus–response compatibility. A model and taxonomy. Psychol Rev 97:253–270

Mushiake H, Inase M, Tanji J 1991 Neuronal activity in the primate premotor, supplementary and precentral motor cortex during visually guided and internally determined sequential movements. J Neurophysiol 66:705–718

Prud'Homme MJ, Kalaska JF 1994 Proprioceptive activity in primate primary somatosensory cortex during active arm reaching movements. J Neurophysiol 72:2280–2301

Sakata H, Taira M, Kusonoki M, Murata A, Tanaka Y 1997 The parietal association cortex in depth perception and visual control of hand action. Trends Neurosci 20:350–357

Scott SH, Kalaska JF 1997 Reaching movements with similar hand paths but different arm orientations: I. Activity of individual cells in motor cortex. J Neurophysiol 77:826–852

Scott SH, Sergio LE, Kalaska JF 1997 Reaching movements with similar hand paths but different arm orientations. II. Activity of individual cells in dorsal premotor cortex and parietal area 5. J Neurophysiol 78:2413–2426

Sergio LE, Kalaska JF 1997 Systematic changes in directional tuning of motor cortex cell activity with hand location while generating static isometric forces in constant spatial directions. J Neurophysiol 78:1170–1174

Sergio LE, Kalaska JF 1998 Changes in the temporal pattern of primary motor cortex activity in a directional isometric force versus limb movement task. J Neurophysiol, in press

Shen L, Alexander GE 1997a Neural correlates of a spatial sensory-to-motor transformation in primary motor cortex. J Neurophysiol 77:1171–1194

Shen L, Alexander GE 1997b Preferential representation of instructed target location versus limb trajectory in dorsal premotor area. J Neurophysiol 77:1195–1212

Snyder LH, Batista AP, Andersen RA 1997 Coding of intention in the posterior parietal cortex. Nature 386:167–170

Tanaka K 1996 Inferotemporal cortex and object vision. Annu Rev Neurosci 19:109–139

Uno Y, Kawato M, Suzuki R 1989 Formation and control of optimal trajectory in human multijoint arm movement. Biol Cybern 61:89–101

Wise SP, Boussaoud D, Johnson PB, Caminiti R 1997 Premotor and parietal cortex: corticocortical connectivity and combinatorial computations. Annu Rev Neurosci 20:25–42

Zhang J, Riehle A, Requin J, Kornblum S 1997 Dynamics of single neuron activity in monkey primary motor cortex related to sensorimotor transformation. J Neurosci 17:2227–2246

DISCUSSION

Ebner: With regard to your idea about specification of information in time, I think we have shown that quite well for different motor parameters (Fu et al 1995). The correlations of the discharge with the movement parameters evolve over time. This is a well established concept.

Kalaska: As I said at the very beginning of my talk, this specification vs. selection model is derivative of many things, including the work done by several participants at this meeting: it is not at all an original idea. Nevertheless, I feel it's necessary to repeat it, because in much of the motor control literature there is still this idea that first a detailed plan of the movement is organized, and then the plan is executed. However, the neurophysiological data suggest that although the planning and execution concept has a certain validity, the plan and its implementation may evolve in parallel, dynamically in real time.

Georgopoulos: I am concerned about the time-varying directional tuning. It is obvious that you cannot compute 'directional tuning' for short time bins because it has been shown clearly that the fine time-course of cell activity reflects several movement parameters, in addition to a constant, stimulus-defined direction, including position, velocity and acceleration (Ashe & Georgopoulos 1994).

Therefore, regressing the time fine course of cell activity against the visually defined direction is practically meaningless and can be very misleading.

Kalaska: First of all, I agree with you that if you just analyse the response properties and represent the response properties of cells only in terms of directionality, you will probably get very misleading results over a short time course. We looked at the evolution of the instantaneous directional tuning of the cell I showed in my talk (Fig. 4) by calculating the preferred direction of the cell activity within a 50 ms window and incrementing that window in 10 ms steps. When you do that for the cell's activity in the isometric task, you find that the cell is strongly tuned to the left throughout the force ramp and the final static force phases of the task. In the arm movement task, however, you get something that looks very peculiar. The cell starts off strongly tuned to the left, as in the isometric task. But about midway through the movement, the cell's directionality appears to snap momentarily around to point almost in the opposite direction for 100 ms or so, before returning rapidly to the left again once the arm stabilizes over the peripheral targets. This is characteristic of many of the cells we have recorded in these tasks so far — their instantaneous directionality remains relatively stable across time in the isometric task but often shows a significant transient deviation and sometimes even a complete reversal during the movement phase of the arm movement task. At face value, one is forced to conclude from that analysis that the cells show highly labile directionality in the reaching task but not in the isometric task.

However, that may be largely an artefact of representing the cell's discharge in a parameter space of hand-centred spatial direction. For instance, when you record the activity of the major prime-mover muscles, they typically show the same combination of response properties in the two tasks as the cells, including an apparent transient 'change' in directionality during limb movement. However, no-one would propose that the muscles possess labile directionality during reaching movements. Their behaviour is clearly reminiscent of the classic 'triphasic burst' pattern of EMG that is well documented in rapid single-joint movements, including a reciprocal antagonist burst to brake movements in directions opposite to the pulling direction of the muscles. If one were to represent muscle activity in an intuitively more appropriate coordinate system of output forces or joint-centred torques or something, one may very well find that EMG directionality in force/torque space is much less variable than in hand-centred directional space. The same may also very well happen when we represent cell activity in other parameter spaces.

We decided to analyse cell activity in handspace coordinates at this first stage of analysis, knowing full well that it could be misleading, because it is the way that data from reaching tasks have usually been represented since we began this type of study more than 15 years ago. Also, it proved useful, because it was a convenient way to capture the often striking differences in temporal pattern of activity between tasks. But as you said, it can be misleading. Obviously, we have to do a systematic temporal regression analysis of cell activity in a variety of parameter spaces, such as handspace kinematics (position, direction, velocity, acceleration of hand motion), force output at the hand (which we measured directly), and maybe even joint-centred forces or torques (which we would have to estimate), among other possibilities. This sort of analysis is fraught with peril and must be done very carefully, so we have not rushed into it yet. Even after all that effort, that analysis may not provide definitive answers about the nature of the coupling between cell activity and motor output. As you said, the force and acceleration profiles will look very similar. Newton's second law of motion, force = mass × acceleration, says that they must. So is the cell signalling a kinematic or a kinetic parameter?

Goodale: When you record from cells in M1, do you know whether those are output neurons or interneurons? It seemed to me that if it is an output neuron it might be coding something rather different than if it were something on the way to becoming an output neuron. Is that a sensible question?

Kalaska: Yes. First, I try to avoid using the word 'coding', because it implies that we know what the cell is doing or what the parameter is. I prefer to use the term 'covariation', because that's really what we are looking at: the covariation of discharge with different parameters. Secondly, I do not know the identity of each of the cells that we've recorded. We intend to study that, at least for corticospinal cells, in the next monkey in the series. But I admit that the majority of these cells are the large cells in intermediate layers in the bank of the central sulcus, so it's likely that a large proportion of these cells are descending output cells, including corticospinal neurons. Simply because it takes quite a while to collect all this data, you need to have a cell that you know you're going to be able to hang on to for a couple of hours, so sampling bias dictates that we will have a lot of large pyramidal cells from layer 5.

Goodale: If you could identify which is which, then you might get some clue as to the nature of the covariation.

Kalaska: We intend to follow-up that problem. Many people have done it, Chris Fromm (Fromm 1983, Bauswein et al 1989) more successfully than any others, and he's found significant differences between these different output populations. Others have not shown that striking a difference. If you only lump them into pyramidal tract versus non-pyramidal track, often the difference between them is not all that impressive.

Andersen: You mentioned this very complete plan and executing the plan. When you think of a plan it is usually a pretty sketchy thing. When you talk of a plan do you include all the parameters of a movement? Doesn't it seem redundant to have that specific a plan? What do you think a plan is? It might be that if the plan is very sketchy, and this would fit with the activity you find in area 5, which is not as specific as activity you find in motor cortex.

Kalaska: The idea of a complete a priori plan (a complete representation of the entire time-course of the movement in some parameter space before movement initiation) is derived from many formal motor control models, especially optimization models. These models say that you produce a movement by first completely defining the entire time-course of a movement in some parameter space and then optimizing it for some cost function. Once you've done that process, which you have to do over the entire envelope of the movement to optimize it, then you execute the movement. These kinds of formal models require that you have a complete description of the movement before you then implement it.

Kawato: We should be careful about this point. As you said, traditional AI style computational models of motor planning and execution explicitly separate a planning stage and an execution stage. For example, Flash (1987) combined the planning in the extrinsic Cartesian space and equilibrium-point control. In this study, for two-joint arm reaching movements the hand equilibrium-point trajectory was planned in the Cartesian space by minimizing the hand jerk integrated over the entire movement duration according to Flash & Hogan (1985). Then, the control was executed in muscle space by using the planned equilibrium point. Thus, planning and execution were completely separate and purely hierarchically arranged in the two different spaces. I called this type of model a unidirectional model since the information flow is only from the visual space to muscle space (Kawato 1996). But in other types of optimal trajectory planning models, such as a minimum torque-change model (Uno et al 1989) or a minimum motor command change model (Kawato 1992), planning and execution are intermingled inseparably and are done online in real time because the smoothness constraint is imposed on motor commands. One example of neural network implementation of this type of dynamic optimization model is the forward-inverse relaxation model (Wada & Kawato 1993). I called this type of model a bidirectional model (Kawato 1996). Furthermore, Flash, in a more recent study (Jordan et al 1994), took an approach in which planning and execution are intermingled in complicated representations which are neither purely visual nor muscle. Thus, I would feel uneasy about your assertion that most of the computational models have separate planning and execution processes.

Kalaska: Your point is well taken. I was unfairly dismissing computational models in general with broad strokes, and I recognize that there are formal models in motor control, including some optimization models, that do not require a complete specification of the plan and that do allow for online planning and execution simultaneously. Again, I repeat that we do not pretend that this idea is entirely original, and claim priority on it. We simply wish to stress that for a proper understanding of the functional architecture of the motor system, one should not assume that 'planning' ends at the moment that muscles begin to contract.

Miller: Apostolos Georgopoulos described the discharge shown in the last slide in your talk in terms of its similarity to acceleration, 'except for the remaining tonic component'. It seems to me that that remaining tonic component is very likely a reflection of force or muscle related activity. Thinking back to the comment you made rather anecdotally at the end of the previous discussion, that you've seen some cells which look just like deltoid and others that look just like some kinematic parameter, are these different types of cells distributed in different layers? Or are they completely co-mingled?

Kalaska: In this particular study we looked mainly for the big cells which we knew we could hold on to for a long time, to increase the probability that we could test the cells in all tasks. In our previous study in which we used external loads (Kalaska et al 1989), we made a greater effort to record from cells across all layers. We reconstructed the penetrations. I can't tell you what the sampling bias is in our current study, but in the previous one we had a clear indication that cells in more superficial layers appear to be less sensitive to external loads. That is, their discharge was not as influenced by the external loads and therefore the kinetics of the task, whereas cells in the intermediate layers were very strongly affected by external loads. Therefore there is evidence for a laminar difference within motor cortex properties.

Kawato: For the last data you showed, which you also presented at the last Neuroscience meeting, the M1 neurons' firing frequency profiles seem to change largely according with the force exerted by the arm both in the isometric force condition and in movement condition (Kalaska & Sergio 1997). Suppose that you apply the inverse dynamics analysis for reconstructing the M1 neurons' firing frequency just like our study for the cerebellum (Shidara et al 1993). That is, if firing frequency is linearly regressed by a combination of hand position, velocity, acceleration and direction of the target, then I'm sure that acceleration should be the main component for reconstructing the firing frequency based on my eye-ball examination of the temporal waveforms which you show. This is consistent with the idea that M1 neurons encode inertia force even in movement condition. However, if this is true, there's a strong discrepancy between your data and Dr Georgopoulos' data, since in Ashe & Georgopoulos (1994) the acceleration was only a small factor in explaining M1 neurons' firing frequency. There are potentially several reasons for this. First, you use a relatively heavy manipulandum in movement conditions, so inertia force is a main force which must be generated by muscles. Second, you were in the most caudal part of the primary motor cortex. Could you comment on this?

Kalaska: I agree. We have to deal with the issue of differences in where we are sampling the cells. In this study we really were in the bank of central sulcus; we never went anterior to the bank. We were in the most caudal part of the primary motor cortex. As to the issue of regression analysis, I'm reluctant to say anything about likely results until we've done the analysis. However, it is quite possible that you are correct. Of the handspace kinematic parameters you proposed, acceleration might account for a significant part of the cell activity, at least during the movement period itself. As you know, that will also probably mean a good correlation with forces as well. Another factor that I suspect might be important is the exact nature of the regression model you use to partition the task-related variance of cell activity amongst the various movement parameters. As a simplistic example, suppose one uses a multifactorial model in which one term is direction, and two other terms are scalar non-directional values of velocity and acceleration. I am sure that the results of this analysis will be very different from a regression model in which the velocity and acceleration terms are vectors with their own directional components. This might account for some of the apparent discrepancies in the conclusions of some studies. It is an issue in which we are interested, and intend to look at it by systematically analysing cell activity using a number of different regression models.

Georgopoulos: I have some comments related to Mel Goodale's question. There are ways to try to identify cells you record from by the destination of their axons but you can't really use the brute force approach. For that purpose you will have to implant a large number of electrodes in different brain areas and stimulate through them to backfire the cell you record from. Now, it is not exactly feasible to cover all the possible projection areas, and the backfiring may not be consistently successful due to potential leakage of current to axonal branches. Cells projecting to the spinal cord can be identified reliably by stimulating the pyramidal tract but backfiring repeatedly a population of pyramidal tract cells may have unknown and untoward consequences on the area of the cortex from which the axons is coming. These effects can be profound and comprise both recurrent inhibitory and recurrent excitatory effects (see, for example, Stefanis & Jasper 1964a, b).

Another common question concerns whether we tend to record more frequently from output cells. Indeed, it is probable that most of the cells we record from are output cells but not necessarily pyramidal tract cells. Every pyramidal cell is an output cell but cells from the upper layers project to other cortical areas instead of the spinal cord to which cells from layer 5 project. The microelectrodes we use for extracellular recording tend to be more selective for larger cells, and pyramidal cells are generally larger than interneurons — hence the bias. Given this bias, the question is, where do these cells project? Although we cannot define the exact projection, we can identify the cortical layer in which the cell was recorded by reconstructing electrode tracts in histologically identified penetrations. For example, we have found similar directional tuning properties for cells in the upper and lower layers (Georgopoulos 1990), and John Kalaska and his colleagues have found some interesting differences with respect to the load sensitivity of cells recorded in the upper or lower layers (Kalaska et al 1989).

Our contribution to the problem of identification of different classes of cells has been a different one. Some years ago we published a paper in which we used a combination of cluster and discriminant analyses of the spike train to classify 1925 available cells to three different types based on (a) the average frequency of discharge, (b) the degree of burstiness in their discharge, and (c) the presence of a high percentage of short interspike intervals (Taira & Georgopoulos 1993). Three classes were thus distinguished: (a) cells with low discharge rate and low bursting (type A, 67.1%); (b) cells with low discharge rate but bursting (type B, 20.2%); and (c) cells with high discharge rate and low bursting (type C, 12.7%). Several considerations discussed in the aforementioned paper led us to propose that type A are pyramidal cells, whereas types B and C comprise both interneurons and pyramidal cells. I believe that this is useful approach to this difficult problem.

Goodale: In the case of the cells John Kalaska is looking at, the ones that show changes in covariation over time, is it known whether the outputs from these cells are driving cells in the ventral horn throughout the whole time that the change in covariation occurs — or whether the outputs drive the ventral horn cells only in the later stages? In other words, could there be differences in the way the outputs are gated at different points in the development of covariation?

Georgopoulos: If the effect of the motor cortical cell is directly on the motoneuron, the ultimate effect on the muscle will depend on the inputs from other systems converging on the same pool. Even when these motor cortical cells are very active, the effect on the muscle might be lost if another system exerts strong inhibition on the same pool.

With respect to differences between our results and those of John and his colleagues, I believe that a likely explanation lies in the different location of the recording sites. Most of our recordings over the years have been in the upper third and the crown of the anterior bank of the central sulcus but not deeply in that bank. I believe that John's recordings have been more in the latter region. Now, there are appreciable differences in the connectivity pattern between the lower bank and crown regions that could account for some of the differences. For example, the projections from area 5 are directed primarily to the crown and exposed part of area 4 and typically spare the lower parts of the anterior bank (Caminiti et al 1985). There could very well be gradients of changing functional properties along the anteroposterior dimension. Another reason for the differences could be selection bias. In our lab, we study all cells that change activity in association with arm movements outside the task (e.g. spontaneous movement, reaching for food, etc.). This is why our 'task-related' cells are a subset of the 'arm-related' cells, and the ratio of the number of cells in the former category over that of cells in the latter category provides a selection-free estimate of the frequency of occurrence of cells with specific functional properties. However, this may not be the case with respect to strategies adopted by other labs. For example, it seems to me that John's sample may be 'enriched' with acceleration-sensitive cells because such cells are specifically sought for study. Of course, this is fine as long as their numbers are not taken (or presented) as unbiased estimates of their true frequency of occurrence: there is a major difference between the statement that 'cells with such-and-such properties exist' and the statement, for example, that 'cells with such-and-such properties are extremely frequent (because only such cells are selected for study)'. This is apparently a *pars pro toto* fallacy, and I am afraid that this distinction is not made clearly in the literature.

Kalaska: Sampling bias is a major issue in any single-unit study. I have already acknowledged a sampling bias towards larger cells, most likely descending output cells in layer 5. There is also unquestionably a sampling bias due to penetration site. Cells like that in Fig. 4 are more prominent in the bank of the sulcus than in the more anterior exposed part of the motor cortex (Crammond & Kalaska 1996). I want to get back to a point that Dr Kawato raised, to re-emphasize that in this task the pendulum has a substantial mass. There is a heavy force transducer at the end of the pendulum, there is the mass of the pendulum itself, and we even added more weight to it for the static equivalence between the two paradigms. We are therefore not just talking about free arm movement anymore: there's an extra constraint. The monkey must generate a force to push that fairly massive object toward the target location. This is different from a free hand movement. We did see cells with these complex temporal waveforms in our earlier tasks (Kalaska et al 1989, Crammond & Kalaska 1996), but they were less common even in the same area. Your comment that not every cell looks like this is true, but about 60% of these cells in the bank of the central sulcus show this behaviour in the task conditions used in this particular study, including a manipulandum with substantially more mass than in the earlier studies. As for an 'enriched' sample, we did our best to avoid experimenter sampling bias. Selection criteria were the same that we have always used, namely a relation to proximal arm movements outside of the task and significant activity changes in either the isometric or movement tasks. How a cell responded in the movement task was never the deciding factor for inclusion in the sample. We did not seek out cells that looked like the acceleration curve or any other temporal profile, or exclude cells because they didn't have the 'right' profile.

Strick: It's important to emphasize that 60% of the cells that you recorded look like the data you presented. I imagine recordings of muscle activity would look very similar to these cells. The neurons in the motor cortex look like they have activity comparable to the agonist burst, antagonist burst, and second agonist burst seen in muscle. Thus, what is the essential difference between these cortical neurons and the muscles they influence?

Kalaska: Qualitatively they may look similar, but there are also quite obvious qualitative differences even before we do a detailed regression analysis. For instance, many motor cortex cells show a prominent brisk initial phasic burst at the onset of response in the isometric task, that overshoots the final tonic activity level of the cell at the final static force level. In contrast, the muscles just show a rapid but smooth ramp-like increase in contractile activity during the force ramp, without any initial dynamic overshoot. In the movement task, phasic response components were also often more prominent in the activity of cells than was evident in muscle activity. For instance, some motor cortex cells showed very exaggerated delayed 'antagonist' busts in the movement task in the direction opposite to their preferred direction, or a strong second burst in their preferred direction just as the movement was ending, that was not seen in any of the prime-mover muscles we studied. Other cells were essentially only phasic in both the isometric and movement tasks, whereas none of the prime-mover muscles were only phasic. This prominence of phasic response components in motor cortex cells compared to muscles has been well documented in many previous studies. Finally, there were a sizeable number of cells that had response components that would appear to have no relation to muscle activity at all. Everyone sees such cells. Whether or not they descend to the spinal cord and influence muscle activity, we cannot say. A cell whose response pattern looks like that of a muscle does not necessarily have a direct role in specifying muscle activity and, conversely, a cell that doesn't look like any muscle may none the less be contributing to the descending motor output command. Eb Fetz's work has shown the latter quite conclusively (Fetz et al 1996). Even cells making monosynaptic connections with spinal motoneurons can have very different response patterns than the motoneurons themselves, and their role in shaping muscle activity may not be intuitively obvious.

Georgopoulos: Any given EMG reflects the integrated inputs to the pool — that is, inputs from many sources.

Kalaska: The muscles do not show the dynamic response components that are quite evident in many primary motor cortex cells. There are many potential explanations for this, one simply being that the muscles work like low-pass filters: a lot of this dynamic response component is simply filtered out at the spinal level. There are many explanations for these differences.

Strick: The results you presented today suggest that neurons in the motor cortex are closer to the implementation end of the spectrum than the planning end.

Kalaska: Many of these cells are strongly affected by the change in the kinetics required to accomplish the overall objective of the task in the two situations. At that level of description they are much closer to the implementation end of the spectrum than to planning. However, that implies that planning can only involve representations of the global visuospatial requirements of the task, i.e. moving the cursor into the target window, independent of what the monkey must do to get it there. By that definition, many of these cells would appear to be implicated in task implementation.

Marsden: I wanted to move out of the motor cortex back into the parietal lobes, before you bury motor planning. We were talking about single motor actions and you said that planning for a single motor action doesn't seem necessary; it is all done online. Go back into the parietal cortex and planning for complex motor acts, like posting a letter, in which you carry out a series of individual motor actions: the human evidence strongly suggests that there are disorders affecting the posterior parietal cortex in which you can carry out each individual component of posting that letter reasonably well but you cannot put them together, because the plan is incorrect — so-called 'ideational apraxia'.

Kalaska: I didn't mean to say we should discount the possibility that there is any planning going on before the movement. On the contrary, there most certainly is some form or other of representation of motor intentions before movement begins. All I'm suggesting is that what is organized before the movement begins is a very rough sketch of the sequence of behaviours required to accomplish the goal, rather than — as some formal models propose — a complete kinematic description of the entire behaviour. What we want to suggest is that the central neural representation of the entire detailed time-course of each movement may only be generated dynamically in real time immediately before and during the movement itself. Furthermore, this representation need not be limited to those parameters that are usually presumed to be related to task implementation, that is, forces, torques and muscle activity. It may also involve neural representations of the temporal evolution of visuospatial constraints, of handspace-centred variables, or other possible information. These are aspects of the motor task that one might be more inclined to label as planning rather than as implementation, even though they are being generated during the response itself, because they do not reflect the biomechanical details of how the animal performs the task. This is why we suggest that these neural events might be better encompassed under the rubric of response specification, which makes no assumptions about the nature or the timing of the movement-related information being processed. The serial dichotomy implicit in planning versus execution or implementation might not be the best conceptual framework within which to interpret neural activity.

Johansson: I understand that your cells show covariance with the dynamics of the task, which is dependent on the mass and the mass distribution of the handle and so on. I also understand that the motion, as such, was rather critically damped. That is, there were no big overshoots in the movements, etc. For the monkey to produce these movements, they would need to rely on a rather qualified internal model of the properties of the manipulandum. Do these cells that you looked at have any relationship to learning of the mechanical properties of the manipulandum? I think that this would be something for the cortex to be involved in. Did you try to change the weight of the manipulandum and analyse the tuning of the behaviour to the new weight?

Kalaska: We haven't looked at adaptation. It's an area that we're increasingly interested in. But let's face it, this is an animal that has done hundreds of thousands of trials before we made the first neural recordings. So he has a very nice internal model of the mechanical properties of the system, and the data we collected were from a highly adapted system.

References

Ashe J, Georgopoulos AP 1994 Movement parameters and neuronal activity in motor cortex and area 5. Cereb Cortex 4:590–600

Bauswein E, Fromm C, Preuss A 1989 Corticostriatal cells in comparison with pyramidal tract neurons: contrasting properties in the behaving monkey. Brain Res 493:198–203

Caminiti R, Zeger S, Johnson PB, Urbano A, Georgopoulos AP 1985 Cortico-cortical efferent systems in the monkey: a quantitative spatial analysis of the tangential distribution of cells of origin. J Comp Neurol 241:405–419

Crammond DJ, Kalaska JF 1996 Differential relation of discharge in primary motor and premotor cortex to movement versus actively maintained postures during a reaching task. Exp Brain Res 108:45–61

Fetz EE, Perlmutter SI, Maier MA, Flament D, Fortier PA 1996 Response patterns and postspike effects of premotor neurons in cervical spinal cord of behaving monkeys. Can J Physiol Pharmacol 74:531–546

Flash T 1987 The control of hand equilibrium trajectories in multi-joint arm movements. Biol Cybernetics 57:257–274

Flash T, Hogan N 1985 The coordination of arm movements: an experimentally confirmed mathematical model. J Neurosci 5:1688–1703

Fromm C 1983 Contrasting properties of pyramidal tract neurons located in the precentral or postcentral areas and of cortical neurons in the behaving monkey. Adv Neurol 39:329–345

Fu Q-G, Flament D, Coltz JD, Ebner TJ 1995 Temporal encoding of the movement kinematics in the discharge of primate motor and premotor neurons. J Neurophysiol 73:836–854

Georgopoulos AP 1990 Neurophysiology of reaching. In: Jeannerod M (ed) Attention and performance XIII, Lawrence Erlbaum Associates Inc, Hillside, NJ, p 227–263

Jordan MI, Flash T, Arnon Y 1994 A model for the learning of arm trajectories from spatial deviations. J Cognitive Neurosci 6:359–376

Kalaska J, Sergio L 1997 Changes in M1 cell activity between isometric and movement tasks. Soc Neurosci Abstr 23:1554

Kalaska JF, Cohen DAD, Hyde ML, Prud'homme M 1989 A comparison of movement-direction related versus load direction-related activity in primate motor cortex, using a two-dimensional reaching task. J Neurosci 9:2080–2102

Kawato M 1992 Optimization and learning in neural networks for formation and control of coordinated movement. In: Meyer D, Kornblum S (eds) Attention and performance XIV. MIT Press, Cambridge, MA, p 821–849

Kawato M 1996 Bi-directional theory approach to integration. In: Inui T, McClelland J (eds) Attention and performance XVI. MIT Press, Cambridge, MA, p 335–367

Shidara M, Kawano K, Gomi H, Kawato M 1993 Inverse-dynamics encoding of eye movements by Purkinje cells in the cerebellum. Nature 365:50–52

Stefanis C, Jasper H 1964a Intracellular microelectrode studies of antidromic responses in cortical pyramidal tract neurons. J Neurophysiol 27:828–854

Stefanis C, Jasper H 1964b Recurrent inhibition in pyramidal tract neurons. J Neurophysiol 27:855–877

Taira M, Georgopoulos AP 1993 Cortical cell types from spike trains. Neurosci Res 17:39–45

Uno Y, Kawato M, Suzuki R 1989 Formation and control of optimal trajectory in human multijoint arm movement — minimum torque-change model. Biol Cybernetics 61:89–101

Wada Y, Kawato M 1993 A neural network model for arm trajectory formation using forward and inverse dynamics models. Neural Networks 6:919–932

The importance of the cortico-motoneuronal system for control of grasp

R. N. Lemon, S. N. Baker, J. A. Davis, P.A. Kirkwood, M. A. Maier and H.-S. Yang

Sobell Department of Neurophysiology, Institute of Neurology, Queen Square, London WC1N 3BG, UK

Abstract. Our recent work has revealed new evidence of the importance of direct cortico-motoneuronal (CM) connections for voluntary control of the hand. Most of these connections are derived from corticospinal neurons located in the M1 hand area, although there are some much smaller contributions from other secondary motor areas, such as the supplementary motor area (SMA). Intracellular recordings show that 75% of upper limb motoneurons in the chloralose-anaesthetized macaque monkey receive a monosynaptic projection from the corticospinal tract; evidence for non-monosynaptic, propriospinal excitatory influences from the corticospinal tract was conspicuously lacking in these anaesthetized preparations. Moreover, in the conscious monkey, hand and arm muscle motor unit responses to corticospinal tract input are dominated by single, brief peaks compatible with monosynaptic excitation. CM excitatory post-synaptic potentials, recorded from a comparable sample of hand and arm motoneurons in anaesthetized macaque and squirrel monkeys, were found to be larger and faster rising in the macaque, which is by far the more dextrous of the two species. CM cells facilitating a given muscle in the conscious macaque are distributed over a wide region of M1 cortex, and each contributes a particular pattern of discharge during a skilled task. In addition to their direct effects on target muscles there may be weaker but potentially important effects that derive from the synchronous binding of assemblies of output neurons. Synchronous oscillations between these neurons are particularly prevalent during steady grip, but disappear during digit movement.

1998 Sensory guidance of movement. Wiley, Chichester (Novartis Foundation Symposium 218) p 202–218

Cortical control and cortico-motoneuronal connections

The corticospinal tract is the major descending pathway through which the cerebral cortex gains access to the spinal machinery for movement. The tract is derived from extensive regions of the frontal and parietal lobes and receives contributions from cortical areas with marked functional differences, including primary (S1) and secondary somatosensory cortex, primary motor (M1), ventral and dorsal premotor areas, supplementary motor area (SMA) and cingulate cortex (Dum & Strick 1991, Porter & Lemon 1993). This suggests that fibres of the corticospinal tract, rather than subserving a single function, are probably involved in a multiplicity of functions. This idea is supported by the different pattern of termination within the spinal grey matter of corticospinal fibres from, for example, S1 and M1. There are some conspicuous differences in the proportion of terminals in different spinal laminae from the different motor areas of the frontal lobe (Dum & Strick 1996, Maier et al 1997a). In the cat there are even differences in spinal termination from different subregions of motor cortex (Martin 1996).

Cortico-motoneuronal (CM) projections form part of the overall corticospinal projection. These projections are particularly well developed in dextrous primates (Bortoff & Strick 1993, Maier et al 1997b), in which they have a striking pattern of postnatal development (Galea & Darian-Smith 1995, Armand et al 1997). There has been widespread interest in these projections because many of the motor responses elicited in humans by transcranial magnetic stimulation can be explained by activation of corticospinal neurons with direct, monosynaptic excitation of motoneurons (Rothwell et al 1991, Edgley et al 1997).

A considerable advance was made when spike-triggered averaging was used to identify CM neurons in the awake, behaving monkey (Fetz & Cheney 1980, Lemon et al 1986). This approach, which depends upon the production of post-spike facilitation (PSF) in the EMG of the neuron's target muscles, demonstrates the direct influence of the CM output. The CM nature of the post-spike effects can be rigorously tested using criteria developed in a recent model of the CM projection (Baker & Lemon 1998). The size of PSF produced by CM cells shows considerable variation (Porter & Lemon 1993); on average it is slightly larger than that produced by peripheral afferent inputs to the same motoneurons or by interneurons located in the same segments as the motoneurons (Fetz et al 1996). The precise proportion of corticospinal neurons that give rise to CM projections is still unknown, although it has been shown that PSF is generated by neurons with slowly-conducting axons, as well as by the larger, faster corticospinal neurons (see Porter & Lemon 1993). CM cells exert a selective influence over a small group of target muscles, their 'muscle field' (Fetz & Cheney 1980). CM cells have been shown to be active during a wide variety of tasks, and there is some evidence for task-specificity (see Porter & Lemon 1993). Those CM cells which exert effects on intrinsic hand muscles are particularly active during tasks such as the precision grip, which are characterized by a 'fractionated' pattern of muscular activity that is necessary for relatively independent finger movements. The cells are recruited in a manner that best exploits their pattern of CM influence, that is they tend to be most active when the muscles which they facilitate most strongly are the most active (Bennett & Lemon 1996). Finally, CM cells receive fast afferent inputs from the hand, involving both cutaneous and muscular receptors.

CM projections from different cortical areas

Both Dum & Strick (1996) and Rouiller et al (1996) have reported anatomical evidence that there are CM projections from motor areas other than M1. Of these areas, the SMA provides one of the largest contributions to the corticospinal projection terminating in the lateral parts of lamina IX in the cervical enlargement (Dum & Strick 1991). There are also some corticospinal terminals in the lateral motoneuronal cell groups originating from the dorsal and ventral cingulate motor areas (CMAd, CMAv) (Dum & Strick 1996).

We have made a quantitative comparison of CM connections from M1 and SMA in a recent anatomical and physiological study in adult macaque monkeys (Maier et al 1997a). Corticospinal projections were labelled by anterograde transport of WGA-HRP. The injection sites were guided by magnetic resonance imaging (MRI) scans to reveal the depth and curvature of the major sulci. In the two weeks prior to the injection, the arm/hand region of SMA was localized by intracortical microstimulation (ICMS) mapping under light sedation with ketamine. The hand regions of either M1 (2 monkeys) or SMA (2 monkeys) were injected. Injection sites were further defined by examination of cortico-cortical and callosal labelling. In one monkey, small injections (c. 1.0 μL) of WGA-HRP were made into M1 and SMA of opposite hemispheres for a direct comparison of the CM projection; this comparison is possible for the projection to lamina IX in the lower cervical segments, since neither M1 nor SMA gives rise to any significant ipsilateral projection to this lamina (Dum & Strick 1996, Armand et al 1997).

Quantitative densitometric analysis of the corticospinal projections (Armand et al 1997) revealed marked differences in the labelling within the hand muscle motor nuclei: projections from M1 occupied the whole area of these nuclei from the caudal C8 to caudal Th1 segment, whereas those from SMA only occupied 20–65% of the same area, depending on the segment. The densest projections from M1 occupied 21–65% of the nuclei, those from SMA only 1–6%.

These anatomical findings were confirmed by electrophysiological studies in which intracellular recordings were made from 30 antidromically identified hand and forearm motoneurons in two monkeys under chloralose anaesthesia. Pairs of intracortical electrodes with a separation of around 1.5–2 mm were placed in the hand regions of M1 and SMA, again guided by previous MRI scans and ICMS mapping. Single stimuli of 100–400 μA (duration 0.2 ms) evoked clear direct (D) and indirect (I) waves recorded from the corticospinal tract (see Fig. 1). The latencies of both D and I waves were clearly shorter from M1 than from SMA, indicating the presence of faster-conducting axons from M1 (typically around

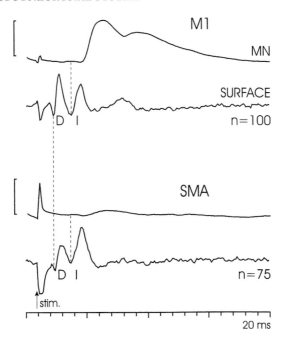

FIG. 1. Comparison of responses to corticospinal inputs from M1 and SMA in the anaesthetized macaque monkey. Intracellular recordings (upper records) from an ulnar motoneuron (MN) in response to local bipolar stimulation of the primary motor cortex (M1) and supplementary motor area (SMA). The lower traces are surface recordings from the dorsolateral funiculus at the same spinal level. Stimulation of M1 and SMA (single shock, 400 μA) evoked a series of descending volleys, the earliest of which reflects direct (D) activation of corticospinal neurons, the later waves being due to indirect (I), transsynaptic activation. Note the shorter latency of the volleys from M1, indicating faster-conducting elements originating from this area than from SMA. M1 stimulation evoked a large EPSP, with a much smaller effect from SMA. Both EPSPs occurred with a delay appropriate for monosynaptic action from the I wave, but not the D wave. Scale bar = 1 mV.

79 m.s^{-1}) compared with SMA (typically 61 m.s^{-1}); this result also suggested that these waves were derived from different populations of corticospinal neurons, i.e. there was no spread of stimulating effects from one region to the other. This was confirmed by showing that there was no occlusion between the volleys evoked by stimulating M1 and SMA simultaneously.

Nearly all (90%) tested motoneurons responded to M1 stimulation with early excitatory post-synaptic potentials (EPSPs), having latencies consistent with CM activation from the I wave (see Fig. 1). Only 57% responded in this way to SMA stimulation, and EPSP amplitudes were much smaller than for M1 (Fig. 1). There were some small, D-wave evoked EPSPs from M1; none were seen from SMA.

This indicates that the corticospinal volleys excited from the SMA to the sampled motoneurons had generally much weaker effects than those from M1.

Thus although corticospinal outputs from M1 and SMA may act in parallel (Dum & Strick 1996, Rouiller et al 1996) the direct CM influence from M1 upon hand and arm movements would appear to be much greater than that from SMA.

Non-monosynaptic effects from the corticospinal tract

Although there may be strong projections from M1 to the ventral horn, it is still the case that the densest and most numerous projections terminate in the intermediate zone (Dum & Strick 1996, Armand et al 1997). Thus it can be argued that there has been too much emphasis upon the importance of the direct CM projection, and there should be more attention paid to other, indirect pathways through which the motor areas of the cerebral cortex might influence spinal motoneurons.

In a recent study, we attempted to look for non-monosynaptic activation of upper limb motoneurons from the pyramidal tract via an upper cervical propriospinal system in the macaque monkey (Maier et al 1996). In the cat this propriospinal pathway is well developed and constitutes an important route for transmission of cortical commands to forelimb motoneurons (Illert et al 1978; see Alstermark & Lundberg 1992). This propriospinal pathway could provide a useful means for rapid updating of the cortical command based on changes in forelimb afferent information or in other descending motor systems (Alstermark & Lundberg 1992). Repetitive stimulation of the pyramidal tract in the cat evokes disynaptic EPSPs in forelimb motoneurons mediated by corticospinal activation of C3–C4 propriospinal interneurons.

We made intracellular recordings from a large sample of upper limb motoneurons in the chloralose-anaesthetized macaque monkey. Segmental delays were measured between the arrival of the corticospinal volley at the segment (recorded with an electrode on the surface of the dorsolateral funiculus) and the onset of postsynaptic potentials. Only 3% of these motoneurons showed evidence of clear-cut disynaptic EPSPs in response to repetitive pyramidal tract (PT) stimulation; 18% showed evidence of oligosynaptic effects (see Table 1). This compares with 77% of motoneurons showing monosynaptic EPSPs, and 65% showing a disynaptic inhibitory post-synaptic potential (IPSP) (a monosynaptic EPSP–disynaptic IPSP sequence was by far the most common response: 55% of motoneurons responded in this way). These results provided little evidence for non-monosynaptic excitation, and suggest that much of the corticospinal input to the intermediate zone could be concerned with other functions, including the segmental inhibition of motoneurons.

However, it could be argued that non-monosynaptic excitation was masked by the IPSPs. To minimize any such masking, a lesion of the dorsolateral funiculus at

TABLE 1 Comparison of corticospinal effects in hand and arm motoneurons in macaque and squirrel monkeys

	No. monkeys	No. motoneurons	% responses to single PT stimuli						% responses to repetitive PT stimuli		Mono EPSP properties	
			Mono EPSP	Mono EPSP+ IPSP	Mono EPSP+ late EPSP	All mono EPSPs	Pure IPSP	No effect	Di-(oligo-) EPSP	Total late EPSPs	Amplitude (mV±SD)	Rise time (ms±SD)
Macaque	10	110	18	55	3	76	10	9	3 (16)	19	2.46±1.52	1.05±0.2
Squirrel	6	93	38	42	0	80	16	4	15 (20)	35	0.74±0.48	1.30±0.37

Comparison of postsynaptic potential responses recorded from arm and hand motoneurons to stimulation of the medullary pyramidal tract (PT) with 200 μA shocks either singly or repetitively (train of three shocks at 300 Hz). Mono EPSP, EPSP appearing after a segmental delay of 1.1 ms or less; late EPSP, EPSP with a disynaptic (>1.2 ms) or oligosynaptic (>2.0 ms) segmental delay. Data from Maier et al (1997a,b).

the C5 segment was made to interrupt the lateral corticospinal tract. The objective was to remove corticospinal input to the lower cervical segments, leaving intact the C3–C4 propriospinal axons that travel in the ventrolateral funiculus (Alstermark & Lundberg 1992). However, in recordings made after such lesions, we found that only 14% of motoneurons showed disynaptic EPSPs after repetitive PT stimulation (Maier et al 1996). As expected, the lesions abolished the fast CM-EPSPs in many motoneurons; in a few they unmasked small monosynaptic EPSPs from slower-conducting corticospinal fibres.

Thus our experiments in the anaesthetized macaque have provided little evidence in favour of transmission of corticospinal excitation to upper limb motoneurons by a C3–C4 propriospinal system in this species. The results cannot be explained by the depressive effects of anaesthesia since it was possible to demonstrate oligosynaptic effects from other central and peripheral sources in the same motoneurons. In addition, it has been observed in the awake macaque monkey that PT stimulation evokes responses in single motor units in hand and arm muscles that are characterized by single peaks of short duration (< 1.0 ms), which are compatible with monosynaptic activation of the motoneuron; similar effects have been observed in cross-correlations between single CM cells and their target motor units (Porter & Lemon 1993, E. Olivier, S. N. Baker & R.N. Lemon, unpublished observations).

Although more complex circuits could be involved, the direct evidence so far suggests that as the CM system has become more developed within the primates, it has come to dominate or even supersede propriospinal transmission of cortical commands. If this were true, we would predict that in humans, where the CM system is most highly developed, propriospinal transmission of corticospinal commands would be of minor importance. There is indirect evidence for propriospinal transmission of cortical commands in humans (see Pierrot-Desseilligny 1996). The interpretation of the results in humans has been strongly influenced by the findings in the cat, and it has been proposed that a C3–C4 propriospinal system in humans is organized along the same lines as that found in the cat. The results described above imply important differences between cat and macaque in the transmission of corticospinal inputs to cervical motor nuclei, and suggest that it is unsafe to interpret results relevant to this transmission in humans on the basis of experiments in the cat.

CM connections in different primates

There are important differences in the extent to which CM connections are developed in different primates, and these differences appear to be correlated with the degree of digital dexterity (Heffner & Masterton 1983). The best-documented example of this is the study of Bortoff & Strick (1993) that compared the corticospinal projections in the New World squirrel (*Saimiri sciureus*) and cebus (*Cebus apella*) monkeys. In the more dextrous cebus monkey, there were abundant projections from the primary motor cortex to the motoneuron pools of the lower cervical cord, including those innervating the intrinsic hand muscles. These projections were extremely sparse in the squirrel monkey, which does not have the capacity to make the precision grip between thumb and index finger, and uses whole hand control for grasping objects (Costello & Fragaszy 1988). As indicated above, the CM projection from M1 in the Old World macaque monkey (*Macaca mulatta*) is also very extensive, in particular the projections to the hand muscle motor nuclei in the C7, C8 and Th1 segments (Armand et al 1997). The densest projections are found in the caudal Th1 segment; this rostro-caudal gradient probably results from the heavier CM projection to the motor nuclei of the intrinsic hand muscles, which are concentrated in the most caudal segments of the enlargement.

We have recently used electrophysiological methods to compare CM effects in the macaque with those in squirrel monkeys (Maier et al 1996, 1997b). Intracellular recordings of postsynaptic potentials were made from spinal motoneurons in response to PT stimulation in chloralose-anaesthetized monkeys. From the anatomical results it might be supposed that CM EPSPs would be rather uncommon in the squirrel monkey recordings, and a few motoneurons were indeed completely unresponsive to single PT stimuli (see Fig. 2B and C). However, as shown in Table 1, motoneurons with monosynaptic EPSPs were just as frequently encountered in the squirrel monkey as in the macaque (80% vs. 77%), with the commonest response being a monosynaptic EPSP–disynaptic IPSP sequence (42% vs. 55%). Here it is worth pointing out that the absence of corticospinal terminations within the motor nuclei in the squirrel monkey is not in itself evidence against the existence of CM connections, since corticospinal neurons could have direct synaptic connections on motoneuron dendrites that extend beyond the boundary of lamina IX. However, the EPSPs were both significantly smaller (mean 0.74 mV vs. 2.46 mV) and more slowly rising (1.30 ms vs. 1.05 ms) than in the macaque (Table 1). These features suggest that, in the squirrel monkey, the CM synapses are located at some distance from the motoneuron soma, which would be consistent with anatomical data (Bortoff & Strick 1993).

These results confirm that the CM system is less well developed in the squirrel monkey than in the macaque. Interestingly, in the squirrel monkey, repetitive activation of the PT evoked late EPSPs in more than a third of the tested hand and arm motoneurons (Table 1); three examples are shown in Fig. 2. This is a greater proportion than in the macaque. The origin of these effects is not yet known; should they prove to be mediated by a C3–C4 propriospinal system, this would support the idea that the corticospinal system in the New World squirrel

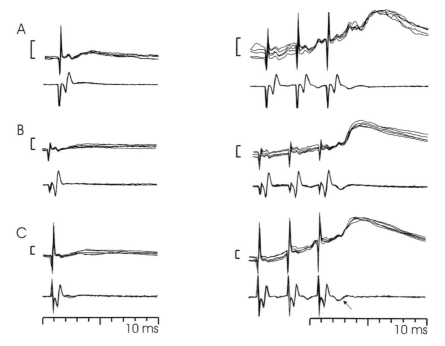

FIG. 2.   Responses of squirrel monkey (*Saimiri sciureus*) motoneurons to stimulation of the
pyramidal tract. These three motoneurons (A, ulnar; B, median; C, radial) were recorded
intracellularly in squirrel monkeys under chloralose anaesthesia. There was little or no
monosynaptic EPSP evoked by single PT shocks at 200 μA (left column), whereas large
EPSPs were observed after three shocks (right column). These EPSPs all had segmental delays
beyond the monosynaptic range (i.e. >1.5 ms), and ranged in amplitude from 1.3 to 2.5 mV.
Scale bars = 1 mV. (Reproduced with permission from Maier et al 1997b.)

monkey occupies an intermediate position between that of non-primates, in which
CM connections are sparse or absent but which possess a well-developed
propriospinal system for delivery of cortical commands, and that of other
primate species, including the macaque (and possibly humans), in which the CM
system is much better developed. The implication here is that the large, fast-rising
CM EPSPs in the more dextrous species is the means by which greater cortical
control of target muscles is achieved. In the hand muscles of stroke patients with
hemiplegia it has been observed that there is never any recovery of voluntary
activation of these muscles without a reappearance of the short-latency EMG
response to transcranial magnetic stimulation; this was not the case for muscles
acting at more proximal joints (Turton et al 1996). Of course, what is important
is selective control of functional synergists, because without this, independent
finger movement would not be possible (Schieber 1995).

Synchronous activity of CM neurons

CM cells with converging facilitatory action on a single motoneuron were referred to by Phillips as a 'colony' (see Phillips & Porter 1977). One of the most challenging organizational features of the CM system is that the members of the colony are distributed over an extensive region of M1, covering at least 6–8 mm^2; the distribution is non-continuous or 'patchy' (see Porter & Lemon 1993). Because CM cells branch and innervate motoneuron pools supplying several different muscles, each CM cell belongs to a number of different 'colonies'. Recent functional magnetic resonance imaging (fMRI) and positron emission tomography (PET) studies demonstrate that large areas of the M1 hand representation are coactivated during the performance of even simple movements (Dettmers et al 1995, Sanes et al 1995).

Recordings of local field potentials from extracellular microelectrodes placed within macaque M1 show bursts of oscillations, with a dominant frequency in the 20–30 Hz range (Baker et al 1997, Murthy & Fetz 1996a,b). These oscillations are coherent across wide regions of motor cortex, and even between M1 in the two hemispheres (Murthy & Fetz 1996a,b). When monkeys perform a precision grip, these oscillations can be readily observed during the hold period of the task (Fig. 3A) during which they are phase-locked with bursts of EMG activity in the contralateral hand muscles (Fig. 3B). We found strong coherence between cortical slow wave recordings and rectified EMG of hand and forearm muscles (Fig. 3C). Studies in humans have also revealed coherence between cortical activity measured with MEG and the EMG of steadily contracting muscles in the contralateral upper limb (Conway et al 1995, Salenius et al 1997).

Spike-triggered averaging of the local field potentials from simultaneously recorded spikes of CM cells and other PTNs has revealed that some of these were phase-locked to the oscillations (Baker et al 1997). This is an important observation because it indicates that cortical output neurons are part of the oscillating network of cells, and that CM connections could mediate the coherence between activity in cortex and in muscle. The oscillatory activity appears to be too weak to have much impact on the spike-triggered averages of rectified EMG compiled with spikes of single CM cells. It can be detected in some averages, but generally gives rise to much slower features than genuine CM effects (see Baker et al 1997, Baker & Lemon 1998).

The function of these oscillations in motor cortex remains unknown; some clues are provided by the observation that the 20–30 Hz coherent oscillations were present mainly during the hold phase of the precision grip task, and disappeared during movement. This is shown in Fig. 3D, which plots changes in the coherence between cortex and muscle during different phases of the precision grip task. The striking increase in coherence in the 20–25 Hz bandwidth during the hold period of the task is evident.

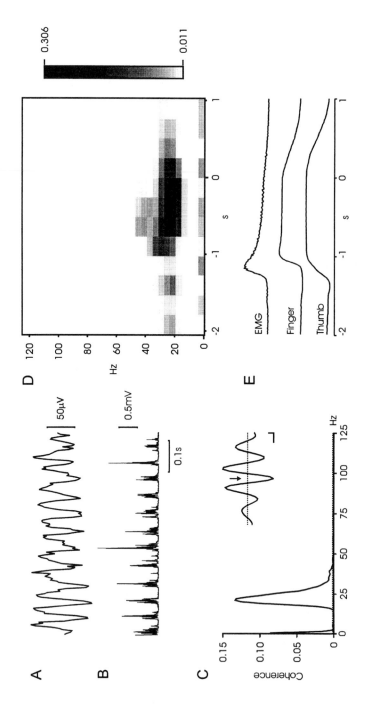

Synchronous oscillations in the CM outflow would act as a stronger input to recruit motoneurons than an asynchronous command having the same overall firing rate (Kirkwood et al 1984, Murthy & Fetz 1996b, Baker 1997). The oscillations might represent an efficient means of maintaining a tonic drive to motoneurons with as little CM activity as possible. Many CM neurons have relatively slow firing rates during the hold period, when compared to other phases of the task (Bennett & Lemon 1996). Thus oscillations could be considered as a stable dynamic state which can be held without excessive computational effort, and this might be advantageous for the maintenance of relatively stable motor states, such as a steady grip force to hold an object. The oscillatory activity may serve to link colonies of CM cells, making them particularly sensitive to common synaptic inputs (Stuart et al 1997).

Conclusions

The results reviewed here strengthen our view that the CM system is likely to make a major contribution to the cortical control of grasp. The evidence is growing that this direct system, which appeared late on the evolutionary scene, has superseded other more indirect corticospinal control mechanisms and is particularly well developed in the more dextrous of the primates. The advent of multiple electrode recording techniques is making it possible to investigate whether the entire colony of CM cells is co-activated during a given task, or whether sub-populations of the colonies function as task groups, facilitating the different combination of muscles that are required to achieve particular postures and movements.

FIG. 3.   Coherence between cortical local field potentials and hand muscle EMG during precision grip performed by a macaque monkey. (A) Cortical local field potential recording from M1 during the hold period of the precision grip task. (B) Simultaneously recorded rectified EMG from the adductor pollicis muscle. Clear oscillations can be seen in the cortical recording, which are phase locked to bursts in the EMG. (C) The coherence calculated between slow wave and rectified EMG, using all data available from one recording session. The peak around 25 Hz indicates consistent phase locking between the two signals in this frequency band. The dotted line just above abscissa is the theoretical significance level for the coherence ($P < 0.05$). Insets show cross-correlations calculated between the signals whose coherence is shown in the main part of the figure. Arrows show time of zero lag; dotted lines the zero correlation level. Peaks to the right of the arrow indicate EMG lagging cortical recordings. Scale bars = 20 ms, $r = 0.01$. (D) Variation in coherence with task performance. The abscissa shows time during task performance: analysis has been time-locked to the end of a successful hold period of the precision grip task (0 s). The ordinate shows coherence frequency. The grey scale map indicates how the coherence between cortical signal and EMG varies with time, using the scale on the right. (E) Variation during the task of the rectified adductor pollicis EMG, and the finger and thumb lever position signals. Parts D and E averaged from 274 successful trials of the task. (Based on data from Baker et al 1997.)

Acknowledgements

The authors would like to thank their colleagues and collaborators: Jean Armand, Michael Illert, Jens Nielsen, Tim Morris and Etienne Olivier. We thank Nora Philbin, Chris Seers, Kully Sunner and Natalia Ogjenovic for technical support. The authors thank The Wellcome Trust, Brain Research Trust and MRC for generous support.

References

Alstermark B, Lundberg A 1992 The C3–C4 propriospinal system: target-reaching and food-taking. In: Jami L, Pierrot-Deseilligny E, Zytnicki D (eds) Muscle afferents and spinal control of movement. Pergamon Press, Oxford, p 327–354

Armand J, Olivier E, Edgley SA, Lemon RN 1997 The postnatal development of corticospinal projections from motor cortex to the cervical enlargement in the macaque monkey. J Neurosci 17:251–266

Baker SN 1997 Quantification of the relative efficacies of asynchronous and oscillating inputs to a motoneurone pool using a computer model. J Physiol 504:116P

Baker SN, Lemon RN 1998 Computer simulation of post-spike facilitation in spike-triggered averages of rectified EMG. J Neurophysiol, submitted

Baker SN, Olivier E, Lemon RN 1997 Coherent oscillations in monkey motor cortex and hand muscle EMG show task dependent modulation. J Physiol 501:225–241

Bennett KMB, Lemon RN 1996 Corticomotoneuronal contribution to the fractionation of muscle activity during precision grip in the monkey. J Neurophysiol 75:1826–1842

Bortoff GA, Strick PL 1993 Corticospinal terminations in two New-World primates: further evidence that corticomotoneuronal connections provide part of the neural substrate for manual dexterity. J Neurosci 13:5105–5118

Conway BA, Halliday DM, Farmer SF et al 1995 Synchronization between motor cortex and spinal motoneuronal pool during performance of a maintained motor task in man. J Physiol (Lond) 489:917–924

Costello MB, Fragaszy DM 1988 Prehension in cebus and saimiri: 1. Grip type and hand preference. Am J Primatol 15:235–245

Dettmers C, Fink GR, Lemon RN et al 1995 The relation between cerebral activity and force in the motor areas of the human brain. J Neurophysiol 74:802–815

Dum RP, Strick PL 1991 The origin of corticospinal projections from the premotor areas in the frontal lobe. J Neurosci 11:667–689

Dum RP, Strick PL 1996 Spinal cord terminations of the medial wall motor areas in macaque monkeys. J Neurosci 16:6513–6525

Edgley SA, Eyre JA, Lemon RN, Miller S 1997 Comparison of activation of corticospinal neurones and spinal motoneurones by magnetic and electrical stimulation in the monkey. Brain 120:839–853

Fetz EE, Cheney PD 1980 Postspike facilitation of forelimb muscle activity by primate corticomotoneuronal cells. J Neurophysiol 44:751–772

Fetz EE, Perlmutter SI, Maier MA, Flament D, Fortier PA 1996 Response patterns and postspike effects of premotor neurons in cervical spinal cord of behaving monkeys. Can J Physiol Pharmacol 74:531–546

Galea MP, Darian-Smith I 1995 Postnatal maturation of the direct corticospinal projections in the macaque monkey. Cereb Cortex 5:518–540

Heffner RS, Masterton RB 1983 The role of the corticospinal tract in the evolution of human digital dexterity. Brain Behav Evol 23:165–183

Illert M, Lundberg A, Padel Y, Tanaka R 1978 Integration in descending motor pathways controlling the forelimb in the cat, 5. Properties of and monosynaptic connections on C3–C4 propriospinal neurones. Exp Brain Res 33:101–130

Kirkwood PA, Sears TA, Westgaard RH 1984 Restoration of function in external intercostal motoneurones of the cat following partial central deafferentation. J Physiol 350:225–351

Lemon RN, Mantel GWH, Muir RB 1986 Corticospinal facilitation of hand muscles during voluntary movement in the conscious monkey. J Physiol 381:497–527

Maier MA, Illert M, Kirkwood PA, Nielsen J, Lemon RN 1996 Lack of evidence for C3–C4 propriospinal transmission of corticospinal excitation to forearm motoneurones in the anaesthetized macaque monkey. J Physiol 494:63P

Maier MA, Davis JN, Armand J et al 1997a Comparison of cortico-motoneuronal (CM) connections from macaque motor cortex and supplementary motor area. Soc Neurosci Abstr 23:502.13

Maier MA, Olivier E, Baker SN, Kirkwood PA, Morris T, Lemon RN 1997b Direct and indirect corticospinal control of arm and hand motoneurons in the squirrel monkey (*Saimiri sciureus*). J Neurophysiol 78:721–733

Martin JH 1996 Differential spinal projections from the forelimb areas of the rostral and caudal subregions of primary motor cortex in the cat. Exp Brain Res 108:191–205

Murthy VN, Fetz EE 1996a Oscillatory activity in sensorimotor cortex of awake monkeys: synchronization of local field potentials and relation to behavior. J Neurophysiol 76:3949–3967

Murthy VN, Fetz EE 1996b Sychronization of neurons during local field potential oscillations in sensorimotor cortex of awake monkeys. J Neurophysiol 76:3968–3982

Phillips CG, Porter R 1977 Corticospinal neurones: their role in movement. Academic Press, London

Pierrot-Deseilligny E 1996 Transmission of the cortical command for human voluntary movement through cervical propriospinal premotoneurons. Prog Neurobiol 48:489–517

Porter R, Lemon RN 1993 Corticospinal function and voluntary movement. Physiological Society Monograph. Oxford University Press, Oxford

Rothwell JC, Thompson PD, Day BL, Boyd S, Marsden CD 1991 Stimulation of the human motor cortex through the scalp. Exp Physiol 76:159–200

Rouiller EM, Moret V, Tanne J, Boussaoud D 1996 Evidence for direct connections between the hand region of the supplementary motor area and cervical motoneurons in the macaque monkey. Eur J Neurosci 8:1055–1059

Salenius S, Portin K, Kajola M, Salmelin R, Hari R 1997 Cortical control of human motoneuron firing during isometric contraction. J Neurophysiol 77:3401–3405

Sanes JN, Donoghue JP, Thangaraj V, Edelman RR, Warach S 1995 Shared neural substrates controlling hand movements in human motor cortex. Science 268:1775–1777

Stuart G, Schiller J, Sakmann B 1997 Action potential initiation and propagation in rat neocortical pyramidal neurons. J Physiol 505:617–632

Schieber MH 1995 Muscular production of individuated finger movements: the roles of extrinsic finger muscles. J Neurosci 15:284–297

Turton A, Wroe S, Trepte N, Fraser C, Lemon RN 1996 Contralateral and ipsilateral EMG responses to transcranial magnetic stimulation during recovery of arm and hand function after stroke. Electroencephalogr Clin Neurophysiol 101:316–328

DISCUSSION

Stein: I want to ask about those thin corticospinal fibres, of which there should be 90%. Where do you think they run in the cord? You cut the lateral cord of your spinal tract, I believe. Secondly, since they conduct so slowly, some of them as slowly as 1 m/s, what do you think they are doing?

Lemon: When we made these lesions, we were basically trying to cut the upper half of the lateral funiculus. If you go too deep, you open yourself to the possibility that that you're also cutting the propriospinal fibres, which are supposed to be in that ventral half of the lateral funiculus. We didn't attempt in any of those lesions to get a complete abolition of the volley that we were recording below the lesion. Typically, we were trying to make the lesion so that we got it down to about 20% of the pre-lesion level. The other possibility is that the surviving fibres travel in the anterior funiculus; we can't dispute that. The slow, monosynaptic effects that we recorded after the CS lesion with latencies of 1.5–3 ms would correspond to fibres conducting down as low as 20 m/s. As you say, there are many that are even smaller than that: we don't know much about these. Some may be involved in autonomic functions. There is good evidence in the rat that there are projections from the limbic areas which are concerned with changing heart rate and vasomotor functions.

Fetz: The simultaneous recordings of many cortical cells that can be correlated with each other and with the target muscles is an exciting development. The fact that CM cells with common target muscles are synchronized again raises the issue of the extent to which the post-spike facilitation might be mediated by a synchrony between cells. Years ago, Wade Smith (1989) also recorded and cross-correlated CM cells: he also found that CM cells with common target muscles often appear to be synchronized. However, the synchrony peaks in cross-correlograms between the cells are usually much broader than the time course of the post-spike effect. So synchrony is not a plausible explanation. In fact, he compiled the spike-triggered averages from the unsynchronized spikes to show that they could independently produce post-spike facilitation (Smith & Fetz 1989). In your records, some of the cross-correlograms look rather sharp, down to several milliseconds. Are you satisfied that this could not be mediating an effect in the post-spike facilitation?

Lemon: The mean width of the cross-correlation effects that we are seeing is around 10 ms, but that includes some much briefer peaks. Obviously, what we need to do is do is exactly what you have done and re-compile the averages, having removed those synchronous spikes. Most of the published examples of large cross-correlation effects are from cells recorded on the same electrode, so we never really knew the true amplitude of the peaks in the resulting 'dead zone' (where both spikes fire close together and cannot be reliably discriminated). It is quite interesting that in the cases where we have found pairs of CM cells with common target muscles, we have always seen cross-correlation effects. We have seen such effects for a pair of CM cells as far apart as 1.6 mm.

Fetz: One of the interesting things Wade Smith found is that CM cells that projected to different muscles were not synchronized. Although they were co-activated and projected to synergistic muscles co-activated, these CM cells didn't show common input synchrony, which was quite surprising. We expected that cells facilitating co-activated muscles would be driven by some higher-order common input; instead, they seem to receive independent input. We'll have to see whether this is borne out by further studies.

Jeannerod: You showed that the degree of coupling between cells changes during the grip. In fact, this is exactly what one would expect, because the grip is not a single trajectory. It would be nice if you could correlate these changes in coupling of cells with the ongoing pattern of muscle contractions.

Lemon: One of the fascinating things is that in the precision grip task, the local field potentials which show this oscillation at 20–25 Hz are almost entirely seen during the steady hold period. One of the things that this could reflect is the fact that during this period, which we would regard as relatively low-level computation of the output system, it may be advantageous to synchronize large numbers of output neurons to support a pattern of target muscle contraction. During maintenance of a steady grip, you actually co-contract a large number of muscles, and all the temporal shaping that occurs during the movement is no longer required. In those conditions the synchronous potentials are clearly present, but as soon as you begin to move that all disappears and there is much more phasic activity, which seems to be necessary to recruit the muscles in a more independent fashion (Bennett & Lemon 1996).

Rizzolatti: 20–25 Hz oscillations can be observed also at rest. I am not sure therefore whether they are to be referred necessarily to a pattern of muscle co-activation.

Lemon: I agree, but one should be careful here. We're talking about a signal that you can detect from the whole cortex, that happens to have a frequency of 20–25 Hz. This doesn't necessarily mean that it's generated by the same system. Of course you can't test whether that signal is coherent with the muscle activity in a completely relaxed subject! But what I would suggest, however, is that the maintenance of a steady co-contracted state is a low-level function for the motor system.

Strick: With regard to the C3–C4 propriospinal system, have you looked at stimulating in the lateral reticular nucleus to see if you actually can get evidence for that system the way it was classically described?

Lemon: We have done extensive mapping of the lateral reticular nucleus (LRN), because it is known from the cat that C3–C4 propriospinal neurons have both a descending axon to the motor nucleus and an ascending one to the LRN. Most of the motoneurons we recorded show an early ESP to stimulation in the LRN. However, many motoneurons with effects from the LRN had no late effects from the pyramidal tract (as one would expect if a propriospinal system mediated corticospinal excitation). If indeed the late EPSPs from the pyramid were conducted by such a system, you would expect that there would be a good parallelism between those two sets of observations, but there isn't. However, there are problems about trying to stimulate the LRN in the monkey: you may activate other ascending (e.g. spinothalamic) and descending systems in the vicinity of the LRN. This is a possible complication. All I can say is that the responses in the monkey from stimulating the LRN are identical to those in the cat. Our conclusion from these experiments in the monkey would be that if there is a propriospinal system in the primate — and it would be very surprising if there weren't — it does not transmit the corticospinal command to any significant extent. It may well transmit commands issued by other descending systems, but the important role it has in the cat of transmitting the corticospinal command may have been superseded because of the existence of direct CM connections to motoneurons.

Miller: I would like to make an additional comment beyond what Mark Jeannerod said about the task-related variation in the level of co-activation between the neurons. At least in the example you showed, the amount of co-activation seemed to be inversely related to the discharge of the cell. This suggests to me that these cells are receiving a lot of other inputs from cells which covary, but are not synchronized at the level of individual action potential. What functional significance does this common input have?

Lemon: Obviously we're very interested in what effect these two different types of connectivity, the stochastic short-term synchrony and the oscillatory synchrony, might have on the shape of the spike-triggered averages. Our results so far indicate that the 25 Hz effect rarely shows itself in the post-spike facilitation. I think the reason for this is that the amount of time that the cell spends in this oscillatory mode is relatively small and therefore concerns only a relatively small percentage of the spikes that the cell is generating. But if you do the averaging just on the hold period of the task, then you begin to see the slow periodic effects come up in the spike-triggered average (STA) of the muscle. But if you take the all of the data during the task performance, it's relatively easy to distinguish from the sharp rise in effects that we think are due to the direct synaptic input to motor neurons as opposed to those which are due to the fact that that CM cell is part of an oscillating network.

References

Bennett KMB, Lemon RN 1996 Corticomotoneuronal contribution to the fractionation of muscle activity during precision grip in the monkey. J Neurophysiol 75:1826–1842

Smith WS 1989 Synaptic interactions between identified motor cortex neurons in the active primate. PhD Thesis, University of Washington, Seattle, WA

Smith WS, Fetz EE 1989 Effects of synchrony between corticomotoneuronal cells on post-spike facilitation of muscles and motor units. Neurosci Lett 96:76–81

Combination, complementarity and automatic control: a role for the cerebellum in learning movement coordination

W. T. Thach

Department of Anatomy and Neurobiology, Washington University School of Medicine, 660 S. Euclid Avenue, St. Louis, MO 63110, USA

Abstract. We have examined several different paradigms of adaptation and of 'acquisition of skill' — skill defined as a movement specialized to meet a certain goal and gained through practice. In each paradigm, change occurs through trial-and-error performance. In some of the tasks, damage of cerebellar cortex impairs adaptation and not performance. The deficits in performance cannot explain the deficits in adaptation. In some of the tasks, the discharge of Purkinje cells and, by inference, the discharge of inferior olive cells and mossy fibres has behaved in a manner consistent with the Marr–Albus theory of motor learning. We extend the theory to show how parallel fibres could implement both the coordination of complex movements and the learning of new movements. The size of the response combinations would be proportionate to the length of parallel fibres. The mechanism proposed here would permit optimized complex movement behaviours to respond to specific behavioural contexts rapidly, stereotypically and automatically. The mechanism would permit storage of many context-response couplings, and many complex responses. The mechanism would permit privacy, individuality and a large number of behavioural responses.

1998 Sensory guidance of movement. Wiley, Chichester (Novartis Foundation Symposium 218) p 219–232

When reaching out to grasp and pluck an apple, we are aware of the apple's location, shape and our intention to move. We are little aware of the movements used to grasp, less those to reach, and not at all of the muscle strategies (Jeannerod et al 1998, this volume). Yet several hundred muscles are active in the correct number, combination, intensity and timing to implement the act. We are quite unaware that the first muscle to contract is the tibialis anterior in the lower leg, which compensates the moving arm's inertial torque on trunk and legs, preventing falling over backwards (Diener et al 1989). Without the cerebellum, single-jointed movements are accurate (Thach et al 1992a,b), but multi-jointed movements lack coordination. As subjects with cerebellar injury reach to grasp an object, the tibialis anterior muscle no longer leads the response (Diener et al 1989). The purpose of this paper is to emphasize the importance of the cerebellum in combination, complementarity and automation of compound movements.

Webster's defines these terms as follows:

- Combination: the result or product of combining: a union or aggregate made by combining one thing with another; a union of mechanical parts so arranged that they interact to produce a practical result.
- Complementarity: the interrelationship — or completion or perfection brought together by interrelationship — of one or more units supplementing, being dependent upon or standing in polar opposition to another unit or other units.
- Automatic: involuntary either wholly or to a major extent so that any activity of the will is largely negligible.

There is evidence for a dissociation in the control of simple movements and compound movements. Unit recording in and inactivation of the deep nuclei of the cerebellum suggested control of compound but not simple movements (Schieber & Thach 1985a,b, Thach et al 1992a,b, 1993, Goodkin et al 1993). By contrast, recording in and inactivation of motor cortex (Schieber et al 1991) suggested control of simple as well as compound movements. We extended the Marr–Albus model (Marr 1969) to propose that the parallel fibre contact on the beam of many somatomotor-coded Purkinje cells could be the mechanism that combines downstream motor nuclei elements and ultimately muscles (Thach et al 1992a,b, 1993, 1995, Bastian et al 1998).

What does the cerebellum learn?

We have previously suggested a cerebellar role in learning the coupling of antagonist with agonist muscle activity in the functional stretch reflex used to hold a position despite perturbations (Gilbert & Thach 1977) and terminating a voluntary ballistic movement to a visual target (Keating & Thach 1990, 1991, 1992). We shall discuss here the coordination of agonists, antagonists and synergists in the adjustment of eye–hand coordination in throwing while adapting to laterally displacing prisms (Martin et al 1996a,b, Greger et al 1996). In throwing, eyes (and head) fixate the target and serve as reference aim for the arm. Coordination between gaze direction and arm throw is a skill: it is developed and maintained by practice. When wedge prism spectacles are placed over the eyes with bases to the right, the optic path is bent to the right, and the

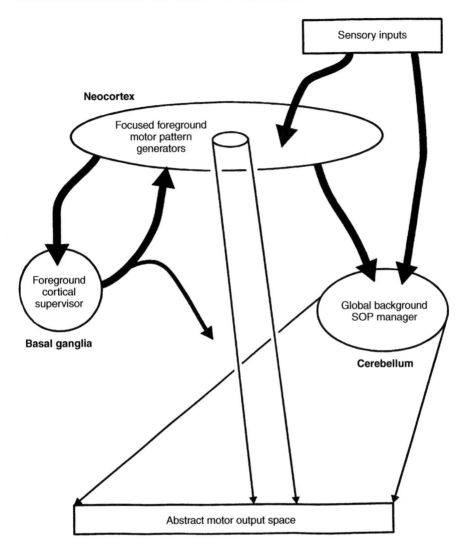

FIG. 1. Scheme showing cerebral cortex and basal ganglia supporting conscious aspects of movement and cerebellum supporting automatic aspects of movement (C. H. Anderson, personal communication).

eyes (and head) move to the left to fixate the target. The arm, calibrated to gaze and the line of sight, throws to the left of the target. With practice, the calibration changes, the gaze–throw angle widens, and the arm throws closer to and finally on-target. Proof that the gaze position is the reference aim for the arm throw trajectory occurs when the prisms are removed and the arm throws. The

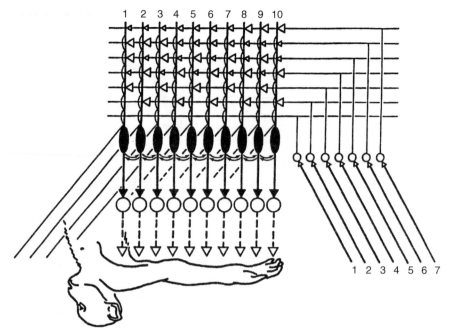

Cerebellar circuitry is a candidate because of:

- *Climbing fibres* — one source, one-to-one contact on Purkinje cells, powerful synapse, low firing
- *Mossy fibres* — many sources and types of information, high frequency firing
- *Granule cells* — multiplex mossy fibre input, $>10^9$ in number
- *Parallel fibres* — spread the context over several motor 'mode' zones, link the response elements across several mode zones

Experimental support

- Ablation of cerebellar cortex impairs/prevents movement adaptation and learning
- Neural recording during movement shows CS (climbing fibre response) firing at low rate, unrelated to movement, while SS (parallel fibre response) fires at high rate, related to movement.
- Neural recording during learning shows CS related to performance error and learning, and SS changing as a function of CS occurrence.
- Paired electrical stimulation of climbing + mossy fibres shows that CS occurrence causes changes in SS response to parallel fibre input (long term depression).

FIG. 2.   Cerebellar theory of motor learning.

calibration of a widened gaze–throw angle, compensating for the previously left-bent gaze, persists: the eyes are now on-target, and the arm throws to the right of target an amount almost equal to the original leftward error. With practice, the angle between gaze direction and throw direction is again recalibrated: each throw moves closer to and finally on-target (Kane & Thach 1989, Martin et al 1996a,b).

Prism adaptation in throwing is specific for arm and type of throw (Martin et al 1996b). Alternating the throwing arm between right and left, subjects threw without prisms with the right then left arm, with prisms with the right arm, then without prisms with the left then right arm. Prism adaptation occurred in all subjects in the right arm, did not influence throws with the left, and readapted only during throws with the right arm. Throwing with the same right arm alternating overhand and underhand, subjects threw underhand then overhand with the right arm, overhand with prisms, and finally underhand then overhand without prisms. With prisms, all subjects adapted the overhand throw. In most (six of eight subjects), subsequent underhand throws showed no influence of prior overhand adaptation. In these subjects, prior overhand adaptation persisted in subsequent overhand throws despite intervening underhand throws, and readapted only with repeated overhand throws. Two subjects showed carryover from overhand adaptation to underhand throws, which then disappeared with underhand throwing, with diminution of the training effect on subsequent overhand throws. Thus, most subjects adapted one task and not another, even though many body parts and muscles participated in both tasks. This implies separate central channels for adaptation of separate tasks.

To test further that the cerebellum is indeed involved in wedge prism adaptation of limb movements to visual targets (Baizer & Glickstein 1974, Weiner et al 1983, Kane & Thach 1989), we studied patients with cerebellar damage (Martin et al 1996a) including generalized cerebellar atrophy, lesions of the superior vermis, damage of the inferior olive, infarcts in the distribution of the posterior inferior cerebellar artery (PICA; possibly with inferior cerebellar peduncle involvement) and focal infarcts in the contralateral basal pons or ipsilateral middle cerebellar peduncle. This group had impaired prism adaptation, with little or no limb ataxia. By contrast, subjects with infarcts in the distribution of the superior cerebellar artery territory (SCA; involving the anterior superior surface of the cortex and the dentate nucleus) or in the cerebellar receiving zones of the thalamus adapted normally, but had marked limb ataxia. These results implicate climbing fibres from the contralateral inferior olive via the ipsilateral inferior cerebellar peduncle, and mossy fibres from the contralateral pontocerebellar nuclei via the ipsilateral middle cerebellar peduncle as being critical for this adaptation.

How many gaze–throw calibrations can be stored (Martin et al 1996b)? Following extended training with the same wedge prism spectacles (12 000 throws, 6 weeks of alternate prism/no-prism throws), subjects stored two eye–hand calibrations (no-prism and learned prism). Trained subjects threw successfully on-target immediately upon donning the learned prisms (gaze away from target) and immediately upon removing them (gaze on target). When donning a novel pair of prisms, subjects adapted as in the naïve state (above): they threw off-target in the same direction as the prism-bent gaze, gradually adapted throws onto target, and then threw off-target in the opposite direction when the novel prisms were removed. This adaptation affected both the no-prisms and learned-prisms calibrations; each calibration had to be re-adapted independently. This showed that two (or more) gaze–hand calibrations can be stored simultaneously. Storage has been maintained without intervening practice for now over 27 months.

What variable(s) are adapted in throwing? To determine what body parts are involved in the long-term gaze–throw recalibration, we video-recorded positions of head-in-space and shoulders-in-space while throwing with and without prisms (Martin et al 1996b). Knowing that eyes foveated the target and that throws hit the target, we computed the angular positions of eyes-in-head, head-on-trunk and trunk-on-arm. We found that gaze adjustment was not confined to any one set of two members (e.g. eyes-in-head, or head-on-body, or body-on-arm), but instead was distributed across all three sets of coupled body parts.

What is coordination?

The coupling of body parts varied from throw to throw despite relative invariance of hits (Greger et al 1996). In long-term prism/no-prism trained subjects, we video-recorded positions of head, shoulders and arm while throwing with and without prisms across trials. Again, the gaze adjustment was not confined to any one set of two members, but was distributed across all three sets of body parts. The coupling changed unpredictably across sessions and trial-by-trial within sessions. The variation in coupling across body parts was larger than the variation of the hits. Thus, the coupling of the body parts changes interdependently (complementarity) to permit the high accuracy of hits.

We have created an anatomic model to account for a cerebellar role in coordinated compound movement and in motor learning (Thach et al 1992a, 1995). In this model, different modes of control are mapped discretely within each of the deep nuclei. Fastigius controls equilibrium, stance and gait under vestibular, somesthetic and visual control. Interpositus controls agonist–antagonist muscle couplings in various somatosensory reflexes. Dentate controls synergists in movements directed into extrapersonal space, under control from frontal, premotor, prefrontal and parietal cortex. Each nucleus appears to contain a complete body map. Body parts within each body map, and adjacent body maps, are coupled by the parallel fibre beam which combines many Purkinje cells, thereby combining muscles. Complementarity may be due to the many different body part configurations all being stored at the level of the parallel fibre–Purkinje cell synapse. Nevertheless, complementarity could be more simply handled by the reciprocal connections between neighbouring (and to some distance) Purkinje cells. Thus, increased activity in cells governing one muscle would automatically and proportionately inhibit cells governing synergist muscles. Such a mechanism would in theory be sufficient to explain complementarity of movements.

Do parallel fibres indeed serve such a function? We have examined the behaviour of children in whom, to remove tumours from the fourth ventricle, neurosurgeons have split the posterior vermis from lobules X and IX to as far anteriorly as V, sparing the deep nuclei and the crossed fastigial output projections (Bastian et al 1998). Within a month following the surgery, these children had been judged normal or nearly so in coordination. We found that their recovery could indeed be remarkable: they could walk, run and even hop on one leg in one place 10 or more times without falling. Yet in the seemingly relatively 'simple' act of walking tandem heel-to-toe along a line, none could make more than three successful single steps without having to side-step voluntarily to prevent falling. We interpret the preservation of ipsilateral leg stance and movement contrasted with the impairment of bilateral leg movement as a loss of cross-body coordination likely due to the midline cut of crossing parallel fibres.

Does the cerebellum store memories?

Damage of the cerebellum prevents control of interaction torques during reaching (Bastian et al 1996). Multi-jointed movement is more complex than a summed combination of single-jointed movements, because interaction torques (inertial, centripetal, Coriolis) are generated by one linkage moving on another. Fast compound reaching movements increase the magnitude of the interaction torques (Soechting & Lacquaniti 1981) and normally require subjects to predict and compensate them. Inverse dynamic equations (Soechting & Lacquaniti 1981) were used to estimate (1) net torques and (2) interaction torques at the elbow and shoulder joints in normal controls and patients with cerebellar lesions performing two-jointed reaching movements. Patients had curved trajectories that overshot the target because of abnormal net torques, in turn due to their inability to control interaction torques. Patients attempted to eliminate the need for control of interaction torques by reducing velocity and by decomposing the reach into movements made at each single joint *seriatim*. As reach velocity increased, the errors increased, consistent with an inability to control interaction torques. Patients made errors in the initial direction of movement, consistent with an inability to predict and compensate interaction torques. EMG of biceps and anterior deltoid showed that onset of all muscle activity was delayed, that the relative timing of composite muscles was normal during early phases of movement, but that the timing broke down as the movement proceeded. The data are consistent with views that the cerebellum both helps to initiate movement and sends predictive signals to prevent errors that otherwise would occur because of uncontrolled interaction torques. We speculate that the cerebellum uses motor commands and somatosensory feedback during early phases of the movement to trigger *ad hoc* learned patterns of muscle activity so selected, scaled and timed as to compensate the interaction torques that develop during later phases of the movement. The predictive compensation is learned (Sainburg et al 1993, Topka et al 1994), and requires somatosensory feedback (Sainburg et al 1993). The learned adjustment is apparently removed by damage to the cerebellar cortex. This suggests to us that the learned programme is stored within the cerebellar cortex.

Conclusions

Cardinal functions of the cerebellum, in contrast to functions of other elements within the motor circuitry, include context–response linkage, combination of downstream motor elements and the provision for their complementarity. Linkage is formed through trial-and-error practice, by inferior olive climbing fibre actions on parallel fibre–Purkinje cell synapses. The capacity for memory storage of different context–response linkages is theoretically proportionate to the number of granule cells and the lengths of the parallel fibre. The size of response combinations is theoretically proportionate to the length of the parallel fibre. Complementarity might most simply be implemented by reciprocal inhibitory interconnections between Purkinje cells. The mechanisms proposed here would permit:

- Automation and speed of context–response coupling.
- Combination of many body parts into complex acts.
- Complementary variation among body parts, at the same time preserving invariance of the goal-oriented resultant.
- Storage of many context–response couplings.
- Privacy and individuality of each context–response coupling, despite the large number of behavioural responses, and the similarity of response components within each.
- Optimization of complex movements through trial and error learning.
- Coordination of both static and dynamic compound movements.
- Stability of storage over time and lack of practice.
- Learning new and adapting old movements.

Such a mechanism might theoretically also link separate motor responses into sequences, in which a prior movement serves as a context for subsequent movements. The mechanism might theoretically underlie 'cognitive' contributions of the lateral cerebellum. The contribution would allow multiple parallel background mental operations (analogous to multiple automatic muscle actions and, paradoxically, 'unconscious') concurrently with conscious foreground mental operations.

Acknowledgements

This work was supported by grants to WTT from the National Institutes of Health (NS12777) and the Office of Naval Research (N00014-92-J-1827); by NIH training grant NRSA 5 T32 GM0700 for T. A. Martin, H. P. Goodkin, S. Kane and M. H. Schieber; and by a grant from the Foundation for Physical Therapy Research (94D-18-BAS-01) to A. J. Bastian.

References

Baizer J, Glickstein M 1974 Role of the cerebellum in prism adaptation. J Physiol (Lond) 236:34–35

Bastian AJ, Martin TA, Keating JG, Thach WT 1996 Cerebellar ataxia: abnormal control of interaction torques across multiple joints. J Neurophysiol 76:492–509

Bastian AJ, Mink JW, Thach WT 1998 Posterior vermal split syndrome. Ann Neurol, in press

Diener HC, Dichgans J, Guschlbauer B, Bacher M, Langenbach P 1989 Disturbances of motor preparation in basal ganglia and cerebellar disorders. Progr Brain Res 80:481–488

Gilbert PFC, Thach WT 1977 Purkinje cell activity during motor learning. Brain Res 128:309–328

Goodkin HP, Keating JG, Martin T, Thach WT 1993 Preserved simple and impaired compound movement after infarction in the territory of the superior cerebellar artery. Can J Neurol Sci 20(suppl 3):S93–S104

Greger BE, Martin TA, Thach WT 1996 Dynamic coordination of body parts during throwing at visual targets. Soc Neurosci Abstr 22:898

Jeannerod A, Paulignan Y, Weiss P 1998 Grasping an object: one movement, several components. In: Sensory guidance of movement. Wiley, Chichester (Novartis Found Symp 218) p 5–20

Kane SA, Thach WT 1989 Palatal myoclonus and function of the inferior olive: are they related? Exp Brain Res Series 17:427–460

Keating JG, Thach WT 1990 Cerebellar motor learning: quantitation of movement adaptation and performance in rhesus monkeys and humans implicates cortex as the site of adaptation. Soc Neurosci Abstr 117:1381

Keating JG, Thach WT 1991 The cerebellar cortical area required for adaptation of monkey's 'jump' task is lateral, localized, and small. Soc Neurosci Abstr 17:381

Keating JG, Thach WT 1992 Adaptation of a ballistic movement to a novel endpoint is enduring. Soc Neurosci Abstr 18:516

Marr DA 1969 A theory of cerebellar cortex. J Physiol (Lond) 202:437–470

Martin TA, Keating JG, Goodkin HP, Bastian AJ, Thach WT 1996a Throwing while looking through prisms: I. Focal olivocerebellar lesions impair adaptation. Brain 119:1183–1198

Martin TA, Keating JG, Goodkin HP, Bastian AJ, Thach WT 1996b Throwing while looking through prisms: II. Specificity and storage of multiple gaze–throw calibrations. Brain 119:1199–1211

Sainburg RL, Poizner H, Ghez C 1993 Loss of proprioception produces deficits in interjoint coordination. J Neurophysiol 70:2136–2147

Schieber MH, Thach WT 1985a Trained slow tracking. I. Muscular production of wrist movement. J Neurophysiol 55:1213–1227

Schieber MH, Thach WT 1985b Trained slow tracking. II. Bidirectional discharge patterns of cerebellar nuclear, motor cortex, and spindle afferent neurons. J Neurophysiol 55:1228–1270

Schieber MH, Kim L, Thach WT 1991 Muscimol in monkey area 4 impairs individuated finger movements, in area 6 produces contralateral neglect. Soc Neurosci Abstr 17:1021

Soechting JF, Lacquaniti F 1981 Invariant characteristics of a pointing movement in man. J Neurosci 7:710–720

Thach WT, Goodkin HP, Keating JG 1992a Cerebellum and the adaptive coordination of movement. Ann Rev Neurosci 15:403–442

Thach WT, Kane SA, Mink JW, Goodkin HP 1992b Cerebellar output: multiple maps and modes of control in movement coordination. In: Llinas R, Soto C (eds) The cerebellum revisited. Springer Verlag, New York, p 283–300

Thach WT, Perry JG, Kane SA, Goodkin HP 1993 Cerebellar nuclei: rapid alternating movement, motor somatotopy, and a mechanism for the control of muscle synergy. Rev Neurol 149:607–628

Thach WT, Martin TA, Keating JG, Goodkin HP, Bastian AJ 1995 Schematic model of short- and long-term adjustments of eye–hand coordination in throwing. Soc Neurosci Abstr 21:917

Topka H, Konczack J, Schneider K, Dichgans J 1994 Analysis at intersegmental dynamics in cerebellar limb ataxia. Soc Neurosci Abstr 712.10

Weiner MJ, Hallett M, Funkenstein HH 1983 Adaptation to lateral displacement of vision in patients with lesions of the central nervous system. Neurology 33:766–772

DISCUSSION

Georgopoulos: Can you speculate on the post-cerebellar signal processing? How is that being processed in brainstem and cortical areas? Do you envisage that, for example, the signal transmitted to the motor and premotor cortices is in the final form of an integrated complex-movement output?

Thach: I'm suggesting that the cerebellum is responsible for these aspects of muscle management — combining and complementarity and context–response linkage. I'm suggesting that this is especially important for complex 'automatic' responses. This frees up one's mind to think about other things, particularly some of these things like target approach and grasping. Lesions of cerebellar thalamus disrupt the pinch and, by extension, possibly also the grasp, but not the reach. In contrast, lesions of the dentate nucleus, which is one of the chief sources of input to the cerebellar thalamus, disturbs both the pinch and the reach. The inference is that the pinch part goes to the motor cortex, and the reach part may go to the brain stem nuclei, and they're coordinated at the level of the dentate lateral cerebellum in a grand plan that is implemented by separate output stages. The interesting thing is what this might do to issuing messages to premotor cortex, prefrontal cortex and parietal cortex. There, the question is whether there is some kind of combination and complementarily which would maintain some kind of uniformity or invariance of the total action of that functioning group. Invariance of precept or concept comes to mind. Another factor would be possible levels at which one thinks about planning. A chess player planning ahead will be thinking strategy in some way. That person will not be thinking the individual moves, but will have to know them and be thinking of them at some level, even, paradoxically, unconsciously — as a subroutine in order to implement the strategy. This would be one way of creating levels of mental operation using these forebrain and associative cortex ensembles in order to enter into that kind of mental activity.

Gibson: In your patients with the vermal split, have you done any tests requiring interlimb coordination, such as using both hands together?

Thach: We haven't looked at that. We want to get back and look at tasks such as knot tying, which involve two hand coordination.

Thier: The children suffering from what you call posterior vermis split syndrome often suffer from mutism after surgery. Is there any explanation of this?

Thach: That was the reason we started this study, wondering about this so-called cerebellar mutism: none of these children had it. The literature on this is variable in that some children have it, some don't. It tends to happen in those that have had complications, such as haemorrhage or infection. When 'mutism' arises, it may come on as long as four days after the surgery. It seems to be a sort of 'remote' effect and it is not reliably reproduced by a definite lesion. Also, these subjects also tend to have dysphagia and other bulbar deficits. I think it's a vasospasm or something in the pons or medulla.

Thier: If I understood you correctly, what you're basically trying to say is that the cerebellum is specifically contributing to the organization of multicomponent movements. What does this mean for people like me who are interested in eye movements? My understanding is that there are large parts of the cerebellum which are specifically devoted to eye movements. You get very basic single component oculomotor deficits if you lesion oculomotor parts of the cerebellum. For instance, if you lesion the flocculus, you get vestibulo-ocular reflex deficits or polysaccadic drifts, whereas lesions of the cerebellar vermis produce saccade dysmetria as well as smooth pursuit deficits. How can you reconcile your concept with the single component nature of these deficits?

Thach: Eye movements are terribly complicated; there are six muscles in each eye. No one has looked at these eye movements at a single muscle level. Jonathan Hore and Titus Vilis created a strabismus in monkeys and the animals slowly regained binocular vision (Snow et al 1985). Was the cerebellum involved in this adaptation? There's a clinical report of this happening in patients who have had strabismus surgery in youth, and then recurrence of the strabismus when they suffer from cerebellar disease later in life. This may be evidence of a cerebellar contribution to the compensatory action of the muscles in order to preserve the alignment.

Thier: In support of your last comment, there was a recent report by David Zee and co-workers which demonstrated that subtle disorders of the binocular control of eye movements can be found in patients suffering from cerebellar dysfunction (Versino et al 1996).

Stein: Many of us feel very happy about the cerebellum being involved in adaptation of eye movements, clearly a sensorimotor control problem. But, as you know, it has now been suggested that much more arbitrary connections between visual or other sensory inputs and motor programming may be set up in the cerebellum. The cerebellum has been involved in conditioning the nictitating membrane reflex in rabbits, which you would think is analogous to Dick Passingham's visual association type of learning. Why might the cerebellum be involved, and do you believe it is involved?

Thach: First, I would emphasize that the cerebellum seems to be a good candidate for this background kind of automatic behaviour. Dick Passingham's task was very different, with a foreground operation in which subjects are consciously thinking about something, and there are long delays between the stimulus and the response. It is known that you don't get eye-blink conditioning if you have too long a delay (Kimble & Reynolds 1967, Finkbiner & Woodruff-Pak 1991). The question about whether it can be associative is an interesting one. Again, one thinks of the cerebellum as having topical input areas of vestibular, somatosensory, and these visual and cognitive inputs. However, the parallel fibres are long: they can carry input information from one area out long distances to adjacent areas. If you look at any one Purkinje cell, you can see potentially a fairly rich mixture of different kinds of information which could be used to create a rather fancy context response coupling.

Passingham: The other question is whether the role of the cerebellum in eye-blink conditioning is in the optimal timing of the eye-blinking so as to avoid the puff. The blink gets more and more efficient in avoiding the puff, and that is a question of specific timing of the response.

Glickstein: If you take away the unconditioned stimulus, you still see the same effect: it's not just simply pushing the timing around. In point of fact, some lesions augment the unconditioned responses; it has got nothing to do with it.

Ebner: To what degree are the computations performed by the cerebellum related to the interactive torques? You alluded to Dr Kawato's work, but that dealt with the eye movements and there are no interaction torques. Yet the Purkinje cells are obviously coding for dynamics. What role would you predict for the cerebellum in an isometric task versus a reaching task? What would you expect to find for cerebellar neurons relative to this interactive torque calculation? You seem to be putting a lot of emphasis on the cerebellum calculating interactive torques.

Thach: Not totally. I'm saying it's needed to combine muscles. One situation would be where they have to respond to interactive torques. I think the eye doesn't have to worry about that, but nevertheless, there are six muscles working on an eyeball and there have to be trade-offs across the muscles if they're not to co-contract too badly. These balances to adjust for the inertia/viscous properties of the eyeball with complementarity from one muscle with respect to the other, or across muscles of the two eyes — that could be something that is controlled by the cerebellum.

Miller: How is that so terribly different from the situation with muscles crossing the shoulder?

Thach: It's not different.

Miller: But the point is, cerebellar deficits don't seem to affect single joint shoulder movements, whereas your hypothesis suggests that the coordination of the multiple shoulder muscles should be abnormal.

Thach: Cerebellar lesions don't appear to impair single joint movements if the load conditions are simple and the movement is made by the action of one muscle only. We haven't looked at single joint shoulder movements in more complicated load adaptations. It is possible that if you study agonist coupling *with antagonist*, you might see deficits. Perhaps it has been wrong to emphasize the sparing of single-joint and the impairment of multiple joint movements. It is really a question of one, or a few, or multiple muscles in combination.

Miall: I wonder if another way of describing the complexity from simple movements to complex ones, is that it is also going more and more towards sensory guided movements. What you're seeing in the cerebellar lesions is that the most impaired movements are sensory guided movements.

Thach: It's true that there are many sensory aspects in the control of movement. But if you are saying that these are movements without sensory guidance, I'm not sure about that.

Miall: I'm not saying there are such things. But certainly if you are reaching for a peanut, for example, you need a lot of online visual guidance to get your hand to the nut.

Thach: Yes, that's correct.

Miles: A propos your experiments with prism adaptation, the subjects appear to have shown considerable variation from trial to trial in the way that they executed the task. In order to compensate the subject must determine that there has been a visual shift. I'm interested in how subjects decide which parameter to modify, given that there might be many potential reasons for inaccurate performance. I suspect that subjects are not very efficient in going about this. When I swing at a baseball and miss, I have little idea which of the many control parameters to modify — the timing of the swing, my estimate of the ball's trajectory, the starting position of my elbow, and so on and so forth. Following such misses, it seems to me that consistency is a key requirement if I'm to be efficient in my attempts to improve my performance. Inconsistency in effect represents a huge source of additional noise. I suspect that the highly ritualized superstitious behaviour of the professional baseball batter is a manifestation of their constant striving for consistency. Presumably, successful batters are highly conservative about altering the parameters of their swing so that, should their average drop, they can deduce the root cause of their problem efficiently and, therefore, quickly.

Thach: What I showed you was a variability among components with a constancy of resultant in those experiments. We had one subject who was an amateur ball player; he was much less variable across components. It looked as though he was adopting a more and more stereotyped pattern in the motions of his throw. This is what Jon Hore has found for overhand throws, where the variation across the joints is minimal. He believes that the main variation determining accuracy, or a lack of it, is timing of release.

References

Finkbiner RG, Woodruff-Pak DS 1991 Classical eyeblink conditioning in adulthood: effects of age and interstimulus interval on acquisition in the trace paradigm. Psychol Aging 6:109–117

Kimble GA, Reynolds B 1967 Eyeblink conditioning as a function of the interval between conditioned and unconditioned stimuli. In: Kimble GA (ed) Foundations of conditioning and learning. Appleton-Century-Crofts, New York, p 279–287

Snow R, Hore J, Vilis T 1985 Adaptation of saccadic and vestibulo-ocular systems after extraocular muscle tenectomy. Invest Ophthalmol Visual Sci 26:924–931

Versino M, Hurko O, Zee D 1996 Disorders of binocular control of eye movements in patients with cerebellar dysfunction. Brain 119:1933–1950

Construction of a reach-to-grasp

A. R. Gibson, K. M. Horn, M. Pong and P. L. E. Van Kan*

*Division of Neurobiology, Barrow Neurological Institute, St. Joseph's Hospital, 350 W. Thomas Road, Phoenix, AZ 85013 and *Department of Kinesiology, University of Wisconsin, Madison, WI 53706-1532, USA*

Abstract. Reaching out to grasp an object requires the coordinated action of many different areas of the brain. Each area probably makes a unique contribution to the control of limb movement. We have studied the discharge of interpositus, the output nucleus of intermediate cerebellum, and magnocellular red nucleus, which connects interpositus to the spinal cord. The neurons in these areas discharge at high rates only if a hand movement is included with the reach, and discharge pattern is similar regardless of reach direction. Therefore, interpositus and magnocellular red nucleus are involved primarily in grasp control during the reach-to-grasp; other areas must be controlling the reach. Several other areas of the brain, including the reticular formation, rostral mesencephalon, superior colliculus and motor cortex, are active during reaching. The output from these descending systems converges on interneurons at spinal level C1 and C2 which, in turn, project to level C6, where motor neurons innervating shoulder muscles are located. We hypothesize that reach control is achieved by the convergence of multiple descending pathways onto a complex spinal interneuronal system.

1998 Sensory guidance of movement. Wiley, Chichester (Novartis Foundation Symposium 218) p 233–251

A complex movement, such as a reach-to-grasp, may be described at many different levels. At one extreme it might be seen as a single action, i.e. picking up an object—at the other, it might be seen as a sequence of contractions by various muscles throughout the body. Every area of the brain involved in the control of a reach-to-grasp probably 'sees' the movement differently. Over the past 20 years my colleagues and I have been trying to understand how neurons in interpositus, the output nucleus of intermediate cerebellum, and its target, the magnocellular red nucleus (RNm), 'see' the reach-to-grasp.

Why choose to study intermediate cerebellum and RNm?

Damage to the cerebellum produces profound deficits in the ability to move smoothly and precisely (Holmes 1939). Interpositus, the output nucleus of intermediate cerebellum, projects to the RNm. RNm has widespread projections to spinal interneurons and a smaller projection to motor neuronal pools. Stimulation of either RNm or interpositus produces movements, so neural discharge in these areas should be closely related to some aspect of movement.

The connections from interpositus to the RNm and then to the spinal cord are arranged in a topographical fashion so that most interpositus neurons related to forelimb movement supply input only to cervical regions of the cord, whereas neurons related to hind limb movement supply input only to lumbar regions (Robinson et al 1987). This topographical arrangement suggests that cells in the system are specific for control of movement of one limb. Indeed, a cell in interpositus or RNm that discharges during movement of the forelimb does not discharge during movement of the hindlimb, and a cell that discharges during movement of the hindlimb does not discharge during movement of the forelimb. At least for most neurons in interpositus and RNm, a reach-to-grasp is a movement confined to one limb or less.

Unfortunately, the anatomical connections are not much help in defining function of the neurons beyond limb specificity. Most rubrospinal axons terminate in Rexed's lamina VII of the cord rather than onto motor neurons directly, and a single rubrospinal axon can terminate at several different segmental levels (Shinoda et al 1977). Therefore, a single cell in forelimb RNm probably plays some role in controlling many muscles of the limb (Mewes & Cheney 1991). However, specificity does exist in the relatively small RNm projection to motor neuronal pools in lamina IX. This projection is selective for motor neurons that innervate muscles that move the digits (Holstege & Tan 1988, McCurdy et al 1987), which suggests that interpositus and RNm may have a special role in the control of hand movements.

The movement should fit the cell

When I (Gibson) learned single-unit recording techniques in the laboratory of Dr Mitchell Glickstein, we were faced with the problem of determining the optimal stimuli for activation of pontine visual cells. Single spots and slits, which are effective stimuli in other parts of the visual system, elicited only weak responses from pontine cells, and it was only when we tried new stimuli that we were able to activate the cells strongly (Baker et al 1976). In an analogous fashion, the study of motor control by a given neural structure requires that the appropriate movement be chosen for study. The reach-to-grasp elicits high discharge rates from neurons in many areas of the brain associated with motor control. Another important advantage of the reach-to-grasp is that it is a highly stereotyped movement that tends to be produced in the same way from trial-to-trial so that discharge related to movement control also will be consistent. The stereotypy of the behaviour allows for comparison between animals and even species. A final advantage of the reach-to-grasp is that it is extremely easy to train animals, since they naturally perform the behaviour.

Figure 1 is a schematic diagram of the testing paradigm used to study the reach-to-grasp in the cat. The cat is trained to stand quietly and, when a tone sounds, to reach out and grasp a lever and pull it in. If the cat responds within a short time following the tone, he is rewarded with puréed chicken extruded from the end of the lever. Figure 2A illustrates discharge of a red nucleus neuron during the reach-to-grasp. Each trial is represented by a line in the

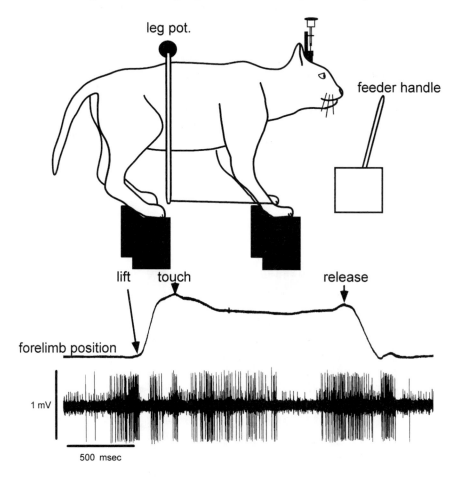

FIG. 1. Behavioural paradigm for cat testing. A record of limb position (middle trace) is obtained from a potentiometer attached with a string at the cat's wrist. The lower trace illustrates discharge from a RNm neuron during the reach, grasp, retrieval and release of the feeder handle.

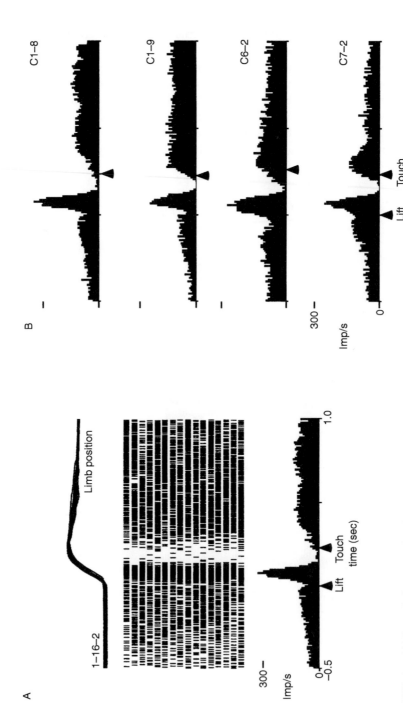

FIG. 2. (A) Records from a single cell over 16 trials. The limb position is overplotted to illustrate stereotypy of the behaviour. Raster display of unit discharge for each trial; note consistency of discharge between trials. Histogram is discharge rate averaged over all trials. (B) Average discharge records of four other RNm cells collected from three cats. The pattern of discharge is very similar to the unit shown in *A*, indicating that RNm cells have common functionality between cats.

raster display, and the limb movement records are overplotted. Notice that both the discharge pattern and movement records are nearly identical from trial-to-trial, and cell discharge has high modulation (during a trial discharge varies from 0–300 spikes per second). RNm neural discharge is tightly related to the reach-to-grasp. For a given cell, the discharge pattern is constant, but the pattern varies between cells indicating individual cells serve specific functions during the movement. Distinct patterns are identifiable, even between cats, and it is possible to group many RNm neurons into a relatively small number of classes. Figure 2B illustrates the discharge patterns of four cells from three cats with essentially the same pattern as the cell illustrated in Fig. 2A. The classes of discharge pattern can be matched to activation patterns of limb muscles during the reach-to-grasp, and it seems likely that RNm neurons are responsible for activation of specific muscles. However, many limb muscles have a similar discharge pattern during the task, so that it is difficult to associate a specific cell with a specific muscle by correlation alone.

Discharge of neurons during fractionated limb movements

The reach-to-grasp elicits consistent discharge patterns and high rates from RNm neurons, but it may be that the neurons are related to movement of only a limited part of the limb rather than to the entire movement. One of the major drawbacks of the cat behavioural paradigm is that it is difficult to train cats to make movements about individual joints in order to break the behaviour into smaller components. Monkeys, on the other hand, can be trained to operate a device that has its pivot point set to correspond to one of the joints of the limb (Thach et al 1982).

In Dr James Houk's laboratory at Northwestern University, we trained monkeys to switch rapidly between a variety of devices so that cells in RNm and interpositus could be tested with movements largely confined to individual joints (Gibson et al 1985, Van Kan et al 1993). Surprisingly, neither RNm nor interpositus neurons fired at high rates during fractionated limb movements, and they showed little preference for movements about a specific joint. Additionally, the discharge that did occur failed to correspond well to parameters such as timing of device movement. Fractionated limb movements never elicited discharge comparable to that seen in the cat RNm during the reach-to-grasp.

Are the neurons in cat RNm simply different from those in monkey RNm and interpositus? Probably not. If a raisin, or any other object, is held in front of the monkey, neurons in RNm and interpositus discharge at high rates during the reach-to-grasp (Gibson et al 1985). Perhaps the cells only participate in the control of coordinated multi-joint movements? Or perhaps they are specialized for the control of hand movements made during grasping? To differentiate between these possibilities, we trained monkeys to make a reach while holding the handle of an articulated arm as well as to reach out and grasp a raisin. The trajectories described by the limb were similar in both cases, but only one movement included a grasp. Comparing reaches with and without a grasp revealed that interpositus neurons fire at high rates during a reach-to-grasp but not during a reach without a grasp (Van Kan et al 1994).

Although it appears that grasping is very important for interpositus cell discharge, it might be that grasping requires visual guidance not involved in moving a device to a fixed location (indeed, the monkeys rarely looked to where they moved the handle). Therefore, we trained another monkey to position a sensor over a visual target by gripping a knob and sliding it over a light target (Gibson et al 1996). Figure 3 illustrates discharge from an interpositus neuron while the monkey moved the knob to the target or while he grasped a raisin presented at the same position as the light target. The left panel illustrates neural discharge during three directions of sensor movement; to the upper left, upper right, and upper left to upper right. No increases in discharge rate can be seen in the spike records corresponding to the three movements. The right panel illustrates the same three directions of limb movement, but in these cases the monkey released the device handle to grasp raisins presented at the same positions as the light targets. Neural discharge reached approximately 250 imp/sec during each reach-to-grasp and peaked just prior to grasping the raisin.

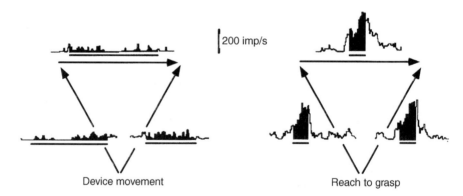

FIG. 3.   Discharge of monkey interpositus cell during forelimb movements with and without a grasp in three directions. The monkeys were trained to position a cursor over a spot of light that moved between three positions arranged in a triangle. (*Left*) Discharge records during movement of the cursor (movement time is marked with dark bar under discharge record). There is little change in discharge rate for movements in any of the three directions. (*Right*) Discharge during movements in the same directions as on left, but in these cases the monkey is reaching to grasp a raisin presented at the different target locations. There are high discharge rate increases during the reaches-to-grasp, and the discharge is similar regardless of the direction of reach.

Neural discharge rate and pattern were essentially the same for each direction of reach-to-grasp.

Although the discharge of only one neuron is illustrated, over half of the neurons recorded in interpositus failed to fire when a grasp was not included in the reach-to-grasp. The other half of the neurons increased discharge to some extent during device use, but they fired much more strongly to the reach-to-grasp. We have never seen an interpositus neuron that fired strongly to a reach without a grasp. Similar observations have been made for monkey RNm neurons during reaches with and without a grasp (McCurdy et al 1997). From these, as well as many other studies, we conclude that interpositus and RNm neurons are primarily involved in the control of grasping, or preparing to grasp, during a reach-to-grasp.

Grasping, however, probably has consequences for musculature of the entire limb. For example, during hand movements the upper arm must be stabilized to provide a steady base, which might account for the widespread interneuronal terminations of rubrospinal fibres. Some support for this possibility comes from an inactivation study by Mason et al (1998): inactivation of posterior interpositus of the monkey produces deficits in the ability to hold the arm steady while grasping food, whereas inactivation of anterior interpositus interferes with forming of the hand to make the grasp.

Together, the findings indicate that the interpositus and RNm are concerned primarily with grasp-related components of the reach-to-grasp. Clearly, to perform the entire movement, there must be areas of the brain concerned with reach-related components.

How is the reach controlled during a reach-to-grasp?

Lawrence & Kuypers (1968a,b) sectioned various descending pathways in the monkey to determine the organization of the motor system. Although the descending pathways have overlapping control of body musculature, different systems focus on specific groups of limb muscles. Monkeys with bilateral lesions of the pyramidal tract are able to reach toward food within a few days of the lesion, but they cannot control the hand to grasp the food and have permanent deficits in hand use. It seems that the pyramidal tract is very important for control of the hand, but much less important for control of proximal limb musculature used for reaching. In contrast, lesions of medially descending pathways produce profound deficits in movements of the shoulder but not of the hand. Principal sources of the medially descending pathways include the reticular formation, vestibular nuclei, superior colliculus and interstitial nucleus of Cajal. For the past several years, we have been studying the discharge in these areas during the reach-to-grasp.

The results from lesion studies (Lawrence & Kuypers 1968a,b), anatomical studies (Holstege & Kuypers 1982) and intracellular recording studies (Peterson et al 1979) indicate that the medullary reticular formation is one of the most likely candidates for control of proximal limb muscles. Indeed, some medullary reticular neurons discharge consistently during the reach-to-grasp, and we have recorded from approximately 50 medullary reticular neurons in the cat with discharge well-related to the movement. About 50% of these neurons discharged during movement of the contralateral limb only, but 35% discharged equally well with use of either limb. The bilateral discharge raises the concern that discharge is related to muscles other than the limb, perhaps those of the neck or back, and discharge did appear to correlate well with contractions of these muscles. It is known that stimulation of medullary reticular formation produces strong bilateral activation of neck muscles (Drew & Rossignol 1990), although limb muscles may also be activated. One interesting possibility is that neurons involved in reaching might be related to either limb, and that the discharge is gated by other inputs for the appropriate side at spinal levels.

Another candidate for control of the reach is the lateral vestibular nucleus (lvn), since lvn cells discharge rhythmically during locomotion (Udo et al 1982) and may have monosynaptic connections to lateral motoneurons at C6 (Shinoda et al 1986), which innervate shoulder muscles. Surprisingly, when we tested lvn cells they showed little modulation in discharge during the reaching task. Discharge related to locomotion but not reaching supports the hypothesis of Lawrence & Kuypers (1968a,b) that independent use of the limbs is controlled by neural circuits different from the ones which coordinate multi-limb movements such as walking and climbing. Organization of motor control is probably based on movements that accomplish a general class of function.

Recordings from more rostral reticular areas in the pons and mesencephalon reveal that there are at least some cells in these areas that discharge strongly during reaching. To date, the most promising area from which we have recorded is the rostral mesencephalon near the red nucleus. We have recorded approximately 60 neurons in the cat mesencephalon that discharge during reaching. Figure 4 illustrates the discharge of two mesencephalic neurons during the reach-to-grasp. The cells have no spontaneous discharge, begin firing before the limb is lifted, and reach a peak of approximately 100 spikes/s during the reach. The mesencephalic neurons only discharge when the cat reaches with the limb contralateral to the side of recording. This is surprising, since the spinal projection from rostral mesencephalic areas is strongest to the ipsilateral cord. Perhaps these cells project to propriospinal neurons that cross to the opposite side of the cord or to other neurons in the brainstem that project to the contralateral cord?

The possibility that at least some reach control is achieved through projections to propriospinal neurons may explain our difficulty in finding a single, compact,

Mesencephalic   Reticular

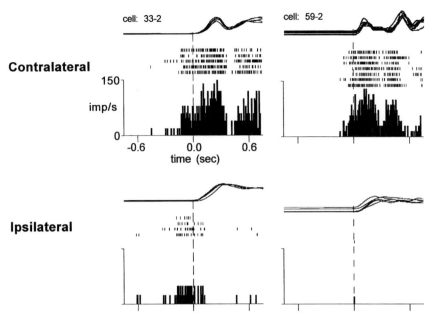

FIG. 4.   Discharge of two neurons in the rostral mesencephalon of the cat during the reach-to-grasp. Records of limb position for the limb contralateral to the recording site indicate angle of elbow joint, whereas ipsilateral limb position was recorded using the potentiometer sensor illustrated in Fig. 1. Discharge is well-related only to contralateral limb movement.

reach-related area in the brainstem. It is clear that neurons in many other areas, such as cerebral cortex (Georgopoulos et al 1982) and superior colliculus (Werner et al 1997), discharge during reaching, and reach control may be achieved by summation of many inputs onto propriospinal neurons. Alstermark et al (1987) have demonstrated that C3–C5 propriospinal neurons located in spinal laminae VII and VIII integrate inputs from cerebral cortex, superior colliculus, reticular formation, red nucleus and cerebellum.

Propriospinal projections to motoneurons innervating shoulder muscles

In order to identify propriospinal neurons projecting to shoulder muscles, we injected WGA-HRP into the ventral horn at spinal level C6. Although shoulder muscles are innervated by motor pools extending from spinal segments C5 to T1 (Horner & Kummel 1993), C6 offers one of the best levels for selectively labelling inputs to shoulder motoneurons: higher cervical levels include motoneuronal pools innervating neck musculature, whereas lower cervical levels include pools innervating distal limb musculature. Figure 5 illustrates the distribution of retrogradely labelled propriospinal neurons from a ventral horn C6 injection on the left side. The spinal cord has been cut in horizontal section, and the level of the section is just ventral to spinal aqueduct. The largest number of propriospinal neurons projecting to C6 are located at C1 and C2. Interestingly, labelled neurons occur on both sides of the cord, but the ipsilaterally labelled neurons are laterally located in the spinal grey, whereas the contralaterally labelled neurons are medially located.

To determine the inputs to the propriospinal neurons, we placed a WGA–HRP injection into C1. The injection resulted in an immense number of retrogradely

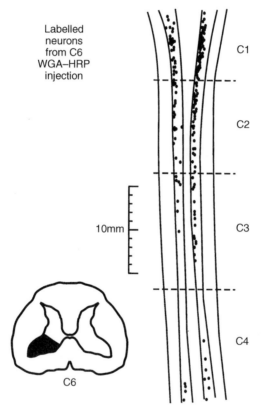

FIG. 5.   Location of retrogradely labelled neurons in cat spinal cord following a C6 ventral horn injection of WGA-HRP. The transverse section through C6 (lower left) illustrates approximate extent of injection site in left ventral horn (dark fill). The spinal cord from C1 to C5 is sectioned in a horizontal plane. The illustrated section is at a level just below spinal aqueduct, and the lateral borders of the cord and spinal gray are outlined in black. Labelled cells are indicated by shaded ellipses.

labelled neurons throughout the brain. Some of the more prominent areas include motor cortex, superior colliculus, magnocellular red nucleus, fastigial nucleus and medial posterior interpositus, and many reticular areas. The terminations of the descending pathways tend to correspond with their functional laterality. For example, projections from superior colliculus (Huerta & Harting 1982), RNm and motor cortex (Holstege & Tan 1988, McCurdy et al 1987) terminate in lateral interneurons at C1, so the projection of cells receiving these inputs to C6 is likely to remain on the same side. Much of the ipsilateral projection from the rostral mesencephalon terminates medially (Holstege & Cowie 1989), so it is likely to cross to the contralateral side, which might explain the contralateral movement relations of mesencephalic neurons. The projection from the cerebellum may be doubly crossed. The projection originates in the contralateral deep nuclei but a large portion of the spinal termination is in medial interneurons (Horn et al 1995), so this output could re-cross to the ipsilateral side in the projection to C6, which would be consistent with ipsilateral movement control by the cerebellum. The large number of crossed projections from propriospinal pathways may be partly responsible for the extensive functional recovery seen after hemisection of the cord (Mettler 1944).

The C1 injection also labelled fibres that project to the lower cervical levels. The projection is not directly to motor neurons but to interneurons lying in laminae VII and VIII. Thus, descending motor pathways access motor neurons for the upper arm via a propriospinal system originating in C1 and C2, as well as via the propriospinal system from more caudal cervical segments (Alstermark et al 1987, Illert et al 1977, 1981). Sectioning of the fibres from propriospinal neurons to lower cervical segments produces deficits in reaching (Alstermark et al 1981), which underscores the importance of propriospinal connections in limb control.

In summary, interpositus and RNm are involved only in the control of grasp-related components of the reach-to-grasp. There are several potential candidates for control of reach-related components of the movement, but it is likely that much of the reach control is achieved by integration of many descending pathways onto propriospinal neurons, as has been suggested by several other investigators (Alstermark et al 1981, Illert et al 1977). It is a challenge for future research to determine the unique contributions that each of the descending systems is likely to make the control the reach-to-grasp.

References

Alstermark B, Lundberg A, Norrsell U, Sybirska E 1981 Integration in descending motor pathways controlling the forelimb in the cat. 9. Differential behavioural defects after spinal cord lesions interrupting defined pathways from higher centres to motoneurons. Exp Brain Res 42:299–318

Alstermark B, Lundberg A, Pinter M, Sasaki S 1987 Long C3-C5 propriospinal neurones in the cat. Brain Res 404:382–388

Baker J, Gibson A, Glickstein M, Stein J 1976 Visual cells in pontine nuclei of the cat. J Physiol (Lond) 255:415–433

Drew T, Rossignol S 1990 Functional organization within the medullary reticular formation of intact unanesthetized cat. II. Electromyographic activity evoked by microstimulation. J Neurophysiol 64:782–795

Georgopoulos AP, Kalaska JF, Caminiti R, Massey JT 1982 On the relations between the direction of two-dimensional arm movements and cell discharge in primate motor cortex. J Neurosci 2:1527–1537

Gibson AR, Houk JC, Kohlerman NJ 1985 Magnocellular red nucleus activity during different types of limb movement in the Macaque monkey. J Physiol (Lond) 358:527–549

Gibson AR, Horn KM, Stein JF, Van Kan PLE 1996 Neural discharge of interpositus during a visually guided reach. Can J Physiol Pharmacol 74:499–512

Holmes G 1939 The cerebellum of man. Brain 62:1–30

Holstege G, Cowie RJ 1989 Projections from the rostral mesencephalic reticular formation to the spinal cord. Exp Brain Res 75:265–279

Holstege G, Kuypers HGJM 1982 The anatomy of brain stem pathways to the spinal cord in the cat. A labeled amino acid tracing study. In: Kuypers HGJM, Martin G (eds) Progress in brain research, vol 57: Anatomy of descending pathways to the spinal cord. Elsevier Science BV, Amsterdam, p 145–175

Holstege G, Tan J 1988 Projections from the red nucleus and surrounding areas to the brainstem and spinal cord in the cat. An HRP and autoradiographical tracing study. Behav Brain Res 28:33–57

Horn KM, Porter CM, Gibson AR 1995 Spinal connections of cat posterior interpositus. Soc Neurosci Abstr 21:1190

Horner M, Kummel H 1993 Topographical representation of shoulder motor nuclei in the cat spinal cord as revealed by retrograde fluorochrome tracers. J Comp Neurol 335:309–319

Huerta MF, Harting JK 1982 Tectal control of spinal cord activity: neuroanatomical demonstration of pathways connecting the superior colliculus with the cervical spinal cord grey. In: Kuypers HGJM, Martin G (eds) Progress in brain research, vol 57: Anatomy of descending pathways to the spinal cord. Elsevier Science BV, Amsterdam, p 293–328

Illert M, Lundberg A, Tanaka R 1977 Integration in the descending motor pathways controlling the forelimb in the cat. 3. Convergence on propriospinal neurones transmitting disynaptic excitation from the corticospinal tract and other descending tracts. Exp Brain Res 29:323–346

Illert M, Jankowska E, Lundberg A, Odutola A 1981 Integration in descending motor pathways controlling the forelimb in the cat. Exp Brain Res 42:269–281

Lawrence DG, Kuypers HGJM 1968a The functional organization of the motor system in the monkey. I. The effects of bilateral pyramidal lesions. Brain 91:1–14

Lawrence DG, Kuypers HGJM 1968b The functional organization of the motor system in the monkey. II. The effects of lesions of the descending brain-stem pathways. Brain 91:15–36

Mason CR, Miller LE, Baker JF, Houk JC 1998 Organization of reaching and grasping movements in the primate cerebellar nuclei as revealed by focal muscimol inactivations. J Neurophysiol 79:537–554

McCurdy ML, Hansma DI, Houk JC, Gibson AR 1987 Selective projections from the cat red nucleus to digit motor neurons. J Comp Neurol 265:367–379

McCurdy ML, Kirsch KA, Boyce CJ, Van Kan PLE 1997 Magnocellular red nucleus discharge in monkey during reaching to grasp in different directions. Soc Neurosci Abstr 23:18

Mettler FA 1944 Observations on the consequences of large subtotal lesions of the simian spinal cord. J Comp Neurol 81:339–360

Mewes K, Cheney PD 1991 Facilitation and suppression of wrist and digit muscles from single rubromotoneuronal cells in the awake monkey. J Neurophysiol 66:1965–1977

Peterson BW, Pitts NG, Fukishima K 1979 Reticulospinal connections with limb and axial motoneurons. Exp Brain Res 36:1–20

Robinson FR, Houk JC, Gibson AR 1987 Limb specific connections of the cat magnocellular red nucleus. J Comp Neurol 257:553–577

Shinoda Y, Ghez C, Arnold A 1977 Spinal branching of rubrospinal axons in the cat. Exp Brain Res 30:203–218

Shinoda Y, Ohgaki T, Futami T 1986 The morphology of single lateral vestibulospinal tract axons in the lower cervical spinal cord of the cat. J Comp Neurol 249:226–241

Thach WT, Perry JG, Schieber MH 1982 Cerebellar output: body maps and muscle spindles. In: Palay SL, Chan-Palay V (eds) The cerebellum — new vistas. Springer-Verlag, Berlin, p 440–454

Udo M, Kamei H, Matsukawa K, Tanaka K 1982 Interlimb coordination in cat locomotion investigated with perturbation. II. Correlates in neuronal activity of Deiter's cells of decerebrate walking cats. Exp Brain Res 46:438–447

Van Kan PLE, Houk JC, Gibson AR 1993 Output organization of intermediate cerebellum in the monkey. J Neurophysiol 69:57–73

Van Kan PLE, Horn KM, Gibson AR 1994 The importance of hand use to discharge of cerebellar output neurones of the monkey. J Physiol (Lond) 480:171–190

Werner W, Dannenberg S, Hoffmann K-P 1997 Arm-movement-related neurons in the primate superior colliculus and underlying reticular formation: comparison of neuronal activity with EMGs of muscles of the shoulder, arm and trunk during reaching. Exp Brain Res 115:191–205

DISCUSSION

Rizzolatti: I liked the beginning of your talk very much. However, it is not clear to me why later on you fell into a kind of cosmic pessimism. It is hard, but not impossible, to distinguish 'grasping' neurons from neurons that code finger movements regardless of their aim. When we found neurons in F5 that fired during opening and closure of the hand we concluded that these neurons were coding neither muscles nor elementary movements. When, subsequently, we observed that the same neurons did not fire when the animal used the fingers for purposes other than grasping, for instance scratching, we decided that these neurons were involved in grasping movements. Why is it so scary to say: 'I found a "grasping" neuron'?

Gibson: The term 'grasp' is too limiting; the cells are not just involved in grasping but in a variety of movements. For example, when RNm is inactivated, the cats not only have difficulty in grasping, but they also fail to position the paw properly during walking. In Jim Houk's laboratory at Northwestern University we trained a monkey to place his fingers into a device that rotated about the metacarpal phalangeal joints. The monkey was required to track a target by flexing and extending his fingers while he rested his forearm on a platform.

Interpositus neurons fired only weakly during these finger movements (Van Kan et al 1993). Perhaps interpositus is only involved in hand movements made in combination with upper limb movement.

Miller: I would like to underscore the point that you made, especially with respect to the function of the red nucleus in opening the digits. We did long timespan cross-correlations between red nucleus and muscle, which indicated the covariation between the signals. We studied cats that were reaching out to grab pieces of food, monkeys that were reaching and grabbing things, and monkeys that were doing the same kind of tracking tasks that you studied. Regardless of whether the monkey was doing the supination/pronation task or a variety of other relatively complex movements of the arm, extensor digitorum communis (EDC) was almost always the most strongly correlated muscle. The red nucleus appears to be strongly organized to open the hand in a variety of different contexts.

The caveat that you made with respect to hand use and motor cortex is an important one. We also found a large number of correlations during these reaching and pressing tasks, with both EDC and flexor digitorum sublimis. I think it may be a large component of what these cells in the arm area are doing.

Lemon: A point about the importance of the EDC muscle. If you look at the way the intrinsic muscles operate, many of them are dependent on what the EDC is doing, because many of them either act at the same joint that the EDC does, or even tug on the EDC tendon when it is unable to move the digits because of the position of the wrist.

Strick: How different is the red nucleus from the motor cortex? EDC is one of a number of muscles in the monkey that receives particularly strong monosynaptic excitation from corticospinal neurons. As such, it is considered one of the 'most preferentially accessible muscles of the hand' in terms of direct cortico-motoneuronal input (Phillips 1968). I wonder whether a very similar arrangement is found in the cat.

Roger Lemon and his colleagues have shown that some neurons in the monkey motor cortex with outputs directed to finger muscles will show dramatic changes in activity when an animal is performing a precision grip. The same neurons, will show only modest changes in activity when the animal is performing a power grip. I wonder whether this type of functional specialization is seen in the cat red nucleus during your reach and grasp task.

Gibson: That's right, there is probably muscle specificity within functional specialization, but it is difficult to parcel these out.

Miller: EDC is strongly active in the grouped digit extension tracking task, and yet you didn't get nearly as strong discharge with that as you did during grasping.

Ebner: I don't want this distinguished audience to go home and think that there are no reach-related neurons in the cerebellar cortex. Fortier et al (1989) showed directionally tuned discharge during a two-dimensional reaching task using a manipulandum. Fu et al (1997) recently demonstrated both directional and distance modulation for cerebellar Purkinje cells. Some of these cells were in the intermediate zone, others were not. The neurons John Kalaska recorded were in the intermediate zone, whereas we've been studying Purkinje cells located more laterally. One also must consider exploring the work space. In your task the animal is performing a simple, one-directional reach with a grasp. Granted the cells fire very strongly with the grasp, but the cells may also fire quite differently if the animal was working in a different part of the work space.

Gibson: The position in work space doesn't seem to be important. An interpositus cell fires in a similar fashion regardless of where the raisin is presented. However, it is likely that cells in different parts of interpositus vary in some way. Mason et al (1998) have discovered that inactivation of posterior interpositus produces a deficit in stabilizing the arm during grasping, whereas inactivation of anterior interpositus produces a deficit in forming the hand to grasp. It is possible that both regions are involved in the control of grasping, but posterior regions influence proximal limb musculature while anterior regions influence distal limb musculature.

Ebner: In a task similar to oculomotor pursuit tracking, our recent work shows that cerebellar Purkinje cells are very modulated during a pursuit tracking task involving the hand. The modulation during tracking is greater than during reaching. Simple spikes are highly modulated, up to 200 spikes/second. Again, the modulation may be task related, or at least related to tasks requiring continuous feedback. I think this goes back to Peter's point: exactly what is it that drives the cells?

Miller: Speaking of firing rates, most of those Purkinje cells that Fortier and Kalaska recorded had modulations around 40 impulses a second, as I recall.

Kalaska: Yes. The amplitude of the average directional tuning curve of proximal arm-related cells in both the cerebellum and the motor cortex was something like 40 impulses per second, so I guess by the Gibson criterion they are not reach related. There are many cerebellar cells that show peak discharges of 100–150 Hz, but in the motor cortex the peak discharge of most neurons is never above 50–60 Hz. You rarely see a discharge of more than 100 Hz in motor cortex, but they are certainly reach related. You can't take some arbitrary value of discharge such as 100 or 200 or 300 Hz as a criterion for whether they are reach related because different cell populations in different structures have different inherent maximal discharge rates.

Gibson: I am not suggesting an arbitrary value for all neurons. All I am suggesting is that each neuron should be tested with a variety of movements to determine which elicits the highest discharge. The brainstem neurons that we believe are reach related have much lower discharge rates than interpositus or RNm neurons.

Stein: Alan, why are you so depressed about not finding a nucleus for reach in the brainstem? Need there necessarily be one? The reticular formation, after all, is the archetypal 'distributed system'. If these cells are in the reticular formation are you surprised to find them all over it?

Gibson: I have been using the term 'reticular system' very loosely. There are cells related to reaching in reticular areas, but some are in identified brainstem nuclei. It is much too simple to say that the movement is composed of a reach and a grasp. For example, axial musculature must make adjustments during the reach-to-grasp, and these muscles are likely to be controlled by separate cells. Also, the biceps and triceps may well be controlled separately from muscles of the shoulder girdle. It is a complicated problem.

Lemon: I appreciate how difficult it is to interpret neuronal discharge as a code or a command signal for behaviour. This has been a problem from the beginning. One has to be aware that when you're studying a particular part of the 'anatomical' map of motor function its behaviour may give you some surprises. The example I like best is the report by Penfield (see Penfield & Rasmussen 1952, p 218). Having mapped the motor cortex of an epileptic patient with his usual method, he found that electrical stimulation of a particular part of the precentral area evoked clear shoulder movement. He wanted to excise this area because it included the epileptic focus. When they examined the behaviour of the patient after surgery, although they expected a lot of paresis and poverty of movement around the shoulder joint, they actually found that the patient could reach perfectly well but that fine control of the hand was destroyed. I believe that much of the motor cortex is devoted to doing something useful with your hand, and its control of more proximal movement subserves this important function. Most, but not all, reaching movements are designed to get your hand into some useful position in space. Thus rather than thinking of motor cortex control of proximal muscles as subserving a totally separate motor system that moves your shoulder, elbow, wrist, etc., we should think of them as a whole nest of control systems that ultimately are subserving the most important thing, which is using your hand to interact with the environment.

Gibson: When a monkey is gripping an object, such as the edge of his testing chair, even very slight hand adjustments elicit high firing rates from interpositus neurons. It is unlikely that these rates translate directly into finger movement. The discharge probably relates to a specific synergy, but it will be very difficult to demonstrate this.

Hoffmann: I would like to give an operational definition of a possible reach nucleus. If you penetrate the monkey colliculus 2–5 mm from the surface you find a lot of reach neurons. It is not that you can aim for a certain location in which every neuron will show the same property. Reach neurons are dispersed and neighbouring neurons have completely different properties. There is an extremely high correlation of these neurons to reaching movements, and there is a strong correlation of the activity of these neurons to the EMGs of proximal arm muscles.

Gibson: Since the superior colliculus doesn't appear to have direct projections to motor neurons innervating shoulder muscles, it is likely that collicular output relays through a brainstem or propriospinal region prior to reaching the appropriate spinal segments. We have tried stimulus-triggered averaging of muscle EMG while activating the superior colliculus in the awake cat. At relatively high current levels we see activation of proximal muscles, but the activation patterns are broad, which suggests also that collicular influences on shoulder musculature are likely to be multisynaptic. We would like to record the activity of neurons between the colliculus and shoulder motor neurons during reaching, but this may not be practical.

Marsden: I'm trying to translate this to humans and I get confused about the present view on the power of the rubrospinal pathway to hand muscles in the human brain.

Gibson: The magnocellular portion of the red nucleus is reported to be small in humans. One interesting possibility is that the largest cells have disappeared in the human, since the largest RNm neurons in monkey project to lumbar cord. Unlike humans, monkeys often use their feet for grasping objects. Of course, humans do have the cerebellar equivalent of interpositus, and it may be that many functions of the RNm have shifted to motor cortex in humans.

Marsden: But it's still the received wisdom that the magnocellular division of the red nucleus is pretty vestigial in humans.

Glickstein: I have one comment on the size of the cells. The retina has the same thickness in virtually every animal. The receptors and the inner nuclear cells are all the same size, but the ganglion cells of an elephant or a whale are huge. This is an example of a cell that must maintain a long axon. Betz, when he first described the Betz cell, noted that they were bigger medially along the central sulcus in humans and smaller laterally.

Miller: I would like to show one picture of the correlations from the superior colliculus to which Klaus-Peter Hoffmann referred (Fig. 1 [*Miller*]). These are long timespan cross-correlations between single-unit discharge and the activity of a large set of limb muscles. The correlations indicate how similar the movement-related modulation in discharge rate of a given neuron is to each of the muscles. The magnitudes of the correlations were similar to those of the red nucleus or motor cortex that we have calculated in the past. This histogram shows the percentage of cross-correlations for each muscle that exceeded a level of 0.25. The figure includes the recent data from the superior colliculus, as well as previous data from primary motor cortex. In both cases, the monkeys were doing a centre–out button pressing task within the vertical plane.

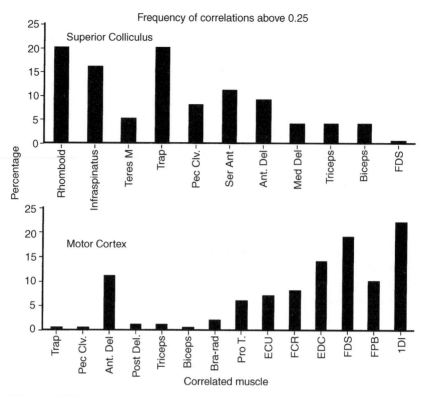

FIG. 1. (*Miller*) Long timespan cross-correlations between single-unit discharge and the activity of a large set of limb muscles. The histogram shows the percentage of cross-correlations for each muscle that exceed a level of 0.25.

I would like to point out that strong correlations between the superior colliculus and the most proximal limb muscles (e.g. rhomboid, infraspinatus and trapezius) were quite frequent, strong triceps and biceps correlations were less common, and those with flexor digitorum superficialis were quite rare. Unfortunately, we lost our extensor digitorum communis recording when someone accidentally clipped a wire during surgery. We don't have a completely overlapping set of muscles by any means. But you can see for those that do overlap, there is a clear trend for strong proximal muscle correlations from the colliculus and relatively few from the motor cortex. The motor cortex distribution is similar to that which we found for red nucleus, although those monkeys were doing a rather different set of tasks. The distribution for motor cortex will obviously have been dependent on the region within M1 from which the recordings were made. Our recordings were made in rostral M1, lateral (and caudal) of the tip of the superior precentral sulcus. This area lies between the classical proximal arm area and the medial hand area recently described by Peter Strick (He et al 1993). Recordings from the centre of the proximal limb area would presumably have yielded more correlations with proximal muscles.

References

Fortier PA, Kalaska JF, Smith AM 1989 Cerebellar neuronal activity related to whole-arm reaching movements in the monkey. J Neurophysiol 62:198–211

Fu Q-J, Flament D, Coltz JD, Ebner TJ 1997 Relationship of cerebellar Purkinje cell simple spike discharge to movement kinematics in the monkey. J Neurophysiol 78:478–491

He SQ, Dum RP, Strick PL 1993 Topographic organization of corticospinal projections from the frontal lobe: motor areas on the lateral surface of the hemisphere. J Neurosci 13:952–980

Mason CR, Miller LE, Baker JF, Houk JC 1998 Organization of reaching and grasping movements in the primate cerebellar nuclei as revealed by focal muscimol inactivations. J Neurophysiol 79:537–554

Penfield W, Rasmussen T 1952 The cerebral cortex of man. Macmillan, New York

Phillips CG 1968 Motor apparatus of the baboon's hand. Proc R Soc Lond B 173:141–174

Van Kan PLE, Houk JC, Gibson AR 1993 Output organization of intermediate cerebellum of the monkey. J Neurophysiol 69:57–73

Cerebellum and the sensory guidance of movement

Mitchell Glickstein

Department of Anatomy and Developmental Biology, Neuroscience and Behaviour Group, University College London, Gower Street, London WC1E 6BT, UK

Abstract. By the end of the 19th century the locations of the primary visual and motor areas of the cerebral cortex were well recognized. At that time it was generally assumed that for the visual control of movement visual areas must be linked to motor areas by way of a series of cortico-cortical fibres. Subsequent experimental evidence showed clearly, however, that skilled visuomotor performance is still possible after complete disconnection of interhemispheric and intracortical fibre systems. Preservation of skilled visuomotor performance after such lesions has often been thought to be mediated by ipsilaterally descending motor pathways. However, the evidence indicates that there must also be subcortical pathways that link sensory to motor areas of the brain. One such pathway involves the cerebellum. There is a massive input from cortical and subcortical visual areas to the pontine nuclei. Cells in the pontine nuclei respond vigorously to appropriate visual targets and they distribute their axonal terminals bilaterally in the cerebellar cortex. A cortico-ponto-cerebellar circuit would have remained intact in all cases in the literature in which there was complete disconnection of cortico-cortical fibres between visual and motor cortex. Lesions of the cortical sensory areas that project to the pons or interruption of the fibres within the internal capsule or basis pedunculi, that link cortical sensory areas with the pontine nuclei, can severely impair the sensory guidance of movement. This paper reviews the evidence for sensory input to the cerebellum and the possible role of a cortico-ponto-cerebellar circuit in the sensory guidance of movement.

1998 Sensory guidance of movement. Wiley, Chichester (Novartis Foundation Symposium 218) p 252–271

The behaviour of humans and animals is under continuous sensory guidance. This symposium addresses the question of how sensory guidance of movement is accomplished by the brain. An earlier question was that of the localization of areas controlling sensation and movement. In this paper I first discuss briefly the history of studies of localization of sensory and motor functions in the cerebral cortex, and go on to consider the ways in which sensory areas are connected to motor areas of the brain. The emphasis is on the linkage between sensory and motor cortical areas, but the same sorts of questions arise about the connections between subcortical sensory and motor structures. One of the major circuits for the sensory guidance of movement involves a pathway from sensory areas of the cerebral cortex to the cerebellum by way of the pontine nuclei. The cerebellum, in turn, exerts a powerful influence on all of the descending motor pathways.

Localization of function in the cerebral cortex

Until the middle of the 19th century there was very little evidence that different regions of the cerebral cortex might be specialized for different functions. The excessive claims of Gall and Spurzheim, the cranioscopists/phrenologists, were contradicted by the careful experiments of Flourens (1824). Flourens made lesions in the forebrain of birds and mammals and reported that no single lesion produced loss of a specific function. Sensation and volition appeared to be controlled by the cerebral cortex acting as a unified whole. The beginnings of modern understanding of cortical localization began with post-mortem study of the brains of patients that had previously lost the power of speech. There were suggestions early in the nineteenth century that deficits in speech might be caused by damage to the frontal lobe. It was the evidence of Pierre-Paul Broca (1861) that directed attention sharply to the role of the frontal lobe in spoken language. Broca's patient, Le Borgne ('Tan') had been incapable of producing any word other than 'tan' for the past twenty years. Tan's case came to Broca's attention shortly before he died at the age of 51. The day after Tan's death Broca gave a preliminary account of his lesion to the Anthropological Society in Paris. Shortly thereafter Broca reported a second case of a patient, Lelong, who had suffered a stroke at the age of 83, and died 18 months later. Like Tan, Lelong had a profound speech impairment. After the stroke he could say only five words: 'Lelo' (for Lelong), 'oui', 'non', 'tois' (for trois) and 'toujours'. Tan's lesion was diffuse with damage to brain structures outside of the frontal lobe. Lelong's brain showed a more definite localization than that of Tan, centred in the left inferior frontal lobe. Articulate speech, Broca concluded, is controlled by the cortex of the frontal lobe.

The beginning of the modern experimental study of cortical localization of function began with the discoveries of Gustav Fritsch and Eduard Hitzig (Fritsch & Hitzig 1870). Fritsch and Hitzig stimulated electrically the frontal cortex of a dog, eliciting movement on the opposite side of the body. If, for example, electrical stimulation at a particular site on the left frontal lobe produced movement of the right forelimb, then a small lesion placed at that same site would cause the animal to be clumsy in using that limb. The cortical motor area that Fritsch and Hitzig found is anatomically distinct. Four years after their report, Vladimir Betz (1874) described 'nests' of very large pyramidal cells in Layer V (his 'fourth layer') of the frontal cortex that are present in those areas of the cortex that produce movement when stimulated. Although there were arguments about the interpretation of Fritsch and Hitzig's discovery, most authors soon accepted the idea that a particular region of the cerebral cortex is specialized for the control of movement.

Finding the location of the visual cortex took a bit longer. The first claim to have identified the visual cortex was summarized by David Ferrier in his book *Functions of the Brain* (1876) (Glickstein 1985). Following Fritsch and Hitzig's example, Ferrier studied the movements that are produced by electrical stimulation of the cerebral cortex. Stimulation of the angular gyrus of a monkey's parietal lobe produced eye movements; bilateral ablation of the angular gyrus appeared to cause blindness. Ferrier concluded that the angular gyrus must be the visual area of the cerebral cortex. In his first experiments Ferrier observed the monkeys for only three days after a lesion was made because of inevitable postoperative infections. Later Ferrier began to practise aseptic surgery and his monkeys could now survive for a much longer time. In his later studies Ferrier reported that the apparent loss of vision caused by angular gyrus lesion was only temporary. Ferrier's descriptions of the symptoms make it clear that the most striking effect of angular gyrus lesions was a profound impairment in the visual guidance of movement.

Ferrier's claim that visual function is localized in the angular gyrus was challenged sharply by Hermann Munk (1881), Professor of Veterinary Physiology in Berlin. Munk made lesions in the brains of dogs and monkeys and observed the deficits produced by those lesions. In a strong attack on Ferrier and his work, Munk asserted that unilateral removal of the occipital lobe in a monkey produces hemianopia; bilateral removal causes blindness. Vision, he asserted, is localized in the occipital, not the parietal lobe. Within a few years after Munk's reports appeared, his experiments were repeated in other labs and were applied by Henschen (1890) to the interpretation of hemianopia in humans that had sustained damage to the occipital lobe.

How is the visual area connected to the motor area?

By the end of the nineteenth century most authorities agreed on the location of the primary visual and motor areas in the cerebral cortex of monkeys and humans. Little thought was given to the question of how the two areas might be linked for the sensory control of movement. The answer seemed to be obvious. There are abundant U-fibres that link adjacent cortical gyri, and long association bundles that interconnect remote cortical areas with one another. Visuomotor coordination was thought to be based on such a system of cortico-cortical fibres. The corpus callosum could serve to link sensory to motor areas across the two hemispheres. Although these assumptions were commonly made, there was little direct evidence that cortico-cortical fibres are necessary for the sensory guidance of movement. In the few cases in which the idea was tested experimentally, the results failed to support it. An indirect test was to study performance of tasks that require bimanual coordination by callosum-sectioned animals. A direct test was to study visually guided movements in monkeys in which all cortico-cortical connections between the occipital and the frontal lobes had been cut.

Hartmann & Trendelenburg (1927) found no impairment in monkeys' performance of bimanual tasks even when they were tested only a few hours after the corpus callosum had been cut. Myers et al (1962) found that monkeys could still perform skilled reaching movements after all cortico-cortical links between the primary visual and motor areas had been severed by deep cuts within the subcortical white matter. Although animals whose vision is restricted to one hemisphere and whose corpus callosum is cut prefer to use the hand opposite to the open eye (Downer 1959), they can easily be trained to use either hand with either eye (Glickstein & Sperry 1963).

Subcortical pathways linking sensory to motor areas of the brain

The skilled performance of monkeys lacking all cortico-cortical links argues that there must be alternative, subcortical routes that connect sensory to motor areas of the brain. There are two massive pathways that might play such a role. One is via the basal ganglia; the other by way of the pontine nuclei and the cerebellum. A surviving parieto-ponto-cerebellar route can explain much of the paradoxical sparing of sensory guided movement in animals in which cortico-cortical connections have been cut.

Nearly all of the fibres in the basis pedunculi are axons of cells in the cerebral cortex. A small percentage of these continue through the brainstem as the medullary pyramids to form the corticospinal tract, but the great majority of peduncle fibres terminate in the pontine nuclei. Even those fibres that go on to become the cortico-spinal tracts send a collateral branch to synapse upon cells in the pontine nuclei (Ugolini & Kuypers 1986). Cells in the pontine nuclei project bilaterally to the cerebellar cortex by way of the middle cerebellar peduncle. In humans, the pontine nuclei are by far the largest source of afferent fibres to the cerebellum. The cerebellum, in turn, has a powerful input on all of the descending motor pathways. One way to appreciate the importance of this route is to compare the effect of bilateral section of the fibres in the cerebral peduncle with that of cutting the corticospinal tract at the level of the medulla. Peduncle lesions produce far more severe and lasting deficits in motor control (Bucy et al 1966) than section of the medullary pyramids (Lawrence & Kuypers 1968).

In order to learn more about the cortico-pontine pathway we studied the areas of the cerebral cortex that project to the pontine nuclei. Which of the large number of cortical visual areas provide an input to the cerebellum? The striate cortex itself sends very few fibres directly to the pontine nuclei and hence to the cerebellum. Nearly all cortical visual information is relayed to the pontine nuclei from adjacent extrastriate visual areas.

The efferent connections of the striate cortex can be divided into two relatively independent streams: one of these has as its final target the inferior temporal cortex; the other the visual areas of the parietal lobe (Ungerleider & Mishkin 1982). In monkeys the dorsal, parietal lobe areas include the cortex at the depth and banks of the superior temporal and intraparietal sulci. Thus Ferrier's lesions of the angular gyrus would have destroyed virtually all of the dorsal stream of extrastriate visual areas.

Cells in the dorsal stream, the parietal lobe visual areas, are responsive to moving visual targets (Zeki 1974, 1978, 1980). Responses to moving targets do not necessarily indicate that a cell is involved in perceiving movement. Equally, such cells are likely to be part of a neuronal circuit that participates in the visual guidance of movement (Glickstein & May 1982).

Behavioural studies of lesions in extrastriate visual areas

In order to compare the behavioural effect of loss of the dorsal and ventral streams, Susan Buchbinder, Jack May and I made lesions in the parietal or temporal lobe visual areas of monkeys and tested them on a visuomotor task first described by Hans Kuypers and his colleagues and on visual discrimination learning (Glickstein et al 1998). On each trial the monkey is presented with a disc which contains a clearly marked groove. The monkey can retrieve a bit of food only by properly orienting its wrist and fingers.

Figures 1 and 2 show the differential effect of parietal and temporal lobe lesions in performance of this task. Parietal lobe lesions produced a profound deficit in the performance of the visuomotor tasks at all orientations. The animal was unimpaired in the acquisition of visual discrimination learning. Although the temporal lobe lesions profoundly impaired visual discrimination learning they had virtually no effect on visuomotor performance (Glickstein et al 1998). The effects of parietal lobe lesions in monkeys are consistent with clinical evidence about the effects of similar lesions in humans. Bálint (1909) described a severe visuomotor deficit in a patient with parietal lobe lesion. Gordon Holmes (1918)

FIG. 1.   (a) Surface reconstruction and representative coronal sections illustrating the parietal cortex lesion in one monkey. Thicker lines in diagrams of the coronal sections mark the extent and site of lesion. (b) Percentage of correct responses in a simple visuomotor task after successive parietal cortex lesions (see text). (c) Percentage of correct responses at each orientation of the slit before and after parietal cortex lesion (see text).

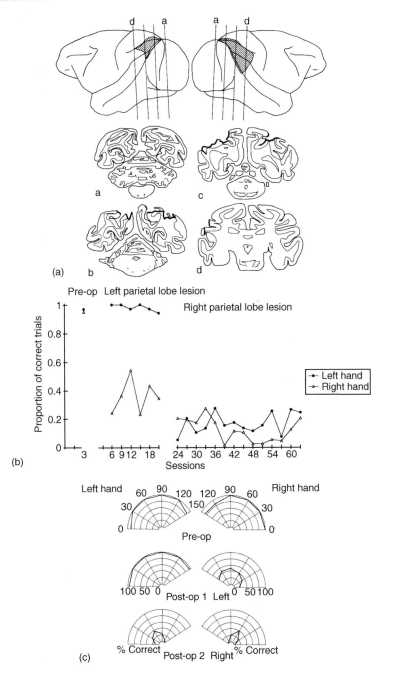

(a)

(b)

(c)

described a similar visuomotor deficit in a series of soldiers of the first World War that had sustained bilateral parietal lobe lesions.

Holmes interpreted the deficits in his patients as a disorder of visual orientation. The most striking symptom in his patients was a deficit in guiding the limbs or the whole body under visual control. The visuomotor deficit that Holmes described was almost identical to that described by David Ferrier in monkeys; so severe that it misled Ferrier to believe that the angular gyrus is the primary visual cortex.

How do parietal lobe visual areas connect to motor structures?

Lesions of the parietal lobe visual areas profoundly impair visually guided movement. In addition to its cortico-cortical connection, one of the major outputs from the parietal lobe visual areas is to the cerebellum by way of the pontine nuclei. We studied the anatomical organization of this pathway by following fibres from the cerebral cortex to the pontine nuclei using degeneration staining and neuronal labelling techniques (Glickstein et al 1980, 1985, 1994). We identified a massive input from the parietal lobe visual areas of monkeys to the dorsolateral pontine nuclei. The temporal lobe visual areas or the striate cortex itself have few or no pontine projections.

Studies using retrograde tracers tell the same story (Glickstein et al 1994). If wheat-germ agglutinin horseradish peroxidase (WGA-HRP) is injected so as to fill either the entire pontine nuclei or if the injection is restricted to the dorsolateral pons, there is dense retrograde filling of lamina V cells in the parietal lobe visual areas. There is little or no retrograde labelling of cells in the temporal lobe or the striate cortex itself. A major output from the dorsal visual stream is to the cerebellum by way of the dorsolateral pontine nuclei.

Cells in the pontine nuclei that receive an input from cortical visual areas are strongly activated by appropriate visual targets. Some years ago we studied visually activated cells in the pons of cats (Baker et al 1976). Visual pontine cells are activated briskly by moving targets. They are sensitive to the direction and velocity but not the precise shape of those targets. The same sorts of receptive fields are characteristic of visually activated cells in the pontine nuclei of monkeys (Thier et al 1988). The response properties of pontine visual cells are consistent with their functioning as a link in the visual control of movement.

FIG. 2.   (a) Surface reconstruction and representative coronal sections illustrating the temporal lobe lesions in one monkey. Thicker lines in the diagrams of the coronal sections demarcate the site and extent of lesions. (b) Proportion of correct responses in a simple visuomotor task after successive bilateral inferotemporal lobe lesions (see text). (c) Percentage of correct responses at each orientation of the slit following temporal lobe lesion (see text).

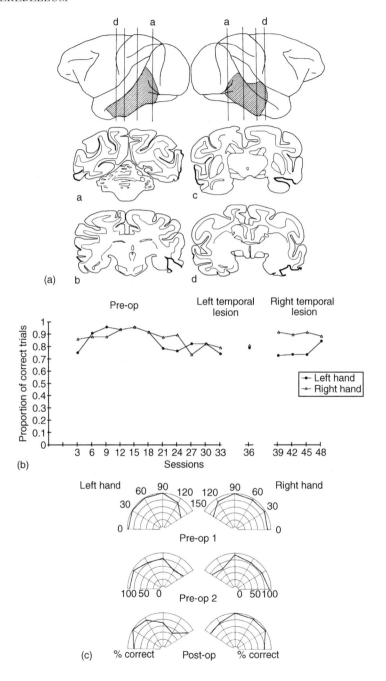

(a)

(b)

(c)

Does interruption of the pathway from sensory cortical areas to the pontine nuclei disrupt sensory guided movement?

Cortico-pontine fibres travel by way of the internal capsule and the cerebral peduncles. The arrangement of fibres on route to the pons is spatially organized. In humans the parietal lobe fibres travel in the caudal limb of the internal capsule.

Direct evidence for a role for the cortico-pontine pathway in the sensory guidance of movement is sparse. The severe deficits that are caused by cutting the fibres of the basis pedunculi (Bucy et al 1966) could have been due to damage to fibres from motor as well as from sensory cortical areas. Two sorts of behavioural evidence demonstrate a role for cortico-pontine fibres as a link in the sensory guidance of movement. One source of evidence comes from study of a patient by Classen et al (1995). This patient had a stroke which resulted in a severe deficit in visuomotor performance. The magnetic resonance imaging (MRI) scans revealed that the patient suffered no damage to the cerebral cortex or its interconnecting fibres. The infarct damaged fibres within the caudal limb of the internal capsule, interrupting the cortico-pontine visual pathway and depriving the cerebellum of a visual input.

There is additional evidence that reflects the importance of the cortico-ponto-cerebellar pathway from an ongoing behavioural study by Ned Jenkinson in my lab. In rats, like humans, cortico-pontine fibres arise from cells in lamina V and travel in the internal capsule and cerebral peduncles. Frontal fibres run in the ventromedial part of the peduncles; occipital and temporal fibres travel in the dorsolateral region. The somatosensory fibres are in the centre (Glickstein et al 1991).

We used a simple behavioural task to study sensory guided movements. In rats the mystacial vibrissae, the large and prominent whiskers on either side of the face, are as important as vision for guiding movement. Rats will jump a gap in the dark if they can feel the distant platform with their whiskers, and refuse to jump if they can not. Removing the barrel fields, the cortical target of the whiskers, is as disruptive as shaving them (Hutson & Masterton 1986).

We cut the fibres of the peduncles of rats on one side, so as to interrupt the cortico-pontine fibres from the barrel fields (Fig. 3). The lesion disconnected almost all of the cortical representation of the whiskers from the pontine nuclei. The lesion was unilateral so the animals still had cortical connections to the pons from one side and thus were not impaired. However, if we shaved the whiskers on the side of the face that retained its connection to the pons, the animal behaved as if the whiskers had been shaved bilaterally. They could not use the input from the surviving whiskers and would now cross the gap only if they could feel the far side with their nose or paw. If we cut the whiskers whose connection to the pontine nuclei had already been interrupted by the peduncle lesion, there was no effect on

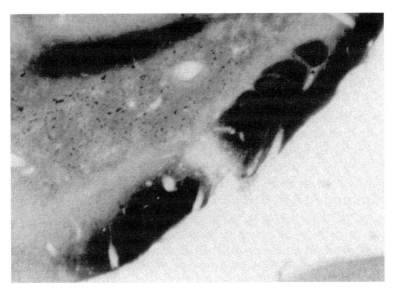

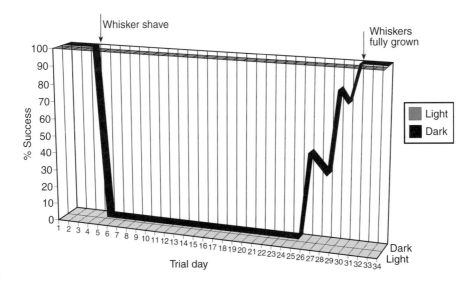

FIG. 3.   (a) Photomicrograph of a fibre-stained coronal section showing the site and extent of a typical peduncle lesion that interrupts connection from the barrel cortex to the pontine nuclei. (b) The success rate of a rat jumping across a gap of 16 cm, following unilateral peduncle lesion and ipsilateral whisker shave. Initially, the unilateral whisker shave disrupts the performance. As the whiskers regrow (from day 25 onward), the animal's performance recovers.

the behaviour. All of the animals recovered normal jumping when the shaved whiskers re-grew and all retained the ability to jump much greater distances when tested in the light.

Localization in the cerebellar cortex

Unravelling the localization of function in the cerebral cortex took many years. Functional localization in the cerebellum remains much more poorly understood. The cerebellar cortex is a deeply folded sheet of cells. Unrolled, its surface area in humans would be over half that of the cerebral cortex. Owing to the dense packing density of cerebellar granule cells the total number of neurons in the cerebellum exceeds that in the cerebral cortex. Despite its anatomical regularity and the known details of its physiology, there is surprisingly little understanding of functional localization in the cerebellar cortex. Lesions of the cerebellum impair the sensory control of movement, motor learning (Yeo et al 1985), and the ability to modify reflexes, but the localization as well as the mechanism of these functions remain unclear. Clinical studies are often vague on possible localization within the cerebellum (Holmes 1917, 1939), and the early physiologists (Luciani 1891) specifically denied its existence. Cerebellar lesions in humans tend to be diffuse, so it is difficult to identify differences in the behavioural effects caused by lesions of different cerebellar subdivisions.

The level of our understanding of cerebellar localization resembles that of the cerebral cortex in about 1850. We know a number of things that the cerebellum must do, but are unclear on where or how it does them. Anatomical studies of the distribution of afferent fibres within the cerebellum, unit activity during movement and behavioural studies of the effects of restricted lesions can all help to further our understanding of cerebellar localization and mechanism.

Where do pontine visual cells project on the cerebellar cortex?

One of the classical symptoms associated with cerebellar lesions in humans is a visuomotor deficit. The cerebellar target areas for visual information are close to vital brain stem structures, so there are relatively few surviving human cases with restricted lesions. Study of the distribution of visual input can help to clarify the general question of localization in the cerebellar cortex. We injected WGA-HRP into the dorsolateral pontine nuclei and studied retrograde labelling of cells in the cerebral cortex and orthogradely labelled fibres in the cerebellum (Glickstein et al 1994). The distribution of retrogradely labelled cells in the cerebral cortex confirmed that this region of the pons receives its input from the visual areas in the parietal lobe. The distribution of mossy fibre terminals in the cerebellar cortex revealed a massive input to a caudal region in the posterior lobe of the cerebellum, particularly the dorsal paraflocculus and adjacent region of the paramedian lobule and rostral uvula. There is a weaker input to lobules VI/VII, the classical vermian visual/oculomotor areas, the ventral paraflocculus, and very little to the flocculus proper.

Cerebellum and short-term motor memory: adaptation to a laterally displacing prism

The cerebellum is known to be necessary for several forms of motor learning and reflex modification. These functions are typically slow to acquire and they persist for a long time once established. The cerebellum may also be involved in types of short-term plasticity. If a person or a monkey looks through a lateral displacing prism they will mis-point in a direction away from the base of the prism. Prism adaptation is not primarily visual but represents a re-calibration of limb position based on a visual error signal (Harris 1965). The prism-induced mismatch between the intended and actual end-point of the reach is corrected within a few trials.

Some years ago, Joan Baizer and I studied the effects of cerebellar lesions in monkeys on prism adaptation (Baizer & Glickstein 1974). Only one of the five animals tested lost the ability to adapt to a laterally displacing prism. At the time we did the study the targets of visual pontine cells were unknown. We recently re-analysed the results of that study. Lesions of the vermian oculomotor area and of lobule V of the anterior lobe did not affect adaptation. It was only in the one animal in which the lesion included the dorsal paraflocculus and adjacent cerebellar visual targets that prism adaptation was lost. The results suggest a possibly important function for the cerebellum as the locus of a short-term 'scratch-pad' motor memory.

Cerebellum and modification of saccadic trajectories

If a person or monkey is asked to look at a target within $20°$ of the fixation point they will typically make an accurate saccade to that target. The usual latency from the time the target is illuminated to the time that the saccade is initiated is on the order of one-sixth of a second. If the original target light is extinguished and re-positioned at a different location, over successive trials people and monkeys will adapt by increasing or decreasing the saccade amplitude appropriately.

Noda and his colleagues mapped saccadic eye movements produced by microstimulation of lobules VI and VII of the vermis (Noda & Fujikado 1987). Although this area has a relatively modest input from cortical visual areas it probably has a much stronger visual input relayed to it from the superior colliculus. Shabtai Barash, Peter Thier and I studied the effect of a small lesion of this region of the monkey cerebellar cortex on the ability of the animal to modify its saccades.

Our preliminary results show that restricted cerebellar lesions impair the normal adaptation to horizontal saccades, without affecting upwards or downward modification. We do not yet fully understand the reason for the asymmetry in the effect of the lesion, but the results illustrate one important and localized function of the cerebellar cortex in short-term modification of a sensorimotor link.

These examples of a specific effect caused by restricted cerebellar lesions suggest that the problem of cerebellar localization is a soluble one. The challenge seems similar to that which faced scientists and clinicians studying the cerebral cortex 150 years ago.

Summary

(1) The cerebellum receives a powerful input from sensory areas of the cerebral cortex. In monkeys, and probably in humans, the visual input arises from a group of dorsal, parietal lobe extrastriate visual areas whose cells are particularly responsive to moving visual targets.

(2) Cells in the pontine nuclei that receive an input from cortical visual areas are powerfully activated by appropriate visual stimuli.

(3) Ponto-cerebellar projections are not completely diffuse, but have definite focal targets on the cerebellar cortex.

(4) Lesions at any point along the pathway from cerebral cortex to the cerebellum can produce deficits in the sensory guidance of movement.

(5) In addition to its known role in motor learning and reflex modification, the cerebellum can also serve as a locus for short-term 'scratch-pad' motor memory used in recalibrating limb position caused by an altered sensory input and the modification of saccadic amplitude.

References

Baizer J, Glickstein M 1974 Role of the cerebellum in prism adaptation. J Physiol (Lond) 236:34–35

Baker J, Gibson A, Glickstein M, Stein J 1976 Visual cells in the pontine nuclei of the cat. J Physiol (Lond) 255:415–433

Bálint R 1909 Seelenlähmung des 'Schauens'; optische Ataxie, räumliche Störung der Aufmerksamkeit. Monatschr E Psychiat u Neurolog 25:51–61

Betz V A 1874 Anatomischer Nachweis zweier Gehirncentra. Zbl Med Wiss 12:578–580; 595–599

Broca PP 1861 Remarque sur la siège de la faculté du langage articulé suive d'une observation d'aphémia (perte de la parole). Bull Soc Anat Paris 36:330–357

Bucy P, Ladpli R, Ehrlich A 1966 Destruction of the pyramidal tract in the monkey. The effects of bilateral section of the cerebral peduncles. J Neurosurg 25:1–23

Classen J, Kunesch E, Binkofski F et al 1995 Subcortical origin of visuo-motor apraxia. Brain 118:1365–1374

Downer J de C 1959 Changes in visually guided behaviour following mid sagittal division of the optic chiasm and corpus callosum in monkey (Macaca mulatta). Brain 82:251–259

Ferrier D 1876 The functions of the brain. Smith Elder, London

Flourens P 1824 Recherches experimentale sur les properiétés et les fonctions du système nerveux dans les animaux vertébrés. Crevot, Paris

Fritsch G, Hitzig E 1870 Über die elektrische Erregbarkcit des Grosshirns. Arch Anat Physiol u Wissenschaftl Med Leipzig 300–332

Glickstein M 1985 Ferrier's mistake. Trends Neurosci 8:341–344

Glickstein M, May J 1982 Visual control of movement. In: Neff W (ed) Contributions to sensory physiology. Academic Press, New York, p103–145

Glickstein M, Sperry RW 1963 Visuo-motor coordination in monkeys after optic tract section and commissurotomy. Fed Proc 22:456 (abstr)

Glickstein M, Cohen J, Dixon B et al 1980 Corticopontine visual projections in macaque monkeys. J Comp Neurol 190:209–229

Glickstein M, May J, Mercier B 1985 Cortico-pontine projections in the macaque: the distribution of labelled cortical cells after large injections of horseradish peroxidase in the pontine nuclei. J Comp Neurol 235:343–359

Glickstein M, Kralj-Hans I, Legg C, Mercier B, Ramna-Rayan M, Vaudano E 1991 The organisation of fibres within the rat basis pedunculi. Neurosci Lett 135:75–79

Glickstein M, Gerrits N, Kralj-Hans I, Mercier B, Stein J, Voogd J 1994 Visual pontocerebellar projections in the macaque. J Comp Neurol 349:51–72

Glickstein M, May J, Buchbinder S 1998 Visual control of the arm, the wrist, and fingers: pathways through the brain. Neuropsychologia, in press

Harris L 1965 Perceptual adaptation to invented, reversed, and displaced vision. Psychol Rev 72:419–444

Hartmann F, Trendelenburg 1927 Zur Frage der Bewegungstörungen nach Balklentrennung an der Katze und am Affen. Ztbl f d ges Neurol u Psychiat 47:149

Henschen SE 1890 Klinische und anatomische Beiträge zur Pathologie des Gehims Pt 1. Almquist and Wiksell, Upsala

Holmes G 1917 The symptoms of acute cerebellar injuries due to gunshot injuries. Brain 40:461–535; 677–681

Holmes G 1918 Disturbance of visual orientation. Br J Ophthalmol 2:449–468; 506–516

Holmes G 1939 The cerebellum of man. Brain 62:1–30

Hutson KA, Masterton RB 1986 The sensory contribution of a single vibrissa's cortical barrel. J Neurophysiol 56:1196–1223

Lawrence DG, Kuypers HGJM 1968 The functional organization of the motor system in the monkey. I. The effects of bilateral pyramidal lesions. Brain 91:1–14

Luciani L 1891 Il Cervelletto. Successori Le Monnier, Firenze

Munk H 1881 Über die Functionen der Grosshirnrinde. A. Hirschwald, Berlin, p 28–53

Myers RE, Sperry RW, McCurdy NM 1962 Neural mechanisms in visual guidance of limb movement. Arch Neurol 7:195–202

Noda H, Fujikado T 1987 Topography of the oculomotor area of the cerebellar vermis macaques as determined by microstimulation. J Neurophysiol 58:359–378

Thier P, Koehler W, Buettner U 1988 Neuronal activity in the dorsolateral pontine nuclei in the alert monkey modulated by visual stimuli and eye movements. Exp Brain Res 70:496–512

Ugolini G, Kuypers HG JM 1986 Collaterals of corticospinal and pyramidal fibres to the pontine grey demonstrated by a new application of the fluorescent fibre labelling technique. Brain Res 365:211–227

Ungerleider L, Mishkin M 1982 Two cortical visual systems. In: Ingle D J, Goodale M A, Mansfield R JW (eds) Analysis of visual behavior. MIT Press, Cambridge, MA, p 459–486

Yeo CH, Hardiman M J, Glickstein M 1985 Classical conditioning of the nictitating membrane response of the rabbit. II. Lesions of the cerebellar cortex. Exp Brain Res 60:99–113

Zeki SM 1974 Functional organization of a visual area in the posterior bank of the superior temporal sulcus of the rhesus monkey. J Physiol (Lond) 236:549–573

Zeki SM 1978 Functional specialisation in the visual cortex of the rhesus monkey. Nature 274:423–428

Zeki SM 1980 The responses of cells in the anterior bank of the superior temporal sulcus in Macaque monkeys. J Physiol (Lond) 308:85

DISCUSSION

Thach: When is the work with Joan Baizer going to be written up and reported in detail? This is the first time I have seen the localization of the one posterior cerebellar lesion that destroyed the prism adaptation or the ability to adapt, whereas the more anterior lesions do not. This is exactly what we have seen and you apparently saw it long before us. All we have from you and Baizer is the abstract in *J Physiol* (Baizer & Glickstein 1974), and that does not mention the critical differential site.

Glickstein: I have written the paper and it sits on my desk, but there's one table I don't like that I keep redoing. I have five cases, I have the pictures and the slides, and a relatively good reconstruction. The paper will soon be submitted.

Thach: We have a monkey who has been trained to adjust his pointing to prisms of three different dioptres. Muscimol is now being injected into various cerebellar sites. We believe that this postero-infero-lateral locator could be critical in storing the learned adjustment.

Gibson: To what extent are cortical contributions to the control of movement mediated by the cerebellum as opposed to direct corticospinal pathways?

Glickstein: If you compare the effects on the monkeys of Bucy's lesions in which he destroyed the entire peduncles in the mid-brain (Bucy et al 1966) with the effects Lawrence and Kuypers described of a corticospinal tract lesion (Lawrence & Kuypers 1968), the results of Bucy's lesion are devastating. Most of the animals were completely incapable of movement for a long time post-operatively. It took months before they had any recovery of their motor symptoms, compared to the relatively mild symptoms from the Lawrence and Kuypers studies in which they had made a clean and precise cut of the corticospinal tract. The other fibres that Bucy cut would have been relaying to the cerebellum by way of the pontine nuclei. When Cajal first began to study this pathway he thought that in 'simple' animals such as rats, as the pyramidal tracts went through the pontine nuclei, they gave off collaterals. Cajal never really had the concept of inhibition. If he saw a fibre going to a cell it had to be an excitatory connection. He therefore thought that these collaterals of the pyramidal tract were something like a power amplifier. Corticospinal fibres do give off collaterals (Ugolini & Kuypers 1986). Thus, in addition to the sensory input to the pontine nuclei, there is also a corollary discharge: if a corticospinal tract fibre is activated it will be registered in the cerebellum.

Goodale: As far as I know, the experiments in which you obtained a double dissociation of deficits in visuomotor control and visual discrimination following parietal and temporal lobe lesions in monkeys are quite unique. I know of no other experiments of this kind. I hope this work will be published soon.

Glickstein: These data will appear in memorial volume for Roger Sperry to be published in *Neuropsychologia*.

Ebner: There is the dorsal stream, which is sending visual information to the motor cortex. Also there is this enormous cerebro-ponto-cerebellar projection which is also providing visual information to the cerebellum. What are the differences and the similarities in the processing provided by these two streams? How is the visual information used in the cerebellum versus in the primary motor cortex and pre-motor areas?

Glickstein: The visual input to the cerebellum can account for paradoxes in the literature; preservation of visuomotor coordination when cortico-cortical fibres are cut. Massive deficits result from interruption along this pathway. We lack any clear understanding of functional localization in the cerebellum; Gordon Holmes was very vague about it. His authority was Luciani, who wrote the definitive book on the cerebellum in 1891. Just as Fritsch and Hitzig, Ferrier and others looked for evidence of functional localization in the cerebral cortex, so Luciani looked for evidence of localization of function in the cerebellar cortex. He said there was none. Gordon Holmes was strongly influenced by Luciani's findings, because his clinical observations mirrored the things that Luciani had described in animals. Gordon Holmes described very clearly that his cerebellar patients had muscle weakness and they had difficulty in carrying through on movements they intended to make. But Holmes doubted that there is any localization of function. The thing that gave localization a bad name was that it was prematurely announced by Lodewijk Bolk. Jan Voogd and I wrote a historical article on his contributions (Glickstein & Voogd 1995). Bolk was a great comparative anatomist and in 1905 he put forward an oversimplified view of cerebellar localization. He reasoned that movements which require collaboration across the mid-line are likely to be coordinated in the vermis. Movements of a limb would be controlled in the hemispheres. I think that's still true. Bolk gave localization a bad name because he assumed a *single* somatotopic map. Giraffes have a big lobulus simplex; that must be the neck. The rest of the head must be controlled by the anterior lobe. He waffled a little bit about paraflocculus and suggested that it is involved in control of the tail.

Thier: You seem to suggest that the pontine nucleus is just a simple relay nucleus handing cerebral information over in a one-to-one fashion to the cerebellar cortex. This view is misleading because it doesn't take into account the complexity of the microcircuitry which we are aware of today. We have been recording from monkey pontine nucleus cells for several years and have seen, for instance in the dorsolateral part of the pontine nuclei, not only visual responses such as you described, but also visuomotor activity such as pursuit-related responses and saccade-related responses (Thier et al 1988, 1996). Recently we have also seen more complex visual responses, such as responses to expanding or contracting visual patterns. The bottom line seems to be that almost every kind of response known to exist at the level of the parietal cortex can also be found at the level of the pontine nuclei. However, there is one difference between parietal and pontine nuclei cell responses in our hands: you can find combinations of response types in the pontine nuclei that don't occur at the level of the parietal cortex. If you look for pursuit- or saccade-related responses in parietal cortex, they seem to be segregated anatomically (Thier & Andersen 1997). In the pontine nuclei, however, there are a large percentage of cells which combine saccade and pursuit related responses (Thier et al 1996). The question is, how is this achieved? One possibility would be simple anatomical convergence. However, our anatomical data seem to rule this out (Schwarz & Thier 1995). In order to understand these combined responses we find in the pontine nuclei, we have to consider more elaborate ways to establish these connections. Our current hypothesis is that these combinations are established by specific elements of the internal circuitry in the pontine nuclei. Two elements could play a role: first, axon collaterals of pontine nuclei principal neurons and, secondly, pontine nuclei interneurons. The existence of axon collaterals of pontine nuclei principal neurons has been suggested by anatomical studies carried out by Mihailoff and co-workers (Mihailoff 1978). Such axon collaterals might contain pontine nuclei neurons in other parts of the pontine nuclei. These axon collaterals would connect the target cells to parts of the cerebral cortex, from which they do not receive direct anatomical input. The same could be achieved by interneurons, which most likely exist at least in the primate pontine nuclei (Thier & Koehler 1987, Cooper & Fox 1976). Finally, a wider dispersion of cerebrocortical signals from a given site in the pontine nuclei, contacted directly by cerebrocortical axon terminals, could also be mediated by way of feedback projections from the deep cerebellar nuclei which receive input from the pontine nuclei, either directly or through cerebellar cortex (Schwarz & Schmitz 1997). If this scenario were correct, one would expect to see not only direct monosynaptic but also late polysynaptic excitatory post-synaptic potentials evoked by stimulation of the cerebrocortical afferents in the cerebral peduncle. This is exactly what we have recently observed in our intracellular recordings from the rat pontine nuclei (Möck et al 1997). Anatomical convergence of cerebrocortical axons originating from different parts of cerebral cortex would result in fixed combinations of functional signals such as the combination of saccade- and pursuit-related signals observed by us. In principal, the indirect pathways outlined before might allow for less rigid convergence, thereby combining visuomotor signals such as saccade-related and pursuit-related signals on the level of single pontine neurons only if appropriate, for instance if catch-up saccades are required in order to compensate for insufficient smooth pursuit. This example prompts the idea that the major function of the pontine nuclei might in general be to combine visuomotor strategies such as saccades or pursuit whose simultaneous activation might be required by the context. We are currently trying to test this hypothesis.

Glickstein: We looked for multisensory units in the pontine nuclei of cats but we never found any. The response properties that we saw seemed to be simply determined by convergence from a large part of the visual cortex. We also looked at the fact that there must be some way of dealing with the difference in receptive field size of cortical and pontine visual cells. I grant your point, but I don't think the internal circuitry of the pons is likely to modify the input greatly.

Georgopoulos: Might the effects of lesions you see from the parietal cortex also be mediated through the cerebellum?

Glickstein: That's the bottom line of what I'm saying.

Passingham: Kuypers cut the fibres from parietal to premotor cortex and showed that the monkeys were impaired on his rosette task (Haaxma & Kuypers 1975), but you have pointed out that this leukotomy also cut the cortico-pontine fibres. If the effect comes from the cerebellum, it should be true that monkeys with cerebellar lesions are impaired in using a visual cue to guide their finger movements on the rosette task. We have tested monkeys with complete excitotoxic dentate and interpositus lesions, and found that they are poor at using the visual cue to guide their fingers into the correct slot (P. D. Nixon & R. E. Passingham, unpublished results). Of course, this does not tell you what the cortico-subcortical unit is doing that is different from the cortico-cortical projection.

Glickstein: One thing about the cerebellum is that it responds quickly. Cerebellar pathways get there quickly. It samples the magnocellular visual system. It receives the fastest of the spinal afferents. Simply put, the cerebellum is involved in the next few seconds of your life. It is particularly specialized for rapid and short-term modification of movement. The evidence is clear that for various kinds of long- and short-term motor learning and visuomotor modifications, the cerebellum is essential. The question is working out the machinery.

Strick: Your illustration of a posterior parietal projection to dorsal paraflocculus is really quite elegant. But I have trouble finding a route from dorsal paraflocculus into a system of that controls arm movements. Do you think that this system influences the portions of the dentate and interpositus that are involved in directing arm movement?

Second, do you think that lesions in the thalamic region that is the site of termination of cerebellar efferents are anyway near as potent in influencing an animal's ability to direct limb movements as lesions of the posterior parietal cortex?

Glickstein: I'll answer the first point simply: I emphasized the dorsal paraflocculus because it looks black when you hold a slide up. But as you see from the cartoon that I showed, the adjacent paramedian lobule also receives a major visual input.

Gibson: Dorsal paraflocculus has a heavy projection to the lateral region of posterior interpositus, which provides input to the superior colliculus (May et al 1990). Although cells in this region of interpositus appear to be related to eye movements (Van Kan et al 1993), they also may provide input to the limb-related cells in the colliculus that Dr Hoffmann and his colleagues have described (Werner et al 1997).

Marsden: To pick up on the second point of Peter Strick's question, there are data to show that parietal lesions in humans produce an order of magnitude greater deficit in visuomotor reaching than is seen in those with cerebellar lesions.

References

Baizer J, Glickstein M 1974 Role of the cerebellum in prism adaptation. J Physiol (Lond) 236:34–35

Bucy P, Ladpli R, Ehrlich A 1966 Destruction of the pyramidal tract in the monkey. The effects of bilateral section of the cerebral peduncles. J Neurosurg 25:1–23

Cooper MH, Fox CA 1976 The basilar pontine gray in the adult monkey: a Golgi study. J Comp Neurol 180:17–42

Glickstein M, Voogd J 1995 Lodewijk Bolk and the comparative anatomy of the cerebellum. Trends Neurosci 18:206–210

Haaxma R, Kuypers HGJM 1975 Interhemispheric cortical connexions and visual guidance of hand and finger movements in the rhesus monkey. Brain 98:239–260

Lawrence DG, Kuypers HGJM 1968 The functional organization of the motor system in the monkey. I. The effects of bilateral pyramidal lesions. Brain 91:1–14

May PJ, Hartwich-Young R, Nelson J, Sparks DL, Porter JD 1990 Cerebellotectal pathways in the macaque: implications for collicular generation of saccades. Neuroscience 36:305–324

Mihailoff GA 1978 Principal neurons of the basilar pons as the source of a recurrent collateral system. Brain Res Bull 3:319–322

Möck M, Schwarz C, Thier P 1997 Electrophysiological properties of rat pontine nuclei neurons in vitro. II. Postsynaptic potentials. J Neurophysiol 78:3338–3350

Schwarz C, Schmitz Y 1997 The projection from the cerebellar lateral nucleus to precerebellar nuclei in the mossy fiber pathway is glutamergic. A study using combinations of immunogold labelling with anterograde tracing in the rat. J Comp Neurol 381:320–334

Schwarz C, Thier P 1995 Modular organization of pontine nuclei: dendritic fields of identified pontine projection neurons in the rat respect the borders of cortical afferent fields. J Neurosci 15:3475–3489

Thier P, Andersen RA 1997 Multiple parietal 'eye fields': insights from electrical microstimulation. In: Thier P, Karnath H-O (eds) Parietal lobe contributions to orientation in 3D space. Exp Brain Res Suppl 25:95–108

Thier P, Koehler W 1987 Morphology, number and distribution of putative GABAergic neurons in the basilar pontine gray of the monkey. J Comp Neurol 265:311–322

Thier P, Koehler W, Buettner UW 1988 Neuronal activity in the dorsolateral pontine nucleus of the alert monkey modulated by visual stimuli and eye movements. Exp Brain Res 70:496–512

Thier P, Dicke PW, Barash S, Ilg U 1996 Demonstration of saccade-related single unit activity in the dorsolateral pontine nucleus (DLPN) of the rhesus monkey. Soc Neurosci Abstr 22:1458

Ugolini G, Kuypers HGJM 1986 Collaterals of corticospinal and pyramidal fibres to the pontine grey demonstrated by a new application of the fluorescent fibre labelling technique. Brain Res 365:211–227

Van Kan PLE, Houk JC, Gibson AR 1993 Output organization of intermediate cerebellum in the monkey. J Neurophysiol 69:57–73

Werner W, Dannenberg S, Hoffmann K-P 1997 Arm-movement-related neurons in the primate superior colliculus and underlying reticular formation: comparison of neuronal activity with EMGs of muscles of the shoulder, arm and trunk during reaching. Exp Brain Res 115:191–205

The cerebellum, predictive control and motor coordination

R. C. Miall

University Laboratory of Physiology, Parks Road, Oxford OX1 3PT, UK

Abstract. I argue that the cerebellum has at least two related roles, both sub-served by its operation as a 'forward model' of the motor system. First, it provides an internal state estimate or sensory prediction that is used for online control of movements; second, these predictive state estimates are used to coordinate actions by different effectors in the normal coordination of eye and hand, reach and grasp, etc. Preliminary electrophysiological data from cerebellar cortical neurons in the monkey supports the hypothesis that a proportion of cells code for the sensory consequences of movement. In a contrast between normal visually guided movement of a cursor and mirror reversed movement, approximately half the sample of 47 directionally sensitive cells were found to code for the movement of the cursor controlled by the monkey's limb, and not the limb movement itself. Functional imaging of the human cerebellum further supports the hypothesis that the cerebellum is involved in motor coordination. Subjects were tested performing ocular tracking, manual tracking without eye movement, or combined eye and hand tracking. Activation of cerebellar areas related to movement of eyes or hand alone was significantly enhanced when the subjects performed coordinated eye and hand tracking of a visual target.

1998 Sensory guidance of movement. Wiley, Chichester (Novartis Foundation Symposium 218) p 272–290

In this paper I will argue that the cerebellum plays an important role in providing predictive information about on-going movements. These cerebellar predictions may be used to help control sensory-guided movements and may also underlie coordinated movement control. I will first briefly describe motor control strategies using predictive signals and provide some evidence that the cerebellum is responsible for the generation of these signals. Finally, I will present some functional imaging data that support these ideas.

Most readers will be aware that robust control can often be achieved using negative feedback or error correction. A comparator determines the difference between the desired 'reference' value of a controlled variable and the present measured value of that variable (a 'state' variable; see Jordan [1994] for an excellent tutorial article). Negative feedback control is simple and useful because it seeks to reduce the measured errors to zero. But it can be compromised if the time delays in the system are too long, so that the relationship between measured errors and the responses become out of phase, or if the measured variables are not an accurate reflection of the state variables. However, simple feedback systems can be greatly improved if some predictive control can be built in. This predictive information might be knowledge of the future values of the reference signal, to be compared with the measured state of the system; or it might be knowledge of how the system will respond to the controller output (the 'motor commands'), i.e. an estimate of the future state of the system.

In a biological setting, reactive, negative-feedback control strategies are common, but there are also many examples of predictive control. When trying to catch a moving ball, the changing target position is predicted and the hand guided to its future position. Even in apparently simple tasks, such as reaching for a stationary coffee cup, predictions of motor actions are used to control the on-going movement. In principle, negative feedback could reduce the positional error between hand and cup, but this would be slow. Alternatively, the movement towards the cup might be pre-programmed and executed without any feedback from the arm or eyes during the reach. But after several spilt cups of coffee, it becomes clear that this 'feedforward' strategy is not effective and some feedback must be incorporated into the control process. It is an interesting question why movements are so inaccurate under these circumstances; possibilities include inaccuracy in target localization, in planning and storage of the motor programmes, and errors in the execution of the programme.

However, it is not a trivial problem to combine feedforward and feedback control systems, as one can destabilize the other. What is required for their combination is predictive information about the outcome of movement, so that these destabilizing effects can be avoided. I have previously argued that the cerebellum provides predictive estimates, based on efferent copies of motor commands (Miall et al 1993). The cerebellum under this hypothesis acts as a 'forward model' (Jordan 1994) in mimicking the forward, causal responses of the motor effectors to the motor command (Fig. 1). Its output is a sensory prediction, a signal estimating the outcome of movement, i.e. the sensory consequences of the motor commands. Note that these sensory estimates are not equivalent to efferent copy. Efferent copy encodes motor commands (e.g. intended muscle forces) and not the result of the command on the effector (e.g. hand motion). The cerebellum as a forward model requires sensory inputs to update its knowledge of the current state of the motor system, an efferent copy of motor commands which are being sent to the motor system, and a learning mechanism to ensure that the forward model accurately reflects the motor system behaviour and adapts over a long time scale (minutes or hours) to its changes. This 'Smith Predictor' hypothesis (Miall et al 1993) allows the motor control system to incorporate feedback and feedforward

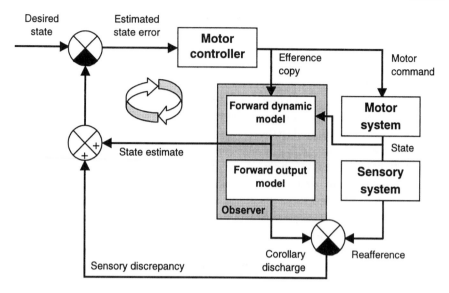

FIG. 1.   Using forward models. The outer loop of this figure indicates a feedback control loop in which motor commands from a motor controller act on the motor system to alter its state, and cause reafferent sensory inputs. To distinguish reafference from exafferent inputs, an observer (a forward model and forward output model; shaded box) generates an internal corollary discharge (an estimate of the sensory consequences of the motor action). The forward model can also produce a state estimate that can be used within an internal (rapid) feedback control loop, indicated by the circular arrow. In a Smith Predictor system (Miall et al 1993), the sensory and motor systems introduce significant feedback delays, so the forward output model is an internal model of these delays. This control scheme based on a Smith Predictor could be modified to include model predictive control, in which the feedback actions take account not only of the estimated state error, but also estimated future errors (Jordan 1994, Towhidkhah et al 1997). The balance between state estimates and sensory discrepancies (indicated by the summing junction on the left) could be modified by a weighting function to form a Kalman filter (Kalman & Bucy 1961). The sensory discrepancies are an appropriate training signal available to maintain the accuracy of the observer models.

control signals: it provides a predictive signal that can be used for updating the on-going motor commands, but it also provides a signal that is timed to synchronise with and cancel out the real feedback expected from the movement (the reafference signal, Fig. 1).

In addition to controlling the arm movement towards the cup, internal predictions based on a forward model may also be vital components of the coordination between thumb and fingers, hand and eye, and arm and trunk which are a normal part of our reaching movements (Miall & Wolpert 1996). The fingers open and reach a maximum aperture just before the hand reaches the cup; the fingers are already closing onto the cup as the hand stops moving forwards (Paulignan et al 1990). As the cup is lifted off the table, the grip force generated between fingers and thumb is synchronously modulated to compensate for the increased load forces (Johansson & Westling 1984). Finally, the eyes follow the moving cup as it approaches the face, and so the target for the oculomotor system is actually provided by the outcome of the arm movement. In this situation, or when tracking an external but predictable target (Barnes & Asselman 1992), ocular tracking responses are superior to those when tracking random targets, and display improved smooth pursuit velocity, reduced response lag and fewer catch-up saccades (Vercher & Gauthier 1988, Koken & Erkelens 1992, Vercher et al 1996). Similarly, the hand can reach for or track targets more accurately if the eyes also track the same target (Abrams et al 1990, Miall et al 1995) implying communication from the oculomotor centres to the manual control system. For all these coordinated and synchronous components of the movement, the effectors cannot each be reacting to feedback signals, but must be using feedforward, predictive, information. Outgoing commands must be based on the current *and* future state of each effector. So the coordination of complex behaviours is also dependent on predictive control, and I would suggest that the cerebellum is involved in this process.

There are several possible organizational schemes for eye and hand coordination. First, there may be a single site that commands separate downstream motor systems in parallel. It was suggested early on that the posterior parietal cortex (PPC) might form such a centre, generating the necessary signals to drive the hand and the eye towards a spatial target. But this scheme cannot explain why coordinated movement is more effective than movement of each effector alone (Biguer et al 1984, Abrams et al 1990, Vercher et al 1994). However, the PPC may have an important role in transformations between different coordinate frameworks. Hence motion of the hand might be translated into craniotopic or retinotopic coordinates in order to provide signals to assist ocular tracking, because its representation in shoulder-based coordinates would not meaningful for oculomotor control.

A second possibility would have separate controllers for each effector, each with access to information about the other. Cortical areas likely to be important are the premotor and supplementary motor areas, and the frontal and supplementary eye fields. In this scheme each controller would 'advise' others of what it was commanding, achieved by relatively direct communication between the relevant motor centres (SEF, FEF and the premotor areas).

However, several results point to the cerebellum having a key role in coordination, which argues against the first two model systems. For hand–eye control, the normal low-latency ocular smooth pursuit of the hand is lost after dentate lesions (Vercher et al 1996); cerebellar patients show abnormal interactions between saccades and hand velocity; and ocular latencies are increased after cerebellar damage in coordinated eye–hand motion (Brown et al

1993, Van Donkelaar & Lee 1994). Interjoint coordination is affected by cerebellar damage (Thach et al 1992) and grip–load force relationships are lost (Muller & Dichgans 1994). The cerebellum may also have a role in interlimb coordination and Thach et al (1992) have stressed the deficits in whole body control.

So, there might be a single site — the cerebellum — maintaining an estimate of the state of the whole body, which updates outward-bound motor commands before sending them onwards to the lower motor centres. Hence the cerebellum might update oculomotor motor commands on the basis of its knowledge of efferent commands to the hand, before these motor commands are sent onwards to the oculomotor nuclei. This hypothesis is close to the idea of the cerebellum as an 'inverse model' (Shidara et al 1993, Jordan 1994), and is analogous to the model of coordination proposed by Thach et al (1992) and Houk et al (1993). One could conceive of a direct translation from efferent copy of arm commands to grip force adjustments or ocular pursuit signals, but for this mapping to generalize across all commanded movements of the arm would imply a daunting complexity of the mapping function.

Finally, a fourth scenario is that a single structure acts as a coordinating hub, receiving from each motor control area and relaying back to the others. Thus the central hub might receive efferent copy from different motor controllers, and return estimates of the state of each system to other controllers. Several groups have suggested that the cerebellum could provide these estimates (reviewed by Miall et al 1993) and this is precisely the role suggested by my Smith Predictor/ forward model hypothesis.

The cerebellum would probably return state estimates in different coordinates for different controllers; for example, providing retinotopic estimates of hand position for the oculomotor system and Cartesian estimates of limb dynamics for the hand system. The cerebellum may also be the locus for adaptive change to these internal estimates, since coordinative information must be updated to reflect changes in the motor system with growth, fatigue, changes in load and even tool use. Effective coordination must allow for these factors because when a load is carried in the hand, the limb dynamics changes; likewise, holding a tool changes the effective limb kinematics.

It is clear that all areas mentioned (PPC, PM, SMA, FEF, SEF) project to the pontine nuclei, and thus to the cerebellum. Cerebellar outflow via the thalamus returns to all the same areas, including SMA and pre-SMA, PPC, FEF and pre-frontal areas. But many of these areas also have cortico-cortical interconnections, and cerebellar outputs do project to descending systems. The four organizational models cannot be distinguished purely on anatomical grounds. We need to turn to more direct tests of these models. It may also not be possible to tell from behavioural measurements alone whether the synchronous control is based on an internal state estimate generated by a forward model as opposed to a feedforward mechanism, but it seems likely to be. For example, in modulating grip forces during lift, it is important to take account of the acceleration of the object against the fingers. These loads act within a Cartesian framework so the planned modulation of grip should be based on an estimate of the Cartesian trajectory of the hand. Basing these modulations on the efferent command would not be appropriate. Likewise, for ocular tracking of the hand, a predictive signal based on efferent motor commands to the shoulder and elbow might be converted by a forward model to a signal describing the hand trajectory in visual space.

Single cell responses in the lateral cerebellar cortex

In order to test the hypothesis that the cerebellum contributes to the sensory prediction of movement, Mr E. Roberston, Dr X. Liu and I have begun to test the responses of cerebellar cortical neurons in a visually guided movement task (Robertson 1998, Robertson & Miall 1997). Two rhesus monkeys were trained to use a 2D manipulandum to control the position of a cursor on a computer screen. The screen was reflected by a mirror, so that a virtual image of the cursor was co-registered with the planar motion of the hidden manipulandum. The monkeys were then trained to follow step movements of a visual target to the left and right of a central start position. They were additionally trained to alternate between this task, in the normal condition, and with a task employing left–right reflection of the cursor movement, such that movement of the hand to the right was displayed as movement of the cursor to the left (Alexander & Crutcher 1990). In this way, we could test the monkeys in step movements of the arm to the left and right, in which the arm and cursor directions were congruent or opposed. The forward model hypothesis predicts that if the cerebellum is estimating the visual consequences of movement, then cells should be found to have sensitivity to the direction of motion of the cursor and not the hand movement. We have recorded so far from 88 cerebellar cortical cells with responses related to arm movement in these two tasks; we have histology from one animal and the majority of the recording sites lie within lobules V and VI, in the territory previously studied by e.g. Ojakangas & Ebner (1992) and Thach et al (1992). We sought to exclude cells with responses to passive manipulation of the arm, and also cells with eye motion-related responses. Of the sample so far recorded, 28 (32%) showed directional specificity during the task, which is a prerequisite for us to be able to test their preferential responses to cursor or hand movement. Of these directional cells, 57% showed a preferential sensitivity for the direction of the cursor (Fig. 2). Only three cells showed preferential responses to the direction of the hand motion, rather than the cursor; the remaining nine cells could not be unambiguously classified (Table 1).

NORMAL TASK

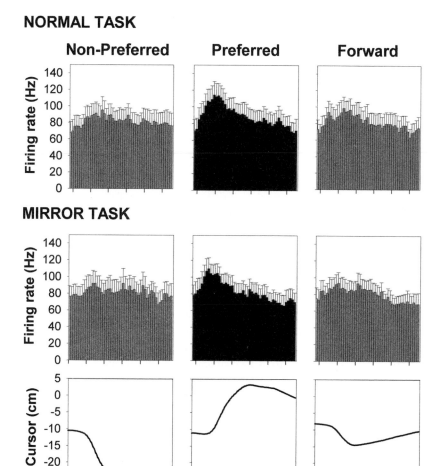

FIG. 2. Cerebellar sensitivity to cursor movement. Each histogram shows the average (± SE) of eight peri-movement time histograms from eight different cells (8–12 trials per cell). (*Top row*) The normal task; (*middle row*) the mirror tracking task. (*Centre column*) Firing patterns during cursor movement in the preferred direction for each cell; (*left column*) movement on the cursor in the non-preferred direction; (*right column*) movement forwards. Average cursor position for one representative cell in the normal task has been plotted at the bottom (horizontal cursor movement for left and centre panels, vertical cursor movement for right panel). Because these cells were selected for their movement direction sensitivity, they were most active during movement in one direction (*top row*). However, the monkey's hand moves in opposite directions in the normal and mirror task and yet the cells' firing pattern was unchanged (*middle row*). Forward movement of the hand is unaffected by the left–right mirroring of the cursor (*right column*).

TABLE 1 Movement-related neurons recorded in the lateral cerebellar cortex during normal and mirror-reversed tracking

	Movement-related neurons 88 (100%)			
	Direction-dependent neurons 28 (32%)			Direction-independent neurons
Cursor related 16 (57%)	Arm related 3 (11%)	Unclear 9 (32%)		60 (68%)

Each entry indicates the total number of cells (and their percentage of the sample). Cells were first classified as showing left–right directional specificity (28 cells) or showing multi-directional or no directional specificity (60 cells). For the detailed breakdown of direction-dependent cells, the percentage figures are given as a proportion of the testable sub-sample of 28 neurons.

Cells that fire preferentially to cursor direction, for example firing more strongly when the cursor moves to the right, may be encoding the target position or the eye movement signal. However, we believe these cell responses do not simply reflect target position or eye movements for two reasons. First, they tend to respond late, well after the target motion and after the reflexive eye movement to follow the target (Fig. 2). Second, by triggering the average from the target motion rather than the monkey's arm movement, the responses become more weakly time locked. It is also unlikely that they reflect eye movements made to follow the cursor. We have previously recorded horizontal eye movements in these tasks, and have seen that the monkeys' eyes follow the target image, rather than the cursor. Of course, many questions still need to be addressed in this work, including testing the responses of the cerebellar nuclear cells receiving from these regions of the cerebellar cortex, distinguishing the responses of Purkinje cells from other cortical cells, and testing the sensitivity of complex spikes to the direction of cursor and arm movement.

Functional imaging of coordinated eye and hand movements

The previous section introduced the possibility that the cerebellar cortex may be coding for the visual consequences of arm movement. This would be an appropriate signal to allow coordinated movement of the eye to track hand movement. I have therefore tested the cerebellar activation in eye and hand coordination using functional magnetic resonance imaging (fMRI). These experiments were performed in collaboration with Dr H. Imamizu and Dr S. Miyauchi (Miall et al 1997).

We tested subjects in three different visually guided movement experiments. The target(s) were provided by a small light-coloured square moving in a slow, smooth and unpredictable trajectory against a black background. In all instances, the target for the eyes was a white square, while the target for the hand movement was a larger red square. In the first two experiments, subjects alternated every 17.6 s between four tasks. For the first experiment these tasks were to mimic the motion of the target with index finger, wrist or forearm movement whilst tracking the target with the eyes; the baseline condition was tracking the target with the eyes without any limb movement. This experiment allowed us to determine cerebellar activation during visually guided movement.

In the second experiment movement of the hand was recorded by a modified computer mouse, and displayed on the screen as a light green square. We also recorded spatial errors and the distance the mouse was moved to monitor tracking performance in the manual tracking conditions. Movement of the eyes could not be monitored during scanning, but was recorded in other subjects outside the scanner during the same tracking tasks. In this experiment, the first baseline task was ocular and hand fixation ('fixation'); the second was ocular tracking of the moving white target ('eyes-only'); the third task was manual tracking, using the mouse to superimpose the green cursor on the moving red target while the eye remained fixed on the stationary white target ('hand-only'). The fourth task was to pursue the moving white target with the eyes, while also tracking the cursor target using the mouse ('eye & hand'). In this last case, the manual tracking task was compensatory, so that the cursor was displaced from the red target by the target waveform, and the subject made compensatory movements of the hand to return the cursor to the stationary red square. We chose to use pursuit tracking in the hand-only condition whilst using compensatory manual tracking in the 'eye & hand' condition so that in all tracking tasks there was equivalent spatial separation of the eye and hand targets, as well as approximately equal retinal input in each case.

Ocular tracking responses detected in Experiment 2 were only just above statistical threshold ($P = 0.01$), hence we also tested subjects as they alternated just between ocular tracking and fixation tasks without hand movement, to double the number of statistical comparisons (Experiment 3). In this experiment, subjects followed the white ocular target with their eyes at all times, without hand movement.

Functional images were collected using an echo planar imaging sequence on a 1.5T fMRI scanner; $1.88 \times 1.88 \times 9.1$ mm voxels, 10 slices per image, TR 4.4 s, 128 acquisitions. Data were analysed with SPM96 statistical parametric mapping software from the Wellcome Department of Cognitive Neurology, London, UK (Friston et al 1995) implemented in Matlab (Mathworks Inc. Sherborn MA, USA),

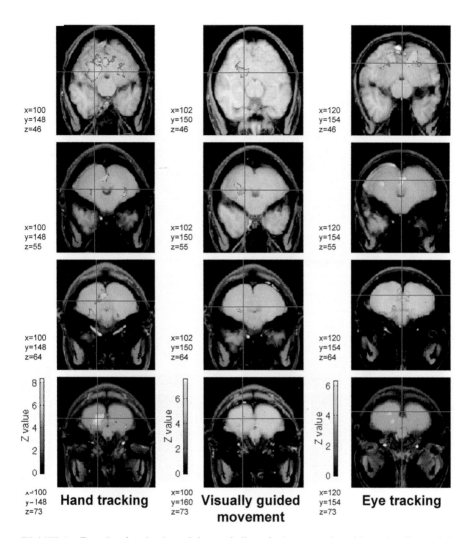

PLATE 1   Functional activation of the cerebellum during manual tracking, visually guided hand movement and ocular tracking tasks. Each panel shows an axial section through the cerebellum with statistically significant activation areas overlaid ($P < 0.001$, corrected). (*Left column*) Contrast of the hand-alone tracking condition against baseline (Experiment 2). (*Centre column*) Contrast of finger, wrist and forearm movement conditions against the baseline condition of ocular tracking (Experiment 1). (*Right column*) Contrast of ocular tracking against the baseline condition of fixation (Experiment 2). Coordinates of the red cross hairs are given in millimetres.

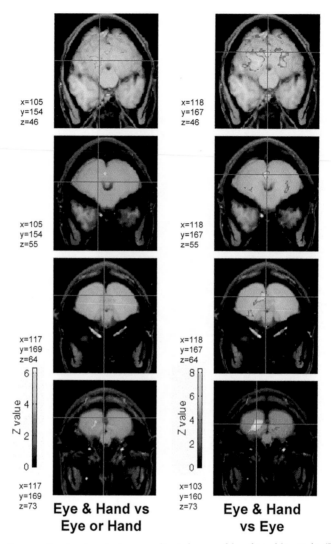

PLATE 2   Increased activation during coordinated eye and hand tracking tasks (Experiment 2). (*Left column*) Contrast of 'eye & hand' tracking with 'eye-only' *or* 'hand-only' conditions. Areas of significance are more activated in the eye & hand condition. The cross-hairs localize the same anterior cerebellar region seen in Plate 1. Notice also the vermal area activated in the second panel. (*Right column*) Contrast of eye & hand tracking against eye-alone conditions. The cross-hairs locate the same vermal region as in Plate 1, right column.

TABLE 2.   Functional activation of cerebellar sites during eye and hand tasks

		Coordinates				Cluster statistics		
Exp	Task contrasts	X	Y	Z	Location	Size k	Z	P
1	Hand vs.	102	150	46	Ant CB	203	7.59	<0.001
	Fixation	88	160	55	Ant CB	—	6.31	<0.001
		94	147	64	Ant CB	—	5.35	0.004
		100	160	73	Post CB	25	6.27	<0.001
2	Hand vs.	111	156	36	Ant CB	1137	8.43	<0.001
	Fixation	149	143	55	Vermis	115	6.68	<0.001
2	Eye & Hand	105	154	36	Ant CB	500	6.26	<0.001
	vs. Eye or Hand	117	169	55	Vermis	—	5.91	<0.001
		105	149	46	Ant CB	—	5.36	0.003
2	Eye & Hand	111	156	36	Ant CB	1258	8.53	<0.001
	vs. Eye	100	149	46	Ant CB	—	8.32	<0.001
		118	167	46	Vermis	—	8.15	<0.001
		100	160	73	Post CB	—	8.00	<0.001
2	Eye & Hand	139	190	46	Ant CB	15	4.80	0.026
	vs. Hand							
3	Eye vs.	105	143	73	Vermis	35	5.54	0.001
	Fixation	139	130	64	PFL	19	5.33	0.003

Table of regional activations characterized by the volume of each region (k), the highest Z value, its corrected significance P, and the location of this primary maximum. The coordinates given are in units of 1.88 × 1.88 × 1.88 mm. Up to three secondary maxima (light font) are included for each region with their associated significance based on the corrected P value. Key to putative locations: Ant CB, ansiform lobule; Post CB, paramedian lobule; PFL, paraflocculus.

combining results from six sessions (three subjects each repeated twice) after 5 mm Gaussian smoothing and spatial normalization to a template of one subject's structural image.

Strong activation of the cerebellar cortex was seen in these visuomotor tasks (Table 2). With this imaging protocol we did not see significant nuclear activation under any condition. Visually guided movement of the hand (Experiment 1) activated two regions most strongly, one close or equivalent to the areas recorded in the rhesus monkeys (lobules V and VI, mainly ipsilateral but with some contralateral activation as well; Plate 1). There was also some activity more caudally, in what is probably paramedian lobe (Plate 1). Visual tracking using the hand-held computer mouse (Experiment 2) activated both these regions more strongly (Plate 1, left column). Ocular tracking (Experiment 3) most strongly activated a site in the vermis, as well as some small sites in intermediate cortex (Plate 2). Contrasting the 'eye & hand' tracking task with eyes-only *or* hand-only tasks within Experiment 2 showed activation in similar sites — the anterior and posterior lateral regions and the vermal area (Plate 2, left column). Thus cerebellar cortical areas activated by eye or hand tracking alone were significantly more activated during coordinated eye and hand tracking. Most interestingly, contrasting the 'eye & hand' condition with 'eyes-alone' (Plate 2, right column) showed that the vermal area activated by ocular tracking was significantly more activated during eye and hand tracking. Thus despite there being similar eye movement in each task, this area was more activated when the hand was used in coordination with the eyes.

Conclusions

Under the hypothesis that the cerebellum acts as a forward model, its input should be an efferent copy of motor commands, and its output should be an estimate of the sensory outcome of the motor systems following those commands. This state estimate is then used as an internal feedback signal to allow rapid and accurate control of the motor system, despite long delays in the feedback loop (Miall et al 1993). A good proportion of neurons in the lateral cerebellar hemisphere appear to fit this pattern of responses. As an additional part of its function as a forward model, the cerebellum could also provide state estimates to other motor systems, e.g. informing the oculomotor system about the predicted motion of the hand. I suggest that this operation allows the cerebellum to coordinate different effectors, and this also seems to be borne out by functional imaging. It will now be important to further dissect the operation of the cerebellar cortex and nuclei, and to study the cerebellar interactions with the cerebral motor areas.

Acknowledgements

This work was funded by a Wellcome Trust Senior Research Fellowship. I gratefully acknowledge the use of the imaging facilities of the CRL Laboratory, Tokyo, and also the facilities of the FMRIB Centre, Oxford, as well as the support of the research teams at CRL, Tokyo and ERATO, ATR, Kyoto.

References

Abrams RA, Meyer DE, Kornblum S 1990 Eye-hand coordination: oculomotor control in rapid aimed limb movements. J Exp Psychol 16:248–267
Alexander GE, Crutcher MD 1990 Neural representations of the target (goal) of visually guided arm movements in three motor areas of the monkey. J Neurophysiol 64:164–178

Barnes GR, Asselman PT 1992 Pursuit of intermittently illuminated moving targets in the human. J Physiol (Lond) 445:617–637

Biguer B, Prablanc C, Jeannerod M 1984 The contribution of coordinated eye and head movements in hand pointing accuracy. Exp Brain Res 55:462–469

Brown SH, Kessler KR, Hefter H, Cooke JD, Freund HJ 1993 Role of the cerebellum in visuomotor coordination. I. Delayed eye and arm initiation in patients with mild cerebellar ataxia. Exp Brain Res 94:478–488

Friston KJ, Holmes AP, Worsley KJ, Poline JB, Frith CD, Frackowiak RSJ 1995 Statistical parametric maps in functional imaging: a general approach. Hum Brain Map 2:189–210

Houk JC, Keifer J, Barto AG 1993 Distributed motor commands in the limb premotor network. Trends Neurosci 16:27–33

Johansson RS, Westling G 1984 Roles of glabrous skin receptors and sensorimotor memory in automatic control of precision grip when lifting rougher or more slippery objects. Exp Brain Res 56:550–564

Jordan M 1994 Computational aspects of motor control and motor learning. In: Heuer H, Keele S (eds) Handbook of motor control. Springer-Verlag, Berlin, p 1–65

Kalman RE, Bucy RS 1961 New results in linear filtering and prediction. J Basic Eng (ASME) 83D:95–108

Koken PW, Erkelens CJ 1992 Influences of hand movements on eye movements in tracking tasks in man. Exp Brain Res 88:657–664

Miall RC, Wolpert DM 1996 Forward models for physiological motor control. Neural Networks 9:1265–1279

Miall RC, Weir DJ, Wolpert DM, Stein JF 1993 Is the cerebellum a Smith Predictor? J Mot Behav 25:203–216

Miall RC, Haggard PN, Cole JD 1995 Evidence of a limited visuo-motor memory used in programming wrist movements. Exp Brain Res 107:267–280

Miall RC, Imamizu H, Miyauchi S 1997 An fMRI study of topographic organisation of the cerebellar cortex in coordinated movement. Soc Neurosci Abstr 23:293.2

Muller F, Dichgans J 1994 Dyscoordination of pinch and lift forces during grasp in patients with cerebellar lesions. Exp Brain Res 101:485–492

Ojakangas CL, Ebner TJ 1992 Purkinje cell complex and simple spike changes during a voluntary arm movement learning task in the monkey. J Neurophysiol 68:2222–2236

Paulignan Y, MacKenzie C, Marteniuk R, Jeannerod M 1990 The coupling of arm and finger movements during prehension. Exp Brain Res 79:431–435

Robertson EM 1998 Some features of motor actions. DPhil thesis, Oxford University, Oxford, UK, submitted

Robertson EM, Miall RC 1997 Neurons in the lateral cerebellum coding for a particular visuo-motor task, but not for the motor commands. J Physiol (Lond) 501P:38–39

Shidara M, Kawano K, Gomi H, Kawato M 1993 Inverse-dynamics model eye movement control by Purkinje cells in the cerebellum. Nature 365:50–52

Thach WT, Goodkin HP, Keating JG 1992 The cerebellum and the adaptive coordination of movement. Annu Rev Neurosci 15:403–442

Towhidkhah F, Gander RE, Wood HC 1997 Model predictive impedance control: a model for joint movement. J Mot Behav 29:209–222

Van Donkelaar P, Lee RG 1994 Interactions between the eye and hand motor systems: disruptions due to cerebellar dysfunction. J Neurophysiol 72:1674–1685

Vercher JL, Gauthier GM 1988 Cerebellar involvement in the coordination control of the oculo-manual tracking system: effects of cerebellar dentate nucleus lesion. Exp Brain Res 73:155–166

Vercher JL, Magenes G, Prablanc C, Gauthier GM 1994 Eye-head-hand coordination in pointing at visual targets: spatial and temporal analysis. Exp Brain Res 99:507–523

Vercher J, Gauthier GM, Guedon O, Blouin J, Cole J, Lamarre Y 1996 Self-moved target eye tracking in control and deafferented subjects: roles of arm motor command and proprioception in arm-eye coordination. J Neurophysiol 76:1133–1144

DISCUSSION

Gibson: I have three questions. First, if your model is predicting cerebellar output, why are you studying Purkinje cells and not nuclear cells? Second, the term 'cerebellum' includes much more than interpositus: are you modelling a function of the entire cerebellum or a specific region of cerebellum such as interpositus? Third, if you cannot define what movements are being controlled by the system, how can you say that the same movements are being studied with different tasks? It seems that your final model might fit better as a model of the processing of cerebellar cortex than of the motor system.

Miall: With regard to the first point, we are of course interested in looking at the output of both the cerebellar nuclei and the Purkinje cells. We started by recording in the cortex — Purkinje cells and other cortical cells — and we have just started shifting to the dentate. It makes a lot of sense to know what's going on in the cerebellar cortex and what's going on in the cerebellar nuclei.

In your second question, you asked which areas of the cerebellum we are concerned with. We have tried to go for exactly the same region that Tim Ebner (Ojakangas & Ebner 1992) and Tom Thach (Thach et al 1992) were recording from. They find cells that are active in these sorts of lever movement tasks, and we find cells which behave in much the same way as these. We're looking at the same sorts of cells in somewhat different tasks.

Concerning your third question about matching movements in the normal and mirror-reversed tasks, I have to accept that all we're recording is the lever movement. The monkeys may be making subtly different finger movements during these tasks.

Gibson: I'm not saying that the cerebellum is only concerned with finger movements, but I am trying to say that different regions may have highly specialized functions in movement control. Just because the task is moving a lever does not mean that lever movement represents the output of the part of the brain being studied.

Miall: No, we can't say that, but what we can say is that is the task that that animal is controlling at that stage. So if you can find cells which are correlated with the behaviour of that task, then you can make the assumption that they may be concerned with that. This is the same in any area: if you're recording in motor cortex, you can't deny the possibility that the monkey is actually twiddling his little toe, but it seems unlikely if he is moving a lever and you are getting correlation of the cells with the lever movement. I accept that in the ideal world you would like to know what every muscle in the animal is doing, so that you could correlate the firing with each muscle, but this is unreasonable and impossible.

Thach: What do you call the process? The term you've given it — a sensory processor — is unfortunately misleading to a lot of people.

Miall: It is processing the sensory consequences of movement. I think that's more precise.

Thach: I have emphasized more the motor controller property, which requires sensory processing. Where I say 'sensory processor', you say 'processing of the sensory consequences of movement' and it becomes semantically complicated. People don't know what we're talking about and think we disagree, whereas in fact I don't think we do. It's a question of terminology.

Many of the things Alan Gibson says are worth emphasizing here. In the human cerebellum there are many inputs which are demonstrably not sensory. In fact there's *no* first-order sensory input: it is all modified. Thus to even call it 'sensory' is stretching the terminology. To many people, when you use the 'sensory' word, they think you mean it's affecting sensation. This clearly is not so, except for certain senses that depend on spindle afferents, as in position of limb detection. Even there, the deficit after sensory damage is so slight as to have taken the strenuous efforts of Steven Grill and Mark Hallett to nail it down (Grill et al 1994). There's another system which has a strong sensory input and is clearly using sensory information to help in its motor control operations, but we call it a motoneuron, because of its more obvious effects on muscle. Would one want to call it a sensory processor? It depends on whether one accepts the *effect* of the signal output or the *process* going on within the structure as the 'label' for it.

Miall: Perhaps the most important distinction I should make is what I mean when I say that it is concerned with sensory consequence of movement and processing that information. I would be very surprised if the cerebellum was involved in primary sensory processing. I don't believe it is doing that. It is trying to generate an internal signal which is used by other systems to tell them what sensory output they can expect from that movement. Now that has a sensory element, because what it is trying to do is match the sensory information that is going to come as a consequence of that movement, but it's not doing primary sensory processing; I am not saying that the cerebellum is involved in visual processing and you'll go blind if you lose your cerebellum. What I'm saying is that it's trying to generate a signal which is vital at some stage in the motor system, and which is an internal estimate of the sensory consequences of your movements. This is done in order to control and coordinate movement.

Jeannerod: I want to bring one observation to challenge what you have said concerning the role of the cerebellum as an indicator of the sensory consequences of movement. We have observed one patient with an anterior parietal lesion, without any motor deficit. When this patient performed complex movements such as grasping, there was virtually no coordination between the grasp and the reach. But this patient was likely to have intact cerebellar circuitry and especially her fast internal feedback loops in her spinal cord and so on were preserved. Do you have any comments on this?

Miall: The only comment that I can make is a rather weak one. In this sort of situation, what I would propose is that the information from those parietal areas is going through to the cerebellum. Although the cerebellum is intact, it is not getting normal inputs.

Georgopoulos: Are you aware of the study of Martin & Ghez (1985)? They recorded cells in the motor cortex of cats performing a task very similar to your task. With the cursor moving in the opposite direction (of the movement), they found that 18/50 (36%) of cells followed the cursor and the remaining 32/50 (64%) followed the direction of force exerted by the arm. I have never recorded in the cerebellum, but I thought that the Purkinje cells would fire at higher rates than some of those you showed.

Miall: Yes, those were slightly lower firing rates than you might expect from Purkinje cells. However, we don't know that all of these cells are Purkinje cells. Although we think that a good proportion are Purkinje cells, we can't at the moment say whether or not there are any differences between them and other cortical cells. The way we have the cells classified at the moment it's not obvious whether the Purkinje cells are doing something different from the other cells.

Marsden: As I understand it, one of your concepts is that the cerebellum is an efficient feedforward motor machine which will generate movement in anticipation of the feedback from the periphery, thus circumventing the delays of the peripheral feedback. I come up against the problem of Friedreich's ataxia. The major pathology of Friedreich's ataxia involves deafferentation of the cerebellum. Its clinical features are identical to those seen in people with cerebellar damage *per se*. Deafferentation produces the same cerebellar deficits as damage to the cerebellum, which to me means that your internal feedforward machine must be highly inefficient or must depend upon the feedback to work.

Miall: I think the latter is the case. It's totally dependent on periodic updating from the real proprioceptive system. Mitchell Glickstein mentioned earlier that the cerebellum is involved primarily in the next 10 seconds of our lives. It is trying to make these predictions on the basis of where you are now and where you may be in 10 seconds time. It then needs updating, because it's such a complex thing that you're trying to predict that you can't let these functions free-run forever. So you predict during the course of the movement and then you need some re-updating of your models.

Stein: I'm pleased you like the idea of the cerebellum predicting the sensory consequences of movement! But it has been expanded by certain people like Ivry to suggest that cerebellum is involved in what everybody would think of as purely sensory processing, for instance timing things or assessing velocity. Do you think this is just wrong?

Miall: No, I don't think it's wrong. One of the very important parts of these sorts of predictions is the timing dimension. These predictions have to be accurate both in the metrics of what they predict and their timing. There's no point in trying to predict a corollary discharge signal if you mis-time it, so that it can't be compared with the true reafferents.

Andersen: In your diagram I didn't notice the massive feedback projections from motor cortical structures back to the sensory cortex. What role do you see them as playing? It seems as if you are having the cerebellum doing all the prediction and updating, and sending efference copies back to the sensory cortical areas.

Miall: I think the general principle that I tried to espouse may be distributed widely throughout the motor system. The motor system generates a lot of sensory information which has to be dealt with. Many of those fibres will therefore be providing information through to the sensory systems.

Lemon: A brief quantitative point. Arthur Prochazka has estimated that one simple flexion or extension movement of the knee joint in the cat generates 10^7 impulses per second of sensory feedback. The amount of sensory input that even a simple movement can generate is therefore a big problem.

Andersen: I guess I was wondering what you think the cerebellum does that isn't being accomplished by the cortico-cortical back projections.

Miall: It does it better!

Ebner: I want to confirm something that Chris Miall is observing. We recently published a paper in which the monkey was trained in a task requiring that the animal perform a visuomotor transformation (Ebner & Fu 1997). The animal was trained to move a cursor on the screen using four different gains. For the first gain the movement of the cursor was appropriate for the hand movement. For the second gain the hand and the cursor movements were completely reversed. For the other two gains the reversal of the hand–cursor relation was limited to either the x or y axis. We recorded the simple spike activity of Purkinje cells, not nuclear neurons. We were surprised that when we examined the 'movement field' of these neurons, it shifted dramatically with the change in gain. That is, the discharge appeared to represent the movement of the cursor on the screen and not only the dynamics or kinematics of the hand movement. Using the temporal regression techniques mentioned by Apostolos Georgopoulos the other day, we asked how firing was correlated with the hand kinematics versus the cursor movement on the screen. The results suggested that the simple spike discharge correlated to movement kinematics actually led the movement. In contrast, the simple spike correlations with the sensory component were later. Would this be consistent with your observations? However, the sensory component may be occurring too late for what your model would predict.

Miall: This is one of the most difficult problems with this sort of work. What you want to try to distinguish is something that's generated by the cerebellum as a sensory prediction, versus the sensation which will be coming in — probably to the same areas — with close temporal alignment. The fact that you get sensation-related activity late on in the movement is predicted from our model, because one of the things that comes out of the cerebellar model is a corollary discharge which should be coincident with the real sensory feedback. Then the problem is: if you're getting this late signal during the course of the movement, how can you distinguish that from something being driven by the sensory inputs? This is very difficult to distinguish. Of course, what you would also like to see is this early predictive signal; maybe that's what corresponds to the activity you say is leading the movement.

Thach: People don't have an intuitive sense of what a predictor is or does. Simple-mindedly, I like to think of the following analogy. In submarine warfare in World War II they had something called an 'is/was machine', where you estimated where the enemy ship *was* and where you were currently and the speed of each, and from this old information you used geometry and time to calculate where to send your torpedo. You needed the 'old' information to make that calculation. To get back to David Marsden's point, you do need sensation as input into the predictor. The sensation that's coming in that's helping to make the prediction is *old* sensory information. This would be a pre-condition prior to the onset of the movement or at the very beginning of the movement. The context in which the movement occurs, including the sensation as to the state of the limb, combined with intent, could lead you to manufacture a signal that would predict and help in the formulation of the movement itself. Friedreich's ataxia patients do have a peripheral neuropathy, and certainly peripheral neuropathies can give ataxias with a normal cerebellum, which are very similar to a 'cerebellar' ataxia. The two — sensation and the cerebellum — work together to predict and make movements.

Miles: The model presented here was a general one and it isn't clear to me how it would be applied to explain the particular experimental data set under consideration. I agree that such general models are an essential first step for the rigorous characterization of biological control problems, but if they are to be successfully tested on actual biological systems they must first be rendered more specific. This transition from generic to particular is not trivial, as evidenced by the many problems encountered during successive attempts to test the general model of cerebellar learning proposed independently by Marr and Albus. One of the most influential of these was the inspired attempt by Ito more than a quarter of a century ago to account for adaptive gain control in the vestibulo-ocular reflex. That the cerebellum was involved in this process was apparent early on, but the exact nature of this involvement was unclear until recently, in large measure I think

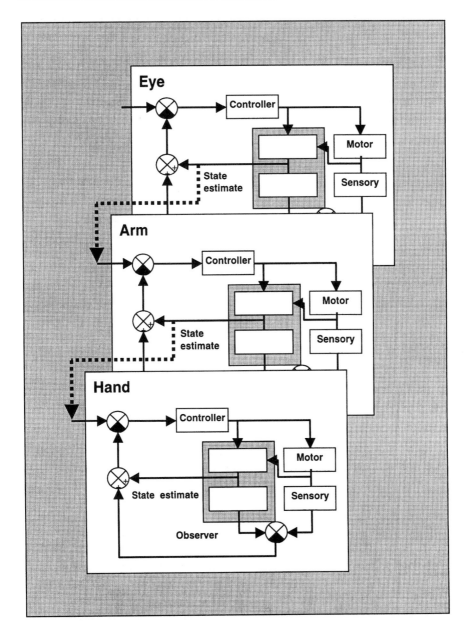

FIG. 3.   A schematic diagram showing how forward models could be used in coordination. The diagram is modified from Fig. 1, and shows three coupled controllers, one for each of the eyes, the arm and the hand. Dotted lines are drawn linking them to indicate how the state estimate provided from one controller could provide predictive information for another controller.

because of the incompleteness of the early models (for recent review see Raymond et al 1996).

Miall: Let me try to justify the use of this sort of diagram (Fig. 3). This is not meant to be an exact simulation of the motor control system, in which we can put in equations into each of those black boxes, put it onto the computer and say this is going to work (but see Miall et al 1993, Miall & Wolpert 1995). This figure is meant to illustrate a principle which the motor system may use in its general operations. For example, you could ask me how the motor system co-ordinates different effectors, or how the hand can track an object that the eye is tracking. We need a general principle to understand that. The principle that I take from this sort of diagram is that, if the eye is following a target, what is important for the hand to be able to follow that same target and perhaps catch it, is some estimate of where the eye is in terms of an egocentric framework. Thus we need an output from the oculomotor system which is in some sort of egocentric representation which the arm control system can then use. Likewise, the arm is carrying the hand, and the fingers will open and close to catch the object: what is important for the hand controller is knowing something about where it is going in real space. The hand may not want to know, if you like, the shoulder angle and the elbow angle and the wrist angle; the grasp may be dependent on the Cartesian movement of the whole arm through space. We need these sorts of translations from motor commands into state estimates in the right sort of framework for the next effector.

References

Ebner TJ, Fu QG 1997 What features of visually guided arm movements are encoded in the simple spike discharge of cerebellar Purkinje cells? Prog Brain Res 114

Grill SE, Hallett M, Marcus C, McShane L 1994 Disturbances of kinaesthesia in patients with cerebellar disorders. Brain 117:1433–1447

Martin JH, Ghez C 1985 Task-related coding of stimulus and response in cat motor cortex. Exp Brain Res 57:427–442

Miall RC, Wolpert DM 1995 The cerebellum as a predictive model of the motor system: a Smith predictor hypothesis. In: Ferrell WR, Proske U (eds) Neural control of movement. Plenum, New York, p 215–223

Miall RC, Weir DJ, Wolpert DM, Stein JF 1993 Is the cerebellum a Smith Predictor? J Mot Behav 25:203–216

Ojakangas CL, Ebner TJ 1992 Purkinje cell complex and simple spike changes during a voluntary arm movement learning task in the monkey. J Neurophysiol 68:2222–2236

Raymond JL, Lisberger SG, Mauk MD 1996 The cerebellum: a neuronal learning machine? Science 272:1126–1131

Thach WT, Goodkin HP, Keating JG 1992 The cerebellum and the adaptive coordination of movement. Annu Rev Neurosci 15:403–442

Internal models for motor control

Mitsuo Kawato and Daniel Wolpert*

*ATR Human Information Processing Research Laboratories and Dynamic Brain Project, ERATO, JST, 2-2 Hikaridai, Seika-cho, Soraku-gun, Kyoto 619-0288, Japan and *Sobell Department of Neurophysiology, Institute of Neurology, Queen Square, London WC1N 3BG, UK*

Abstract. The process of moving the hand to a target in space involves a series of sensorimotor transformations that translate visual and other sensory information about the location of the target object and the limbs into a set of motor commands that will bring the hand to the desired position. Recent work at various laboratories has provided strong support for the hypothesis that the CNS learns and maintains internal models of sensorimotor transformations. An internal model is a neural system that mimics the behaviour of the sensorimotor system and objects in the external environment. Internal models enable the CNS to predict the consequences of motor commands and to determine the motor commands required to perform specific tasks. In this chapter, we first summarize recent computational, behavioural and neurophysiological studies that address the theoretical necessity of internal models, the locations of internal models, and the neural mechanism for acquiring internal models through learning. Then, we propose a new computational model of multiple internal models.

1998 Sensory guidance of movement. Wiley, Chichester (Novartis Foundation Symposium 218) p 291–307

Many recent computational studies in sensorimotor control have addressed the following three questions regarding internal models of a motor apparatus and the external world in visuomotor transformations. (1) Why are internal models necessary for visuomotor transformation? (2) Where might internal models be located in the brain? (3) How can internal models be acquired in the brain? We first briefly summarize several studies done at ATR while addressing these questions in the following two sections.

Movements are performed within a wide range of visuomotor environments. For example, when controlling chopsticks, we must learn the mapping between the finger joint angles and torques and the distance and force exerted between the tips of the chopsticks. In everyday life we manipulate a variety of objects with different kinematic and dynamic properties, e.g. a cup, a car, a computer mouse or a pencil. We also behave in qualitatively different visuomotor environments such as an office, a road, a garden, a tennis court, a downhill skiing slope or a video game. To deal with these wide variety of behavioural paradigms associated with different objects and environments, we need to employ specific sensorimotor transformations that are tailored to particular situations.

Given these considerations, it seems reasonable to suggest that the CNS maintains multiple internal models of sensorimotor transformations. In the fourth section, we propose a computationally coherent model of how the human brain learns and switches between multiple internal models.

Computational and behavioural reasons for the necessity of internal models

The problem of controlling goal-directed limb movements can be categorized conceptually into information-processing sub-processes: trajectory planning, coordinate transformation from extracorporal space to intrinsic body coordinates, and motor command generation. These sub-processes are required to translate the spatial characteristics of the target or goal of the movement into an appropriate pattern of muscle activations. Each of the three problems is computationally difficult in the sense that its solution cannot be uniquely determined because the number of control variables that must be determined is much larger than the number of input variables that specify the motor task. For example, in the visuomotor coordinate transformation, the degrees of freedom of the arm and body trunk are much larger than the degrees of freedom specifying visual location of the target. In a trajectory planning problem, the CNS must specify an infinite number of variables for a continuous temporal pattern of arm trajectory given only the final state of the arm. In motor command generation, the number of joint torques, muscle tensions, motor neuron activations, and firing patterns of motor cortical neurons are much more extensive than those of joint angles, angular velocities and acceleration, which are sufficient to specify arm trajectory. A computationally coherent approach that can resolve this computational difficulty, often called *ill-posedness*, *redundancy*, or *indeterminacy*, necessitates internal models (Kawato 1996). Here, let us concentrate only on the motor command generation problem.

Fast and coordinated arm movements should be executed under feedforward control since biological feedback loops are slow and have small gains. Two major feedforward control schemes have been proposed in the computational study of motor control. The first is the equilibrium-point control hypothesis (Fel'dman 1966, Bizzi et al 1984, Hogan 1984, Flash 1987), some versions of which advocate that the CNS can avoid complicated computations by relying on spring-like properties of muscles and reflex loops. For this mechanism to work efficiently, the mechanical and neural feedback gains, which can be measured as mechanical stiffness and viscosity in perturbation experiments, must be quite high. The second proposed feedforward control mechanism assumes that the CNS needs to acquire an internal inverse dynamics model of a controlled object through motor learning and to utilize it in fast and well coordinated movement control (Kawato et al 1987). In the latter hypothesis, the arm's mechanical stiffness during movement could be quite low. Gomi & Kawato (1996) recently measured the stiffness of the arm during multijoint movements by using a novel mechanical device called PFM (Parallel link direct drive air and magnet Floating Manipulandum). Their finding of low stiffness suggests that fast and coordinated movements cannot be executed by relying solely on intrinsic mechanical properties of muscles or on neural feedback loops. Therefore, an inverse dynamics model of the arm is necessary.

Neurophysiological characterization of internal models

Internal models may be located in many places in the CNS. However, the cerebellar cortex is one of the few places where the existence of such models is experimentally well supported. Acquiring an inverse internal model through motor learning is computationally difficult. Kawato and colleagues proposed a cerebellar feedback-error-learning model to resolve this difficulty (Kawato et al 1987, Kawato & Gomi 1992). In this model, climbing fibre inputs, one of the two major synaptic inputs to the cerebellar cortex, are assumed to carry a copy of the feedback motor commands generated by a crude feedback control circuit. Thus, the complex spikes (CS) of Purkinje cells (P cells) activated by climbing fibre inputs are predicted to be sensory error signals in motor command coordinates. This scheme was recently experimentally supported for the ventral paraflocculus (VPFL) of the monkey cerebellum during ocular-following responses (OFRs). OFRs are tracking movements of the eyes evoked by movements of a visual scene and are thought to be important in the visual stabilization of a gaze. The model schematically depicted in Fig. 1 was supported by a number of studies by Kawano and his colleagues (Shidara et al 1993, Kawano et al 1996a, Kobayashi et al 1998, Kawato et al 1997), including an inverse dynamic analysis of the simple spike (SS) and CS firing frequency of VPFL P cells.

Shidara et al (1993) reconstructed complicated SS firing patterns of VPFL P cells during OFRs by using an inverse-dynamics representation of eye movement (i.e. linear combination of eye acceleration, velocity and position). They found that SS firing frequency temporal profiles were fairly accurately reproduced by this model: the determination coefficient was larger than 0.7 for more than 80% of the neurons studied (19/23). The mean ratio of acceleration coefficient to velocity coefficient of the P cells was 72.1, which was close to that of motoneurons (67.4). These results provide evidence for the proposition that the cerebellar cortex constitutes a dynamic part of the inverse dynamics model of the eye motor plant: first, because

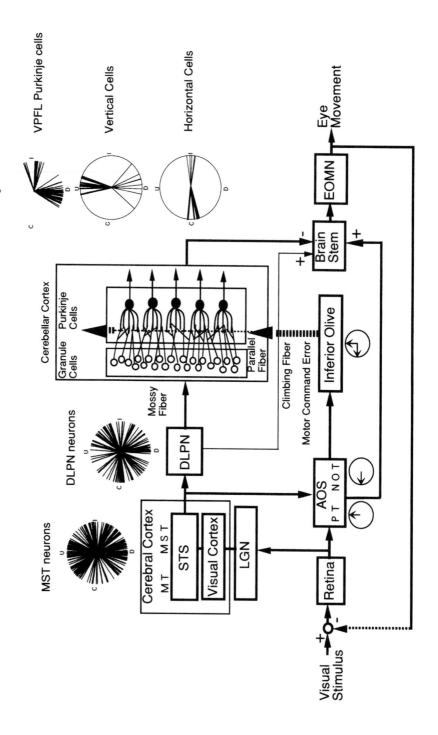

the SS of P cells can provide a motor command that compensates both the inertia and viscous forces necessary for OFR; second, because it was revealed that neural firing patterns were not well reconstructed by the inverse dynamics model for the area MST neurons or for the dorsolateral pontine nucleus (DLPN) neurons, which provide visual mossy fibre inputs to the VPFL. That is, while the parallel fibre inputs to the cerebellar cortex most probably provide the desired trajectory information, the SS outputs from the cerebellar cortex provide the dynamic part of the necessary motor command. This is equivalent to the definition of the inverse dynamics model.

The circuit diagram shown in Fig. 1 was modified from the scheme of Kawano et al (1996b) to correspond to the block diagram of the cerebellar feedback-error learning model (CFEL). The phylogenetically older crude feedback circuit of CFEL corresponds to the lower negative feedback loop of Fig. 1, comprising the retina, the accessory optic system (AOS) and the brain stem. The phylogenetically newer, more sophisticated feedforward/feedback pathway and the inverse dynamics model of CFEL correspond to the cerebral and cerebellar cortical pathway and the cerebellar cortex of Fig. 1, respectively.

Insets in Fig. 1 show the preferred directions of neurons in different brain regions in response to large visual stimulus motion that induces OFR. The data for DLPN and MST were taken from Kawano et al (1992, 1994). SS data were from Shidara & Kawano (1993). Pretectum (PT) and nucleus of optic tract (NOT) data were based on Kawano et al (1996b). The pairwise preferred directions of the SS (thin line) and the CS (thick line) of individual P-cells were taken from Kobayashi et al (1998). The preferred directions of MST and DLPN neurons were evenly distributed over 360°. Thus, the visual coordinates for OFR have an uniform distribution in all possible directions. On the other hand, projections of the 3D spatial coordinates of the extraocular muscles become oriented in either the horizontal or vertical direction, and they were entirely different from the visual coordinates. Shidara & Kawano (1993) demonstrated that the preferred direction of P cell SS was either downward or ipsilateral, and at the site of each recording, electrical stimulation of a P cell elicited eye movement toward the preferred direction of the SS of that P cell. These data indicate that the SS coordinate framework is already that of the motor commands. Thus, a drastic visuomotor coordinate transformation occurs at the

---

FIG. 1.   Schematic diagram of main neural pathways and neural networks responsible for control of ocular following responses in monkeys. STS, superior temporal sulcus; DLPN, dorsolateral pontine nucleus; AOS, accessory optic system; PT, pretectum; NOT, nucleus optic tract; EOMN, extraocular motor neurons. Different brain regions are arranged so that the overall figure resembles the feedback-error learning model of the cerebellum.

parallel fibre–P cell synapse. What, then, is the crucial information for this sensorimotor transformation (in other words, inverse dynamics model)? The CFEL model proposes that the CS and, eventually the AOS are the source of this motor command spatial framework. The preferred directions of PT neurons are upward and those of NOT neurons are contralateral; they are inherited by the inferior olive neurons and ultimately by the CS of P cells. If long-term depression and potentiation occur at the parallel fibre–P cell synapse controlled by the high and low CS firing rates, respectively, the CS preferred directions could determine the opposite preferred directions of the SS on a cell-by-cell basis. A much more sophisticated analysis using a generalized linear model of CS and SS firing probability combined with the inverse dynamics model revealed that the CS temporal firing probability carries very-high frequency, accurate information with its ultra-low firing rate (1–2 spikes/second); furthermore, there exist cell-to-cell negative correlations between SS and CS firing characteristics on an individual cell basis (Kobayashi et al 1998, Kawato et al 1997). All of these recent findings strongly support the CFEL, and consequently, neural implementation of the inverse dynamics model.

Multiple paired forward-inverse model

In the previous sections we reviewed both the computational theories and behavioural and physiological studies that support the assertion that the brain, especially the cerebellum, acquires internal models of the motor apparatus. There are three potential advantages to employing multiple inverse models, with their inherent modularity, over a non-modular single inverse model. First, the world is essentially modular, in that we interact with multiple qualitatively different objects and environments. By using multiple inverse models, each of which might capture the motor commands necessary when acting with a particular object or within a particular environment, we can achieve an efficient coding of the world. In other words, the large set of environmental conditions in which we are required to generate movement requires multiple behaviours or sets of motor commands, each embodied within an inverse model. Second, the use of a modular system allows individual modules to participate in motor learning without affecting the motor behaviours already learned by other modules. Such modularity can therefore reduce interference between what is already learned and what is yet to be learned, thereby speeding up motor learning while also retaining previously learned behaviours. Third, many situations we encounter are derived from a combination of previously experienced contexts, such as novel conjoints of manipulated objects and environments. By modulating the contribution to the final motor command of the outputs of the inverse modules, an enormous repertoire of behaviours can be generated. With as few as 32 inverse models, in which the outputs of each model either contributes or does not contribute to the final motor command, we have 2^{32} or 10^{10} behaviours — sufficient for a new behaviour for every second of a person's life. Therefore, multiple internal models can be regarded conceptually as motor primitives, which are the building blocks used to construct intricate motor behaviours with an enormous vocabulary.

Assuming that multiple internal models are present within the brain, several questions naturally arise. Since inverse models are not expected to be genetically inherited, how are they acquired during motor learning? In such acquisition, it would be necessary to divide up the repertoire of behaviours for different contexts while preventing new learning from corrupting previously learned behaviours. At any given time we are usually faced with a single environment and a single object to be manipulated, so the brain must solve the selection problem of issuing a single set of motor commands from its large vocabulary. Therefore, how can the outputs of the inverse models be appropriately switched on and off in response to different behavioural contexts to generate a coordinated final motor command? In this section, we propose a new model that answers these fundamental questions in a computationally coherent manner from a single principle. Empirical data supporting this model will be presented later.

The basic idea of the model is that each inverse model is augmented with a corresponding forward model. The brain therefore contains multiple pairs of corresponding forward and inverse models (Fig. 2). Within each pair, the inverse and forward internal models are tightly coupled during both their acquisition, through motor learning, and their use, through gating dependent on the behavioural context. Key to this model are responsibility signals, which reflect, at any given time, the degree to which each pair of forward and inverse models should be responsible for controlling the current behaviour. A responsibility signal is derived from the comparison of the errors in prediction of the forward models. This signal couples the inverse and forward model pairs, guides learning in each pair of the inverse and forward models, and gates the contribution of each inverse model's output to the final output.

In our specific computational model, which embodies this general idea, we use multiple competing forward models to partition experience. Our assumption is that at least one forward model will provide an accurate prediction given any context. The prediction errors of the forward models are used to calculate the responsibility signal λ_i by the soft-max function (Equation 3). This responsibility signal is used in three ways: to gate the learning of the forward models (Equation 8), to gate the learning of the inverse models (Equation 9), and to gate the contribution of the inverse models to the final motor command (Equation 7).

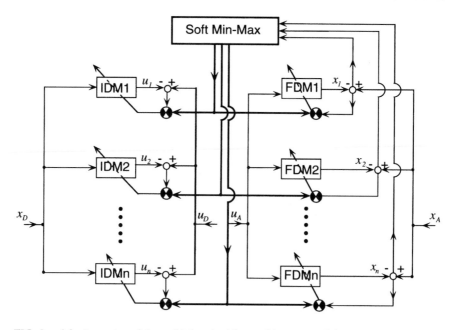

FIG. 2.   A basic version of the multiple paired forward-inverse model.

$$x_A(\cdot) = f[u_A(\cdot)] \tag{1}$$

$$x_i(t) = \phi\{w_i(t), x_A(t - \Delta), u_A(t)\} \tag{2}$$

$$\lambda_i(t) = \frac{\exp\{-\parallel x_A(t) - x_i(t) \parallel^2\}}{\Sigma_{j=1}^n \exp\{-\parallel x_A(t) - x_j(t) \parallel^2\}} \tag{3}$$

$$x_E(t) = \sum_{i=1}^n \lambda_i(t)x_i(t) = \sum_{i=1}^n \lambda_i(t)\phi\{w_i(t), x_A(t - \Delta), u_A(t)\} \tag{4}$$

Here we consider a motor system we wish to control by motor command $u_A(t)$ at time t. The resulting (actual) movement trajectory, $x_A(t)$, is determined by Equation 1, which describes the causal relationship between the motor command and the movement governed by the functional f, which describes the forward dynamics of the motor apparatus. In most cases, f is represented by a set of non-linear differential equations with time delays. We now consider a set of forward models with outputs $x_1, x_2, \ldots, x_n$ representing the predictions made by the

1st, 2nd, . . ., and n-th forward models, respectively. The prediction $x_i(t)$ of the state of the motor apparatus $x_A(t)$ by the i-th forward model is calculated through the non-linear function ϕ, which depends on three variables (Equation 2): the synaptic weights w_i of the neural network comprising the i-th forward model, the previous state of the motor apparatus $x_A(t-\Delta)$, and the motor command $u_A(t)$. On the basis of the prediction errors of the forward models, the responsibility signal λ_i for the i-th forward model–inverse model pair is calculated by the soft-max function of Equation 3. The final state prediction is given by the summation of the outputs from the whole set of n forward models weighted by λ_i (Equation 4).

$$u_D(\cdot) = f^{-1}[x_D(\cdot)] \tag{5}$$

$$u_i(t) = \psi\{\alpha_i(t), x_D(t)\} \tag{6}$$

$$u_E(t) = \sum_{i=1}^{n} \lambda_i(t)u_i(t) = \sum_{i=1}^{n} \lambda_i(t)\psi\{\alpha_i(t), x_D(t)\} \tag{7}$$

For the inverse models, x_D and u_D, denote the desired trajectory and the desired motor command, respectively. Each inverse model produces a motor output with $u_1, u_2, \ldots, u_n$ denoting the outputs from the 1st, 2nd, . . ., n-th inverse models. The output of the i-th inverse model is calculated through the non-linear function ψ, which depends on two variables (Equation 6): the synaptic weights α_i of the neural network comprising the i-th inverse model and the desired state of the motor apparatus $x_D(t)$. For simplicity, we assume that the motor command of each module is calculated purely by feedforward mode from the desired trajectory; however, this can be directly extended to also include the feedback of the current state. The total motor command generated by the whole set of n inverse models is given as the summation of outputs from these inverse models weighted by the responsibilities (Equation 7).

$$\frac{dw_i}{dt} = \varepsilon\lambda_i(t)\frac{d\phi_i}{dw_i}(x_A(t) - x_i(t)) = \varepsilon\frac{dx_i}{dw_i}\lambda_i(t)(x_A(t) - x_i(t)) \tag{8}$$

$$\frac{d\alpha_i}{dt} = \varepsilon\lambda_i(t)\frac{d\psi_i}{d\alpha_i}(u_D(t) - u_i(t)) = \varepsilon\frac{du_i}{d\alpha_i}\lambda_i(t)(u_D(t) - u_i(t)) \tag{9}$$

In summary, each forward model receives the total motor command, and each model's prediction is compared with the actual outcome. Only those forward models with small errors should adapt, and those with large errors should learn little. This is mediated through the responsibilities λ_i. Conceptually speaking, if one forward model's prediction is good, its corresponding inverse model receives the major part of the motor error signal and its output contributes significantly to the final motor command. On the other hand, if the forward model's prediction is poor, its corresponding inverse model does not receive the full error and its output contributes less.

The simpler model described above (Fig. 2) assumes that the desired motor command is available to train multiple inverse models. This assumption is implausible for biological motor learning, and a more sophisticated physiological computational model is shown in Fig. 3, which combines the feedback-error learning model (Kawato et al 1987, Kawato & Gomi 1992) with the simple model described above.

$$u_A(t) = u_E(t) + u_F(t) \tag{10}$$

$$u_F(t) = g\{x_D(t) - x_A(t)\} \tag{11}$$

$$\frac{d\alpha_i}{dt} = \varepsilon\lambda_i(t)\frac{d\psi_i}{d\alpha_i}u_F(t) = \varepsilon\frac{du_i}{d\alpha_i}\lambda_i(t)u_F(t) \tag{12}$$

The total motor command fed to the motor apparatus is the summation of the total feedforward motor command $u_E(t)$ and the feedback motor command $u_F(t)$. The feedback motor command can be calculated from the difference between the desired movement pattern $x_D(t)$ and the actual movement pattern $x_A(t)$ through an appropriate function g (usually a PID controller or a PAD controller is assumed appropriate). In the learning (Equation 12), the feedback motor command is used as the error signal for the motor command.

We will briefly review some of the psychophysical studies showing that multiple behaviours can be learned, switched on the basis of context, and even mixed. Several studies have shown that the motor system is able to adapt to multiple different environments. Context-dependent adaptation can also be seen if cued by gaze direction (Kohler 1964, Hay & Pick 1966, Shelhamer et al 1992), body orientation (Baker et al 1987), arm configuration (Gandolfo et al 1996), an auditory tone (Kravitz & Yaffe 1972) or the feel of prism goggles (Kravitz 1972, Welch 1971, Martin et al 1996). In general, de-adaptation is quicker than adaptation (Welch 1986), suggesting that de-adaptation may be mainly a switching process while adaptation represents learning a new module. Similarly, adaptation becomes increasingly rapid when subjects are repeatedly presented with two different prismatic displacements separated temporally (McGonigle & Flock 1978, Welch et al 1993), suggesting that a retained module can be quickly switched on again in response to the behavioural context. Data for mixing two

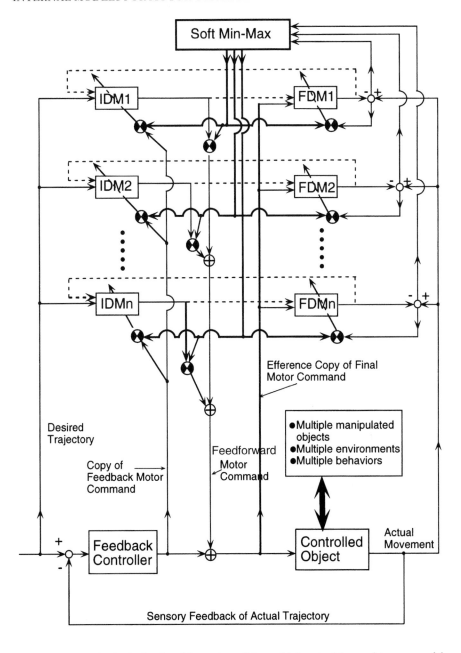

FIG. 3.   A more biologically plausible version of the multiple paired forward-inverse model. Here, the error signal for multiple inverse models is provided by the feedback-error learning mechanism.

new learned modules based on prism work (Ghahramani & Wolpert 1997) suggests a specific way in which multiple modules are integrated.

We now compare the current model with the previous computational model, in which multiple modules can be acquired through learning the mixture of experts controlled by a gating network (Jacobs et al 1991, Gomi & Kawato 1993, Jacobs & Jordan 1993). In this algorithm, either back propagation or an EM algorithm is necessary to train one gating network and many experts. The new model does not require a gating network, back propagation or an EM algorithm. Furthermore, inverse and forward model pairs are simultaneously acquired.

While theoretically it is possible to gate the outputs of the inverse models without prediction, we now give reasons why we prefer the predictive mechanism. First, consider a grand discriminator which determines context based on sensory and motor information. While such a mechanism would seem appropriate for a few contexts, it would not scale well to many thousands of contexts, especially if the output from this one discriminator needed to be distributed to this many inverse modules. An alternative is to have individual discriminators, one for each module, where each discriminator solves its job without use of prediction. The difficulty here is in linking the outputs from many discriminators to the inverse models. The second shortcoming of this approach is that we cannot judge objectively which individual discriminator is signalling the correct responsibility and which is false-alarming. However, by using predictive forward models and by comparing errors in their prediction, it is trivial to compare different modules' capabilities objectively. While calculation of the denominator in Equation 3 is trivial for the forward models, it would not be for the individual discriminators. In summary, our proposition is that the best way to train and switch multiple inverse models is to train and use multiple paired forward models.

Conclusion

Ten years ago, in biological disciplines, internal models were generally thought of as an engineering or purely computational concept which had little relevance to real biology. Today, we have a flood of psychological and physiological data supporting this idea. In a similar manner, the computational model of multiple paired forward and inverse models currently appears to be too computational and biologically implausible. However, we expect to extend it to a more biologically plausible neural network model and also obtain experimental data which more directly support it in a near future.

References

Baker JF, Perlmutter SI, Peterson BW, Rude SA, Robinson FR 1987 Simultaneous opposing adaptive changes in cat vestibulo-ocular reflex directions for two body orientations. Exp Brain Res 69:220–224

Bizzi E, Accornero N, Chapple W, Hogan N 1984 Posture control and trajectory formation during arm movement. J Neurosci 4:2738–2744

Fel'dman AG 1966 Functional tuning of the nervous system during movement control or preservation of stationary posture. III. Mechanographic analysis of human performance of the simplest motor tasks. Biofizika 11:667–675

Flash T 1987 The control of hand equilibrium trajectories in multi-joint arm movements. Biol Cybern 57:257–274

Gandolfo F, Mussa-Ivaldi F, Bizzi E 1996 Motor learning by field approximation. Proc Natl Acad Sci USA 93:3843–3846

Ghahramani Z, Wolpert DM 1997 Modular decomposition in visuomotor learning. Nature 386:392–395

Gomi H, Kawato M 1993 Recognition of manipulated objects by motor learning with modular architecture networks. Neural Networks 6:485–497

Gomi H, Kawato M 1996 Equilibrium-point control hypothesis examined by measured arm-stiffness during multi-joint movement. Science 272:117–120

Hay J, Pick H 1966 Gaze-contingent prism adaptation: optical and motor factors. J Exp Psychol 72:640–648

Hogan N 1984 An organizing principle for a class of voluntary movements. J Neurosci 4:2745–2754

Jacobs RA, Jordan MI 1993 Learning piece-wise control strategies in a modular neural network architecture. IEEE Trans Syst Man Cybern 23:337–345

Jacobs RA, Jordan MI, Nowlan SJ, Hinton GE 1991 Adaptive mixtures of local experts. Neural Comput 3:79–87

Kawano K, Shidara M, Yamane S 1992 Neural activity in dorsolateral pontine nucleus of alert monkey during ocular following responses. J Neurophysiol 67:680–703

Kawano K, Shidara M, Watanabe Y, Yamane S 1994 Neural activity in cortical area MST of alert monkey during ocular following responses. J Neurophysiol 71:2305–2324

Kawano K, Shidara M, Takemura A, Inoue Y, Gomi H, Kawato M 1996a Inverse-dynamics representation of eye movements by cerebellar Purkinje cell activity during short-latency ocular-following responses. Ann NY Acad Sci 781:314–321

Kawano K, Takemura A, Inoue Y, Kitama T, Kobayashi Y, Mustari MJ 1996b Visual inputs to cerebellar ventral paraflocculus during ocular following responses. In: Norita M, Bando T, Stein B (eds) Progress in brain research, vol 112. Elsevier BV, Amsterdam, p 415–422

Kawato M 1996 Bi-directional theory approach to integration. In: Inui T, McClelland J (eds) Attention and performance XVI. MIT Press, Cambridge, MA, p 335–367

Kawato M, Gomi H 1992 The cerebellum and VOR/OKR learning models. Trends Neurosci 15:445–453

Kawato M, Furukawa K, Suzuki R 1987 A hierarchical neural-network model for control and learning of voluntary movement. Biol Cybern 57:169–185

Kawato M, Kobayashi Y, Kawano K et al 1997 Cell-to-cell negative correlations between the simple spike and the complex spike firing characteristics of individual Purkinje cells. Abstr Annu Meet Soc Neurosci 23:1299

Kobayashi Y, Kawano K, Takemura A et al 1998 Temporal firing patterns of Purkinje cells in the cerebellar ventral paraflocculus during ocular following responses in monkeys. II. Complex spikes. J Neurophysiol 80:832–848

Kohler I 1964 The formation and transformation of the visual world (translated by H Fiss). Psychol Issues 3:1–173

Kravitz J 1972 Conditioned adaptation to prismatic displacement. Percept Psychophys 11:38–42

Kravitz J, Yaffe F 1972 Conditioned adaptation to prismatic displacement with a tone as the conditional stimulus. Percept Psychophys 12:305–308

Martin TA, Keating JG, Goodkin HP, Bastian AJ, Thach WT 1996 Throwing while looking through prisms. II specificity and of multiple gaze-throw calibrations. Brain 119:1199–1211
McGonigle B, Flock J 1978 Long-term retention of single and prismatic adaptation by humans. Nature 272:364–366
Shelhamer M, Robinson DA, Tan HS 1992 Context-specific gain switching in the human vestibuloocular reflex. Ann N Y Acad Sci 656:889–891
Shidara M, Kawano K 1993 Role of Purkinje cells in the ventral paraflocculus in short-latency ocular following responses. Exp Brain Res 93:185–195
Shidara M, Kawano K, Gomi H, Kawato M 1993 Inverse-dynamics model eye movement control by Purkinje cells in the cerebellum. Nature 365:50–52
Welch R 1971 Discriminative conditioning of prism adaptation. Percept Psychophys 10:90–92
Welch RB 1986 Adaptation to space perception. In: Boff KR, Kaufman L, Thomas JP (eds) Handbook of perception and performance, vol 1. Wiley, Chichester, p 24–45
Welch R, Bridgeman B, Anand S, Browman K 1993 Alternating prism exposure causes dual adaptation and generalization to a novel displacement. Percept Psychophys 54:195–204

DISCUSSION

Gibson: The inferior olive is extremely sensitive to sensory stimulation: its response probability is essentially 1.0 to appropriate stimulation. This is when the animal is not moving. As soon as he begins to move the response probability drops to a low level (Horn et al 1996). It seems that the function of the inferior olive is to provide information about specific sensory events when the animal is not moving.

Kawato: It's difficult to reconcile your findings. Today I talked about the ventral paraflocculus of the cerebellum. Also, Dr Kitazawa recently reported beautiful data showing that even for whole-arm reaching, the endpoint error signal is represented by the complex spikes (Kitazawa et al 1998). I think it depends on behavioural paradigms as well as which part of the cerebellum you are talking about.

Gibson: Complex spikes represent endpoint error only after a large number of trials are averaged. Certainly mossy fibre inputs provide much better information about error.

Miller: I don't understand how you're suggesting that an LTP or LDTD mechanism, which presumably could account for an updating of synaptic weights at the end of a trial or upon repeated errors, could account for a negative correlation between simple spikes and complex spikes in real time during the trial.

Kawato: It is probably better to use equations to show this. If you write down an equation based on long term depression and long term potentiation, you could predict after millions of trials that the temporal profile of the simple spike should be roughly the mirror image of the complex spikes in this system.

Miller: But this assumes that the complex spikes are occurring consistently, rather than being driven by some kind of random error.

Kawato: Actually, this is a feedback-controlled system. It could not predict the motion of the visual stimulus beforehand. So even if you have a very elegant feedforward-controlled system, you always have some retinal slips at the beginning of the ocular following responses. The complex spike cannot get to zero for this feedback-controlled system. Within this framework you could predict that complex spike waveform and simple spike waveform should be approximate mirror images of each other on an individual cell basis. Then it is straightforward to derive negative cell to cell correlations on all aspects of the firing frequency.

Miles: The finding that, when averaged over many trials, the probability of firing of the simple spikes during early ocular following is the mirror image of that of the complex spikes is nicely in accord with the idea that complex spikes have a teaching role, gradually sculpting the simple spike profile. Dr Kawato has shown how the inverse dynamics approach can be used to uncover several signals that are simultaneously encoded (that is, multiplexed) in the temporal discharge patterns of the individual neurons. Krauzlis & Lisberger (1991) have also attempted this during pursuit eye tracking, using a multi-channel model that parses the simple spike discharges of floccular Purkinje cells into eye velocity and various derivatives of the retinal slip signals. Dr Kawato, what do you see as the major difference between your approach and that of Krauzlis and Lisberger?

Kawato: The essential difference between Krauzlis and Lisberger's model and ours is that in their model the feedback of the eye velocity is essential to simulate the simple spike firing and eye movement behaviour. This difference might be ascribed to the different Purkinje cell types which are activated and examined during smooth pursuit and ocular following responses, because we are just looking at 400–500 ms of the eye movement after the stimulus motion onset whereas they look at it over a much longer interval. In the case of smooth pursuit with longer durations, maybe feedback signal or efference copy of the motor command could contribute significantly.

Gibson: The same afferents that provide input to the rDAO (rostral dorsal accessory olive) provide input also to the cuneate nucleus. During movement the cuneate nucleus is sensitive to somatosensory stimuli that would activate olivary cells at rest. Since the cerebellum receives information from the cuneate (as well as from the spinocerebellar system) as mossy fibre input, there appears to be a rich signal about movement and disturbance of movement arriving via mossy fibre input but not via climbing fibre input.

Stimuli that activate the olive report on body movement, but not necessarily self-produced movement. Visual stimuli that excite the olive produce the sensation of falling over, vestibular stimulation reports on being rocked or moved, and somatosensory stimuli report on being touched. I think that the secret of the olive is that it is telling you that something happened to your body that was *not* the result of your movement. Possibly, the olive provides a signal that planned actions may no longer be appropriate due to external events.

Kawato: From our viewpoint, the theory which you said you like most is similar to our models.

Wolpert: What the cell could be signalling is that my present control strategy is no longer responsible for something that has happened and I have to switch responsibility to something else.

Gibson: Correct. It doesn't seem likely that climbing fibre activity is appropriate for feedback about self-produced error. Another effective stimulus for the olive is pain, which produces tonic discharge of olivary cells. The tonic discharge would not be useful information about movement error but might result in an alteration of the movements influenced by a particular region of the cerebellum. Finally, climbing fibre pathways are slow in comparison to mossy fibre pathways, which would not seem to be a particularly desirable feature for feedback needed for error correction.

Miller: Alan Gibson, you keep making arguments based on the part of the olive that you have studied. Does the sensitivity of the olive decrease during eye movements like it does for the somatosensory system or not? I think that is an important question.

Gibson: That experiment has not been done. The proper experiment is to compare the threshold for activation of olivary cells with retinal slip when the eye is still to the threshold when the eye is moving.

Kawato: Simpson and colleagues and Sato and colleagues have already done experiments examining complex spikes in anaesthetized rabbits whose eyes do not move. The complex spike firing frequency has a significant positive correlation with the magnitude and direction of retinal slips which are in accordance with our awake monkey data. I think the firing frequencies of rabbit complex spikes are lower than our monkey data in ocular following responses. This is against what you said.

Gibson: Retinal slip appears to be a very effective stimulus for activating olivary cells in the anaesthetized cat in the absence of eye movements.

Hoffmann: Are you saying that there are no climbing fibre spikes during eye movements? That is wrong.

Gibson: I am not saying that, although I am saying response probability during movement appears to be low. Why would you have a system that provides information about movement be most sensitive when you are not moving? Wouldn't feedback about movement other than your own error produce inaccurate movement?

Miall: I'll give you one answer. One of the things that we should think about, if you accept my idea that the cerebellum is a forward model, is that it is predicting sensory consequences of actions, which includes posture. If you're predicting the sensory consequences of standing still, then if somebody touches you, that's an enormous prediction error, which is why the olive fires. You are predicting that nothing should happen and something happened.

Thach: But you cannot learn to do anything about it.

Lemon: Motor error that is bad enough to produce a C fibre input is a pretty severe form of error. Most of us would want to believe that our controllers are better than having to go all the way to actually generating C fibre input before realizing something is wrong.

Miles: Alan Gibson, what do you make of the mirror image temporal profiles?

Gibson: I do not have a good model for the olive. All that I am saying is that a model of olivary function should attempt to account for the properties known about olivary cells.

References

Horn KM, Van Kan PLE, Gibson AR 1996 Reduction of rostral dorsal accessory olive responses during reaching. J Neurophysiol 76:4140–4151

Kitazawa S, Kimura T, Yin PB 1998 Cerebellar complex spikes encode both destinations and errors in arm movements. Nature 392:494–497

Krauzlis RJ, Lisberger SG 1991 Visual motion commands for pursuit eye movements in the cerebellum. Science 253:568–571

The apraxias are higher-order defects of sensorimotor integration

C. D. Marsden

University Department of Clinical Neurology, Institute of Neurology, The National Hospital for Neurology and Neurosurgery, Queen Square, London WC1N 3BG, UK

Abstract. The classical features of motor disorders due to neurological disease affecting the pyramidal pathways, cerebellum and basal ganglia in humans are well known. What is less understood is the clinical world of apraxia — 'inability to perform purposeful skilled movements in the absence of any elementary motor (weakness, akinesia, abnormal posture or tone) or sensory deficits, or impaired comprehension or memory'. Much of what clinicians call apraxia is a failure of gesture production to command, due to problems of transcoding language into motor action, without motor deficit in ordinary life. However, damage to premotor regions and superior parietal lobules provokes devastating spontaneous higher-order motor deficits, including limb-kinetic apraxia, diagnostic apraxia, visuomotor apraxia and ideational apraxia.

1998 Sensory guidance of movement. Wiley, Chichester (Novartis Foundation Symposium 218) p 308–331

The goal of this symposium is stated to be the understanding of the functional links between sensory and motor areas of the brain. My assigned task is to attempt to use the findings from basic science to interpret relevant human movement disorders. The most interesting, and most complex, of these fall within the rubric of what neurologists and neurophysiologists call apraxia, so one must start with a review of these higher-order motor disorders.

Apraxia

All discussions of apraxia start and depart from the concepts of Liepmann (1900, 1908, 1920). Liepmann identified higher-order motor disorders, not explained by weakness, ataxia, akinesia, sensory deficit or cognitive impairment, which were often but not necessarily linked to aphasia. Geschwind & Damasio (1985) refined the definition of apraxia into 'an impairment of the execution of a learned movement in response to a stimulus which would normally elicit the movement, subject to the condition that the afferent and efferent systems involved are intact, and in the absence of inattentiveness or lack of cooperation'. They went on to state that 'For the overwhelming majority of clinical situations, however, one can use the following operational definition: apraxia is (a) failure to produce the correct movement in response to a verbal command, or (b) failure to imitate correctly a movement performed by the examiner, or (c) failure to perform a movement correctly in response to a seen object, or (d) failure to handle an object correctly. Thus defined, apraxia is a disorder of the high level control of the execution of some classes of movement, as requested by an observer in the verbal or visual mode. The movements fail to be carried out entirely or are performed defectively'.

Liepmann identified *ideational apraxia* (Ideatorische Apraxie) as the inability to conceive appropriate movement, so that the patient does not know what to do, particularly how to organize complex sequential motor activity. Such patients cannot perform a complex motor task (e.g. make an espresso coffee) to command, or in response to the request to imitate or pretend (pantomime) the motor act, or at will. As a result they have major motor disability in everyday life. Yet the single actions in a complex sequence of movements can be executed reasonably well, and the provision of the objects involved does not improve performance.

Liepmann attributed ideational apraxia to disruption of a hypothetical *motor plan* (Bewegungsentwurf). The motor plan has to be translated into its component *motor programmes* (movement formulae — Bewegunsformel — or visuo-kinaesthetic motor engrams in the terminology of Heilman [1979]).

Roy & Square (1985) subsequently refined a praxis model into a conceptual system and a production system (Fig. 1). The conceptual system was conceived to contain knowledge of (1) object and tool use; (2) actions independent of tools; and (3) organization of single actions into a sequence. Lesions affecting the conceptual system cause ideational apraxia.

Ideational apraxia is probably the least commonly recognized type — perhaps because 90% or so of such patients have concomitant aphasia or dementia.

CONCEPTUAL SYSTEM contains knowledge of:

1. Object and tool use
2. Actions independent of tools
3. Organization of single actions into a sequence

PRODUCTION SYSTEM represents knowledge of sensorimotor action

1. Action programmes or movement formulae
2. Translation of 'time–space' representations into innervatory patterns

---

FIG. 1.   The Roy & Square (1985) praxis model.

However, ideational apraxia is a discrete entity, which is distinct from ideomotor apraxia (see below). There is no correlation between tests for ideational apraxia (multiple object use) and ideomotor apraxia (manual gesture imitation) (De Renzi & Lucchelli 1988).

There is debate as to the nature of the key deficits in ideational apraxia. Some authors focus on a deficit of carrying out a sequence of motor acts to complete a complex motor behaviour or coherent motor plan (e.g. Liepmann 1908, Heilman 1973). Others interpret the breakdown of movement as due to an inability to perceive the correct use of objects (agnosia of usage) (De Renzi et al 1968a,b), because those with ideational apraxia not only fail on tests of multiple object use (e.g. open and close a lock with a key, or prepare and post a letter), but also on use of single objects (e.g. employing a toothbrush). Even if carrying out a series of motor acts is the fundamental deficit, some hold that the sequencing itself is not in error (Poeck 1983, De Renzi & Lucchelli 1988). The lesions responsible for ideational apraxia usually involve the left (dominant) posterior temporoparietal regions, but often the condition is seen in those with diffuse degenerative brain disease.

Liepmann's second form of higher-order motor deficit was *ideomotor apraxia* (Ideokinetische Apraxie). Here the patient understands the action required but cannot carry out the motor act to verbal command. Whereas in ideational apraxia the patient does not know *what* to do, in ideomotor apraxia the patients does not know *how* to do it, but makes spatiotemporal errors in gesture production (pantomime) to command. The errors are in the posture of the limb, its spatial orientation and joint coordination, as well as in the timing of the action (Poizner et al 1995, Clark et al 1994, Poisner et al 1990). The deficit is worse for transitive gestures (e.g. show me how to use a tool, such as a screwdriver or hammer), than for intransitive gestures for non-verbal communication (e.g. show me how to wave goodbye [representational gesture] or raise your arm and wiggle your fingers [non-representational gesture]). Performance improves if the subject is asked to mimic a pantomime or imitate an action, and even more so if the actual tool is provided. The patient can carry out the act spontaneously and automatically, but not to command (automatic–voluntary dissociation), so is not disabled in everyday life. Accordingly, the motor plan and motor programmes are intact, but cannot be engaged in response to command.

Liepmann conceived ideomotor apraxia as due to disconnection of the motor plan/programmes from those brain areas responsible for translation of motor programmes (time–space visuokinaesthetic motor engrams in the terminology of Heilman [1979]) into innervatory patterns which define the muscle activation (distribution, forces and timing) required to execute the act.

Roy & Square (1985) considered ideomotor apraxia as due to damage to their *production system*, which represents knowledge of sensorimotor action in the form of movement formulae (motor programmes), and translation of the time–space representations of movement formulae into innervatory patterns.

Ideomotor apraxia is the commonest and most widely studied form of apraxia. It usually is attributed to damage to the posterior parietal regions of the cerebral cortex.

Finally, Liepmann referred to *limb-kinetic (melo-kinetic) apraxia* (Gliedkinetishe Apraxie) as a loss of kinetic memories of innervatory patterns due to damage to the 'senso-motorium'. Such patients understood the action, engaged the appropriate motor programmes, but all actions were performed clumsily because the muscle activity was incorrectly specified. The deficit is unilateral, usually affects the arm, and is manifest as a difficulty in manipulation of small objects and with fine finger movements, despite normal or near normal strength. All types of movement are affected; there is no automatic–voluntary dissociation.

Limb-kinetic apraxia is the most controversial of Liepmann's three types of apraxia. Many have dismissed it as merely the expression of basic motor deficits. Geschwind (1965a,b) stated '... my feeling had been that "limb-kinetic" apraxia has not been defined clearly enough to separate it from mild pyramidal disturbance'. Faglioni & Basso (1985), in their review of the literature, found only seven cases that conformed to the description of classical limb-kinetic apraxia. However, others including this author, would agree that limb-kinetic apraxia is a true entity, over and above pyramidal deficit. Luria (1966), for example, emphasised the slowness, clumsiness and awkwardness of movements, with loss of the kinetic melody, decomposition of movement, and disordered timing in those with limb-kinetic apraxia. Heilman & Rothi (1985) described limb-kinetic apraxia as an inability to make fine precise movements, although selection of the motor pattern, sequencing and spatial orientation are intact. Kleist (1907) attributed this type of apraxia to damage to premotor frontal lobe areas.

Liepmann identified the dominant (usually left) hemisphere as being the repository of motor planning and programming. He also speculated that the posterior (parietal) cerebral cortical regions were most concerned with the planning and programming of motor activity, while the anterior (frontal) cortical regions were involved in translating motor programmes into innervatory patterns.

Development of concepts of ideomotor apraxia

Liepmann's basic concepts have stood the test of time, but have been refined, and have been increasingly mapped to neuroanatomical and neurophysiological properties of the cerebral cortex. Heilman et al (1982), for example, have identified two types of ideomotor ataxia for gesture to command (Fig. 2). Lesions of the left posterior inferior parietal lobule in the region of the supramarginal or angular gyrus (Brodmann areas 40 and 39) cause inability to

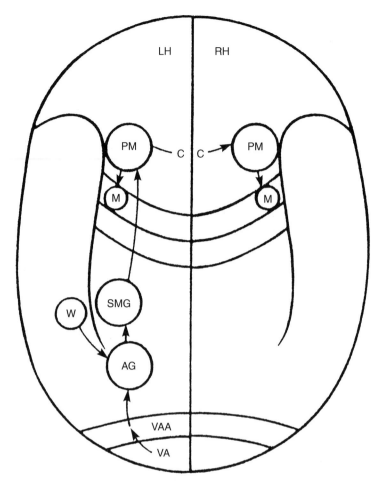

FIG. 2.   Heilman et al (1982) schema to explain two types of ideomotor apraxia. (1) A lesion in the dominant left inferior parietal lobe affecting the supramarginal gyrus (SMG) and angular gyrus (AG), which receive input from Wernicke's area (W), and visual area (VA) via visual association areas (VAA) causes ideomotor apraxia, with additional loss of the ability to recognize correct performance of pantomimes performed by the examiner. (2) A lesion disconnecting the inferior parietal regions from premotor cortex (PM) causes ideomotor apraxia, but recognition of the correct act is preserved. LH, left hemisphere; RH, right hemisphere; CC, corpus callosum; M, motor area.

perform gestures to command, and inability to recognize a correct performance when pantomimed. Lesions more anterior in the dominant anterior inferior parietal region or frontal lobe cause a similar inability in producing gestures to command, but recognition of correct pantomime is preserved.

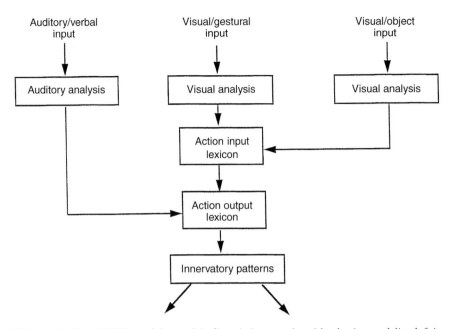

FIG. 3.   Rothi et al (1991) model to explain dissociation apraxias with selective modality deficits in gestural production to command. An Action Lexicon is proposed (by analogy with models of language production) in which visuokinaesthetic motor engrams program skilled movements. To account for patients who have no problem with comprehension of pantomimes, but who could not imitate gestures, they divided the action lexicon into an Action Input-Lexicon and an Action Output-Lexicon; a lesion at some point after egress from the input-lexicon could explain spared gesture reception in the presence of impaired imitation. Other patients exhibit more severe impairment of gesture imitation than gesture to verbal command. So, auditory/verbal language input must gain direct access to the output-lexicon. Impairment both to verbal command and visual imitation would be due to dysfunction at or after access to the action output-lexicon. Finally, some patients cannot pantomime the function of pictured objects, but can respond to verbal command so separate channels for auditory/verbal, visual/gestural and visual/object input are shown.

Rothi et al (1991) have also identified a range of patients with dissociations of gestural responses to specific sensory inputs. All these individuals had ideomotor apraxia for specific commands via different input channels. All could describe the desired act, recognize correct pantomime, imitate the examiner and use objects faultlessly. So motor plans and programmes were preserved, and they could be transformed into correct innervatory patterns. However, some could not carry out a gesture in response to spoken command (verbal–motor dissociation), others to visual stimuli (visuomotor dissociation), and others to somaesthetic stimuli (tactile–motor dissociation). This led Heilman and his colleagues to propose specific dissociations of verbal, visual or tactile inputs into the intact parietal lobe repository of gestural motor plans and programmes (Fig. 3; Rothi et al 1991).

Thus, Ochipa et al (1994) described a patient who had no difficulty with pantomime recognition, but could not imitate movements, yet could carry out the same movements better to verbal command. They called this syndrome conduction apraxia, and deduced that verbal instructions must be able to engage motor programmes downstream of the processes involved in imitation. Heilman et al (1973), conversely, described three cases who could imitate gestures flawlessly, but who could not pantomime to command. Rothi et al (1986) described two patients who could not comprehend or discriminate gestures, but could perform them to command. They deduced that the responsible left-occipital temporal lesion had prevented access of visual stimuli to motor programming regions. Rothi et al (1986) also described a patient who could pantomime the function of a named object to command, but who could not pantomime the function of pictured objects. So visual object input must utilize a pathway to motor programmes separate from language-based verbal gestural input.

Apraxia, aphasia and motor disability

A striking theme running throughout the literature of apraxia is the close relationship of the disorder to aphasia. This is not surprising, for the brain regions in the dominant hemisphere responsible for the understanding of language and the production of speech are closely mapped to those areas concerned with the planning and programming of movement. In general, right hemisphere lesions in right-handers do not induce apraxia (Geschwind 1965a,b). Hécaen (1962), for example, found that amongst 415 patients with parietal, temporal or occipital lesions, all those with apraxia had dominant (left hemisphere) or bilateral damage. Likewise, De Renzi et al (1982) found ideational or ideomotor apraxia in around 50 cases out of 150 left hemisphere lesions, but in only about 10 cases amongst 110 right hemisphere lesions. Yet apraxia can certainly can occur independent of aphasia (De Renzi et al 1980, 1982).

A second and related theme is the description of the commonest and most widely studied type of apraxia, namely ideomotor apraxia, in terms of failure of gesture production to command. Classical ideomotor apraxia is just such a deficit, yet these patients have no motor disability in everyday life. Their apractic disorder is unearthed by specific testing. How often do we face the need to 'show me how you use a hammer'. We use the hammer!

Yet there are other apraxias which cause major disruption of normal motor activity. In the context of integration of sensation and motor action, the most important of these are the unimodel apraxias of visuomotor apraxia and tactile apraxia, and the syndromes of primary progressive apraxia and diagonistic apraxia. All are attributed to damage to the superior parietal regions.

Visuomotor apraxia

The first major paper on this syndrome was that of Bálint (1909), who described a single patient with a triad of psychic paralysis of gaze, optic ataxia (Optische Ataxie), and a spatial disorder of attention. This patient had normal eye movements and no visual field defect, but could not orientate his eyes onto objects on the left, even though he could see the objects and could look around spontaneously. He also could see only one object at a time in a panorama. (The deficits in eye movements and visual attention will not be considered further here.) Movements of the left hand were normal, but those of the right hand when reaching into space to objects were grossly inaccurate due, Bálint surmised, to defective visual control of that limb. Position sense in the right hand was normal, but Bálint noted that the movement deficit resembled tabetic ataxia due to proprioceptive loss, hence the term 'optic ataxia'. Post-mortem examination revealed bilateral posterior parietal lesions.

Subsequently, Holmes (1918) described similar cases due to gunshot wounds. Holmes described the motor deficit as a loss of 'the power of localizing the position in space and the distance of objects by sight alone'. Some had left-sided lesions, others right-sided brain damage, with corresponding visual field defects but intact visual acuity and visual recognition of objects. The patients would project their arm in the wrong direction to targets, then grope and search ineffectively for them, even though they could see the objects. The responsible lesions were deduced to be in the posterior parietal lobe.

Although the designation of optic ataxia was favoured by Bálint and others (Rondot et al 1977, Perenin & Vighetto 1988), the motor deficit does not resemble that seen with sensory (deafferentation) ataxia or cerebellar ataxia (Rothwell et al 1982, Day et al 1998). Certainly the movement is imprecise but, in addition, it is misdirected and inappropriate in its execution. Furthermore, those with sensory or cerebellar ataxia can improve their reaching and grasping performance with visual feedback, whereas those with visuomotor apraxia cannot. Accordingly, such visuomotor deficit is better classified as visuomotor apraxia (Freund 1992). Visuomotor apraxia (defective reaching and grasping) is quite different from the motor behaviour seen in adults with acute blindness. Those with visuomotor apraxia cannot improve their performance with training. Their trajectory of reaching and their shaping of the hand for grasping are persistently disturbed.

A distinction can be made between lesions affecting cognitive visuospatial perception (inferotemporal cortex) and visuomotor behaviour (posterior parietal lobules). For example, Goodale et al (1991) described a patient with a striking dissociation between accurate guidance of the hand towards objects whose qualities she failed to perceive. Conversely, the typical patient with visuomotor apraxia cannot reach accurately objects that are perceived correctly.

Classical Bálint's full syndrome turns out to be relatively rare, perhaps because it requires bilateral symmetrical posterior parietal lesions. However, visuomotor apraxia is a more frequent deficit (for a review see Rondot et al 1977), and in itself comprises a variety of complex disorders.

In general, operations dealing with the outside world, such as visuomotor control, have equal representation in both hemispheres. It has become apparent that there are subtle, but important, variations in the motor performance or arm reaching and grasping into extrapersonal space in different patients with posterior parietal lesions sparing simple visual function. A right hemisphere posterior parietal lesion produces cognitive and visuomotor spatial disorientation in left hemispace, and vice versa. However, this issue is more complicated. Classically, patients with visuomotor apraxia misreach for objects in the visual field contralateral to the lesion (Rondot et al 1977). Some misreach only with the contralateral hand, but others misreach with either hand into contralateral space (the 'visual field effect'). A subtle visual field deficit does not account for such motor deficits, for the visual fields in such patients are normal, and spatial discrimination of position of objects or orientation of lines is preserved in the affected hemifield. Other patients may exhibit misreaching of the hand contralateral to the lesion in both hemifields (the 'hand effect'). The visual field effect can be combined with the hand effect especially in left dominant posterior parietal lesions, causing misreaching with both hands in the contralateral hemifield, and with the contralateral hand in both hemifields, but not with the ipsilateral hand in the ipsilateral hemifield.

Visuomotor ataxia used to be attributed to a cortico-cortical disconnection between visual and motor areas. This view followed the experiments of Haaxma & Kuypers (1975), and Moll & Kuypers (1977) who described defects of visual guidance of hand and finger movements in monkeys after lesions in the cortico-cortical connections between parieto-occipital visual and frontal premotor areas. However, Glickstein & May (1982), on the basis of data showing that cuts interrupting all cortico-cortical fibres between occipital and frontal cortex in monkeys did not impair visually-guided limb movements (although hand and finger use were disturbed), proposed an alternative explanation. They suggested that subcortical projections from the parietal lobe reach the motor cortex (and brainstem motor structures) via descending projections to pontine nuclei, the cerebellum and thalamus (see Glickstein 1998, this volume). There is abundant evidence for such a pathway, and now there is suggestive evidence from human pathology.

Classen et al (1995) described a single patient with a large right thalamic haemorrhage producing a permanent contralateral visuomotor apraxia. The lesion caused a left-sided hemianopsia, loss of proprioception and cutaneous sensation, hemineglect and hemidystonia, but no pyramidal deficit. There was no visual agnosia. MRI of the brain revealed no cortical lesion. Although he had left limb deafferentation, the visuomotor apraxia was quite different from that seen in patients with peripheral deafferentation, in that he could not compensate with visual information. Although this case had multiple sensory and visuomotor deficits, it adds weight to the concept that a subcortical lesion can cause visuomotor apraxia.

Tactile apraxia

Peripheral deafferentation grossly interferes with motor function (Rothwell et al 1982, Sanes et al 1985), as does loss of proprioception due to posterior column lesions in the spinal cord, or to thalamic sensory lesions. Anterior parietal lobe lesions (areas 1, 2 and 3) affecting the targets of afferent input to somatosensory cortex produce similar motor disturbances (Nathan et al 1986). Jeannerod (1984) described a patient with an infarct affecting the post-central gyrus, but sparing the motor areas and thalamus, whose motor deficits were strikingly similar to those observed in patients with peripheral deafferentation. Lesions of posterior superior parietal cortex (areas 5 and 7 in the human), however, cause more complex impairments of somatosensorimotor function (Pause et al 1989).

Such patients have grossly disturbed hand and finger movements when palpating or manipulating objects. They cannot engage the digital actions required to sample the properties of objects, so cannot recognize form or texture (astereognosis). There is a breakdown in the transformation of somatosensory information into the motor programmes required to explore objects, so they cannot execute the purposive actions required to extract information. The responsible lesions lie in the contralateral superior parietal lobule (areas 5 and 7). Such patients can carry out many normal movements, but cannot use the hand as a sense organ. They have lost the ability for active manual touch and manipulation.

Diagnostic apraxia

This describes a peculiar behaviour of the left hand after lesions of the posterior corpus callosum (Tanaka et al 1996). The left hand appears to act at cross-purposes to the right; in particular, the left hand interferes with voluntary right hand action, a form of intermanual conflict. Such patients do not exhibit the pathological grasp or forced groping seen with frontal lobe lesions. Tanaka et al (1996) attributed this phenomenon to the effect of the posterior corpus callosum lesion disrupting connections between the right superior parietal lobule and its counterpart in the left hemisphere. As a result, voluntary movement of the right hand involving the left (dominant) superior parietal lobule is not able to transfer inhibitory control to the right superior parietal lobule. The abnormal behaviour of the left hand was often elicited by tasks involving visual or tactile information which would reach both hemispheres. If such patients reached for an object in space with the dominant right hand, the left would interfere.

Primary progressive apraxia

Finally, a small number of patients have been described with a syndrome of apparently isolated limb apraxia, at least in the initial stages of their illness (De Renzi 1986, Dick et al 1989, Rapcsak et al 1995, Green et al 1995). Such patients cannot carry out movements of the arm to will or in response to commands, and have severe motor disability. They 'know what they want to do, but cannot do it'. They exhibit major errors in the spatial and temporal aspects of voluntary movements, particularly of the arm and hand. Their concept of movement is intact, as is language, they can describe the action and recognize correct pantomimes. Initially, the condition is unilateral, but it progresses to become bilateral, affecting both arms but sparing oro-facial movements. The likely pathology is that of Alzheimer's or Pick's disease.

Rapcsak et al (1995), described a particularly instructive case of primary progressive apraxia and attributed the condition to initial focal degenerative pathology in the superior parietal lobules. This patient developed slowly progressive bilateral limb apraxia. She could not make her hands do what she wanted, and even simple routine motor tasks were no longer automatic. She could recognize gestures, could identify tools and their use, and had preserved conceptual knowledge of single or complex sequential actions. There was no aphasia, but she had considerable spatial disorientation. She was unable to produce gestures with either hand to verbal command or imitation. MRI revealed striking focal bilateral atrophy of the posterior superior parietal lobes.

Apraxia and the parietal lobules

A consistent theme concerning the site of pathology in visuomotor, tactile, diagonistic and primary progressive apraxia is a focus on the superior parietal lobules (areas 5 and 7 in the human). In all these syndromes, the patients have severe motor disability in everyday life. This contrasts dramatically with classical ideomotor apraxia and the disconnection or dissociation apraxias, which are attributed to lesions affecting the inferior parietal lobules. Patients with the latter have a problem transcoding verbal or visual language-based instructions into motor action, but have no problem with spontaneous everyday motor activity. A reasonable explanation for this dissociation is that the classical ideomotor and selective dissociation syndromes are due to interruption of the pathways to and from the posterior inferior parietal lobule and inferotemporal cortex, which decode language-based visual and verbal instructions for gestural action, from the true motor programming areas in the more rostral posterior parietal lobules.

Vision and movement

Many of the tests for apraxia involve the presentation of visual (as well as verbal) stimuli requesting movement. This raises the issue as to how the brain deals with visual input and, in particular, how visual input is transformed into motor action.

Ungerleider & Mishkin (1982) proposed two cortical visual systems: (1) A *dorsal stream* of visual information processing from striate cortex to posterior parietal cortex which subserves object localization (the 'where' system); and (2) A *ventral stream* from striate cortex to inferotemporal cortex mediating perceptual and cognitive aspects of vision (the 'what' system). The dorsal stream codes the spatial characteristics of the visual scene and analyses motion. The ventral stream is concerned with the conscious cognitive analysis of the visual scene and with the perception of form, colours and features. Both the dorsal and ventral visual information streams project to the frontal lobes, but to different regions for spatial memory and object memory respectively (Wilson et al 1993). How the two streams interconnect is a matter for debate (see Passingham et al 1998, this volume).

Subsequently, Goodale & Milner (1992) suggested that the dorsal stream is concerned with the unconscious spatial analysis of visual information relevant to the programming of motor commands for visually guided movements (see also Goodale 1998, this volume). Such movements are directed to objects whose characteristics are identified in the ventral pathway. Single-unit recordings in the parietal cortex of primates have revealed neurons whose activity is related to the actions of reaching and grasping (Mountcastle et al 1975, Sakata et al 1995).

The dorsal stream itself may be divided into two subsystems, one for reaching towards objects in extrapersonal space (via the superior parietal lobule to dorsal premotor cortex), and the other for shaping the hand for grasping the object (via the inferior parietal lobule to ventral premotor cortex) (Gallese et al 1994, Jeannerod et al 1995). Arbib (1981) proposed an influential model of how reaching and grasping could be achieved (Fig. 4), with separate but interacting input and output channels for the reach and the grasp. Neurons in the superior parietal lobule of the monkey behave in a way consistent with the concept of a body-centred or egocentric frame of reference for arm reaching (Lacquaniti et al 1995). The activity of some neurons in the inferior parietal cortex is related to the

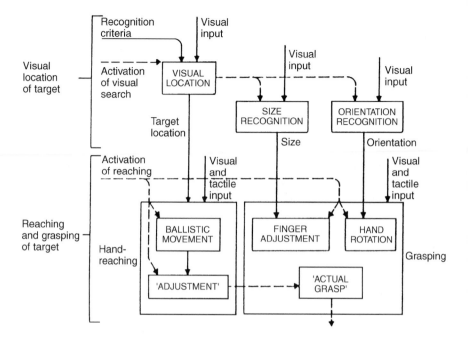

FIG. 4. The Arbib (1981) model for the organization of reaching and grasping an object. Separate (but interacting) channels are employed to visualize the location of the object in space to produce the ballistic reach movement towards the target, and to recognize the size and orientation of the object in order to formulate the hand position and finger adjustment appropriate to grasp the object.

pattern of hand manipulative movements or the characteristics of the manipulated object (Sakata et al 1995).

In humans, the inferotemporal cortex (areas 20 and 21) appears to be concerned with the perception and cognitive processes of visual recognition. Other areas of temporal cortex in the dominant hemisphere are responsible for the decoding of language-based instructions. In contrast, the posterior parietal lobules (areas 5 and 7) appear to be involved in the integration of visuospatial information, and tactile/proprioceptive data, with motor programmes required to execute limb movements in response to visual targets, tactile exploration and perhaps verbal instruction.

The superior parietal lobules seem more concerned with arm reaching (area 7m) and tactile exploration (area 5), while the inferior parietal lobules (areas 7a and 7b, equivalent to areas 39 and 40) are involved with extracting visual information from objects for generating the motor commands required for hand manipulation.

The operations conducted by the dorsal stream to achieve movement to a visual target require planning or conception of the visual goal in extrapersonal space, and then the computation of the arm reach and hand actions required to capture and manipulate the target. Such visuomotor transformation requires parallel processing of transport of the arm to the object location and configuration of the hand shape appropriate to the size, orientation, 3D characteristics and weight of the object (see Jeannerod et al 1998, this volume). Such transformations appear to be undertaken by the posterior parietal regions.

The appropriate parameters for arm reach and hand position must then be transferred to frontal motor cortical areas (see this volume: Strick et al 1998, Rizzolatti & Fadiga 1998, Georgopoulos 1998, Kalaska et al 1998, Lemon et al 1998). Two parallel pathways probably are engaged, direct cortico-cortical connections and descending cortical projections to cerebellum (see this volume: Glickstein 1998, Thach 1998), and basal ganglia (see Passingham et al 1998, this volume), brainstem including the superior colliculus and reticular formation.

A neurophysiological concept of apraxia

The traditional interpretation of apraxia in humans with neurological lesions has been based upon 'black box' models of motor organization (see Fig. 5 for a modification of the Roy & Square [1985] praxis model). It is now possible to attempt to translate such theoretical concepts into neurophysiological principles.

Commands to move, whether visual or verbal have to be understood. The decoding and understanding of visual and verbal instructions is achieved in the posterior parietotemporal cortex. Such language-based instructions then have to be translated into appropriate motor action (the motor plan or goal). The overall motor plan then must be transferred into specification of the motor parameters required to achieve the motor plan or goal. Such transformation requires the specification of appropriate motor programmes. This is the provenance of the more rostral posterior parietal cortex, with perhaps the parameters of appropriate arm movement being transformed in the superior parietal lobe and those of hand conformation in the inferior parietal lobe. At this stage, such general motor programmes are conditional, that is they will not necessarily be delivered, but are available for use if selected for action. Stimulation of parietal cortex does not evoke movement.

Conditional motor programmes formulated in parietal cortex are transferred to appropriate motor areas of frontal motor cortex, both by direct cortico-cortical connections and by descending projections to cerebellum, brainstem (superior colliculus and reticular formation) and basal ganglia. These latter descending projections engage further motor processing in the cerebellum, brainstem and basal ganglia, which sets the motor scene for action by returning instructions to

CONCEPTUAL SYSTEM	IDEATIONAL APRAXIA
Knowledge of: 1. Object and tool use 2. Actions independent of tools 3. Organization of single actions into a sequence	Loss of concept of action and sequencing Do not know *what* to do Motor handicap
PRODUCTION SYSTEM	IDEOMOTOR APRAXIA
Knowledge of: Movement programmes 1. Inferior parietal lobule 2. Superior parietal lobule	Normal concept of action Loss of gesture production No motor handicap Motor handicap
DECODING INTO INNERVATORY PATTERNS Translation of programmes into muscle kinetics and dynamics	LIMB KINETIC APRAXIA Loss of fluency of all movement

FIG. 5.   Modified Roy & Square (1985) praxis model.

the motor regions of frontal cortex and by engaging other brainstem and spinal cord motor machinery.

The stage is now set for movement, but the decision to act is still required. Response selection and the trigger to action is the provenance of the frontal lobes. Working memory in prefrontal regions, for example area 46 for spatial working memory, may be engaged in such selection of the appropriate motor response.

Finally, the specified and selected motor action programme is transformed into the required muscle forces and timing by premotor and motor cortical areas.

Thus, the route to motor action involves the general specification of a possible motor plan or goal in posterior parietal regions ('the rough sketch'), the transformation of that plan into conditional motor programmes in more rostral parietal areas ('the first drawings'), the selection of the response and decision to act in the pre-frontal lobes, and the final shaping of the conditional motor programmes into the kinematics of movement in the premotor and motor areas ('the finished picture').

Ideational apraxia would be an inability to put together a coherent motor plan. Ideomotor apraxia, in its various forms, would be an inability to specify the conditional motor programmes required to execute the motor plan.

Limb-kinetic apraxia would be the inability to translate those conditional motor programmes into the muscle contractions required to achieve the action required.

References

Arbib MA 1981 Perceptual structures and distributed motor control. In: Brooks VB (ed) Handbook of physiology, section 1: The nervous system, vol II: Motor control. Williams & Wilkins, Baltimore, p 1449–1480

Bálint R 1909 Seelenlähmung des 'Schauens', optische Ataxie, räumlische Störung des Aufmersamkeit. Monatsschr Psychiatr Neurol 25:51–81

Clark MA, Merians AS, Kothari A et al 1994 Spatial planning deficits in limb apraxia. Brain 117:1093–2106

Classen J, Kunesch E, Binkofski F et al 1995 Subcortical origin of visuomotor apraxia. Brain 118:1365–1374

Day BL, Thompson PD, Harding AE, Marsden CD 1998 Influence of vision on upper limb reaching movements in patients with cerebellar ataxia. Brain, in press

De Renzi E 1986 Slowly progressive visual agnosia or apraxia without dementia. Cortex 22:171–180

De Renzi E, Lucchelli F 1988 Ideational apraxia. Brain 111:1173–1185

De Renzi E, Faglioni P, Scotti G 1968a Tactile spatial impairment and unilateral cerebral damage. J Nerv Ment Dis 146:468–475

De Renzi E, Pieczuro A, Vignolo LA 1968b Ideational apraxia: a quantitative study. Neuropsychologia 6:41–52

De Renzi E, Motti F, Nichelli P 1980 Imitating gestures: a quantitative approach to ideomotor apraxia. Arch Neurol 37:6–10

De Renzi E, Faglioni P, Sorgato P 1982 Modality-specific and supramodal mechanisms in apraxia. Brain 105:301–312

Dick JPR, Snowden J, Northe B, Goulding PJ, Neary D 1989 Slowly progressive apraxia. Behav Neurol 2:101–114

Faglioni P, Basso A 1985 Historical perspectives on neuroanatomical correlates of limb apraxia. In: Roy EA (ed) Advances in psychology, vol 7: Neuropsychological studies of apraxia and related disorders. Elsevier Science BV, Amsterdam, p 3–44

Freund H-J 1992 The apraxias. In: Asbury AK, McKhan GM, McDonald WI (eds) Diseases of the nervous system, vol 1: Clinical neurobiology. WB Saunders, Philadelphia, p 751–767

Gallese V, Murata A, Kaseda M, Niki N, Sakata H 1994 Deficit of hand preshaping after muscimol injection in monkey parietal cortex. Neuroreport 5:1525–1529

Georgopoulos AP 1998 Online visual control of the arm. In: Sensory guidance of movement. Wiley, Chichester (Novartis Found Symp 218) p 147–170

Geschwind N 1965a Disconnexion syndromes in animals and man. I. Brain 88:237–294

Geschwind N 1965b Disconnexion syndromes in animals and man. II. Brain 88:585–644

Geschwind N, Damasio AR 1985 Apraxia. In: Devinsky O, Schachter SC (eds) Selected publications on language, epilepsy and behaviour. Butterworth-Heinemann Inc, Newton, MA, p 195–208

Glickstein M 1998 Cerebellum and the visual guidance of movement. In: Sensory guidance of movement. Wiley, Chichester (Novartis Found Symp 218) p 252–271

Glickstein M, May JG 1982 Visual control of movement: the circuits which link visual to motor areas of the brain with special reference to the visual input to the pons and cerebellum. In: Neff WD (ed) Contributions to sensory physiology, vol 7. Academic Press, New York, p 103–145

Goodale MA 1998 Vision for perception and vision for action in the primate brain. In: Sensory guidance of movement. Wiley, Chichester (Novartis Found Symp 218) p 21–39

Goodale MA, Milner AD 1992 Separate visual pathways for perception and action. Trends Neurosci 15:20–25

Goodale MA, Milner AD, Jakobson LS, Carey DP 1991 A neurological dissociation between perceiving objects and grasping them. Nature 349:154–156

Green RC, Goldstein FC, Mirra SS, Apazraki NP, Baxt JL, Bakay RAE 1995 Slowly progressive apraxia in Alzheimer's disease. J Neurol Neurosurg Psychiatry 59:312–315

Haaxma H, Kuypers HGJM 1975 Intrahemispheric cortical connexions and visual guidance of hand and finger movements in the rhesus monkey. Brain 98:239–260

Hécaen H 1962 Clinical symptomatology in right and left hemisphere lesions. In: Mountcastle VB (ed) Interhemispheric relations and cerebral dominance. Johns Hopkins University Press, Baltimore, p 215–243

Heilman KM 1973 Ideational apraxia — a re-definition. Brain 96:861–864

Heilman KM 1979 Apraxia. In: Heilman KM, Valenstein E (eds) Clinical neuropsychology. Oxford University Press, New York, p 159–185

Heilman KM, Rothi LJG 1985 Apraxia. In: Heilman KM, Valenstein E (eds) Clinical neuropsychology. Oxford University Press, New York, p 131–150

Heilman KM, Hammer LC, Wilder BJ 1973 An audiometric defect in temporal lobe dysfunction. Neurology 23:384–386

Heilman KM, Rothi LJG, Valenstein E 1982 Two forms of ideomotor apraxia. Neurology 32:342–346

Holmes G 1918 Disturbances of visual orientation. Br J Ophthalmol 2:449–506

Jeannerod M 1984 The timing of natural prehension movements. J Mot Behav 16:235–254

Jeannerod M, Arbib MA, Rizzolatti G, Sakata H 1995 Grasping objects: the cortical mechanisms of visuomotor transformation. Trends Neurosci 18:314–320

Jeannerod M, Paulignan Y, Weiss P 1998 Grasping an object: one movement, several components. In: Sensory guidance of movement. Wiley, Chichester (Novartis Found Symp 218) p 5–20

Kalaska JF, Sergio LE, Cisek P 1998 Cortical control of whole-arm motor tasks. In: Sensory guidance of movement. Wiley, Chichester (Novartis Found Symp 218) p 176–201

Kleist K 1907 Das Kortikale (innervatorische) Apraxie. Jahrb Psychiatr Neurol 28:46–112

Lacquaniti F, Guigon E, Bianchi L, Ferraina S, Caminiti R 1995 Representing spatial information for limb movement: role of area 5 in the monkey. Cereb Cortex 5:391–409

Lemon R, Baker SN, Davis JA, Kirkwood PA, Maier MA, Yang H-S 1998 The importance of the cortico-motoneuronal system for cortical control of grasp. In: Sensory guidance of movement. Wiley, Chichester (Novartis Found Symp 218) p 202–218

Liepmann H 1900 Das Krankheit der Apraxie ("motorische Asymbolie"), auf Grund eines Falles von einsetger Apraxia. Monatsschr Psychiatr Neurol 8:182–197

Liepmann H 1908 Drei Aufsätze aus dem Apraxiegebiet. Karger, Berlin

Liepmann H 1920 Apraxie. In: Brugsch's Ergebnisse der Gesamten Medizin. Urban & Schwarzenberg, Berlin, p 518–543

Luria AR 1966 Higher cortical functions in man. Basic Books, New York

Moll L, Kuypers HGJM 1977 Premotor cortical ablations in monkeys: contralateral changes in visually guided reaching behaviour. Science 198:317–319

Mountcastle VB, Lynch JC, Georgopoulos A, Sakata H, Acuna C 1975 Posterior parietal association cortex of the monkey: command functions for operations within extra-personal space. J Neurophysiol 38:871–908

Nathan PW, Smith MC, Cook AW 1986 Sensory effects in man of lesions of the posterior columns and some other afferent pathways. Brain 109:1003–1041

Ochipa C, Rothi LJG, Heilman KM 1994 Conduction apraxia. J Neurol Neurosurg Psychiatry 57:1241–1244

Passingham RE, Toni I, Schluter N, Rushworth MFS 1998 How do visual instructions influence the motor system? In: Sensory guidance of movement. Wiley, Chichester (Novartis Found Symp 218) p 129–146

Pause M, Kunesch E, Binkofski F, Freund H-J 1989 Sensorimotor disturbances in patients with lesions of the parietal cortex. Brain 112:1599–1625

Perenin M-T, Vighetto A 1988 Optic ataxia: a specific disruption in visuomotor mechanisms. Brain 111:643–674

Poeck K 1983 Ideational apraxia. J Neurol 230:1–5

Poizner H, Mack L, Verfaellie M, Rothi LJG, Heilman KM 1990 Three-dimensional computerographic analysis of apraxia. Brain 113:85–101

Poizner H, Clark MA, Merians AS, Macauley B, Gonzalez Rothi LJ, Heilman KM 1995 Joint coordination deficits in limb apraxia. Brain 118:227–242

Rapcsak SZ, Ochipa C, Anderson KC, Poizner H 1995 Progressive ideomotor apraxia: evidence for a selective impairment of the action production system. Brain Cogn 27:213–236

Rizzolatti G, Fadiga L 1998 Grasping objects and grasping action meanings: the dual role of monkey rostroventral premotor cortex (area F5). In: Sensory guidance of movement. Wiley, Chichester (Novartis Found Symp 218) p 81–103

Rondot P, de Recondo J, Ribadeu Dumas JL 1977 Visuomotor ataxia. Brain 100:355–376

Rothi LJG, Mack L, Heilman KM 1986 Pantomime agnosia. J Neurol Neurosurg Psychiatry 9:451–454

Rothi LJG, Ochipa C, Heilman KM 1991 A cognitive psychological model of limb praxis. Cogn Neuropsychol 8:43–58

Rothwell JC, Traub MM, Day BL, Obeso JA, Thomas PK, Marsden CD 1982 Manual motor performance in a deafferented man. Brain 105:515–542

Roy EA, Square PA 1985 Common considerations in the study of limb, verbal and oral apraxia. In: Roy EA (ed) Advances in psychology, vol 23: Neuropsychological studies of apraxia and related disorders. North Holland, Amsterdam, p 111–161

Sakata H, Taira M, Murata A, Mine S 1995 Neural mechanisms of visual guidance of hand action in the parietal cortex of the monkey. Cereb Cortex 5:429–438

Sanes JN, Mauritz KH, Dalakas MC, Evarts EV 1985 Motor control in humans with large-fiber sensory neuropathy. Hum Neurobiol 4:101–114

Strick PL, Dum RP, Picard N 1998 Motor areas on the medial wall of the hemisphere. In: Sensory guidance of movement. Wiley, Chichester (Novartis Found Symp 218) p 64–80

Tanaka Y, Yoshida A, Kawahata N, Hashimoto R, Obayashi T 1996 Diagonistic dyspraxia: clinical characteristics, responsible lesion and possible underlying mechanism. Brain 119:859–873

Thach WT 1998 Combination, complementarity and automatic control: a role for the cerebellum in learning movement coordination. In: Sensory guidance of movement. Wiley, Chichester (Novartis Found Symp 218) p 219–232

Ungerleider LG, Mishkin M 1982 Two cortical visual systems. In: Ingle DJ, Goodale MA, Mansfield RJW (ed) Analysis of visual behavior. MIT Press, Cambridge, MA, p 549–586

Wilson FAW, O'Scalaidhe SP, Goldman-Rakic PS 1993 Dissociation of object and spatial processing domains in primate prefrontal cortex. Science 260:1955–1958

DISCUSSION

Glickstein: How complete is the cerebellar loss in the cerebellum patients that you describe? A little bit of cerebellum goes a long way. There was a myth some years ago that the cerebellum isn't really necessary and that patients in whom the cerebellum fails to develop do fine without it. I scoured the literature to find the origin of this and was unable to find it, until I found the one case in Cambridge that seemed to have been the source of the myth (Glickstein 1994). A cadaver was found not to have a cerebellum. On the death certificate the man's occupation was given as 'building worker'. This was steadily elaborated over 40 years — every generation had a more skilled occupation for him, until finally he became a carpenter or a skilled brick layer.

Marsden: The degree of deficit in the patients studied on that visual reaching task was moderately severe cerebellar disease. These were patients who used sticks to walk and were disabled in terms of arm function, but not devastatingly so.

Passingham: We have made confirmed excitotoxic lesions in the interpositus and dentate nuclei of the cerebellum, and have compared the degree of misreaching with that shown by monkeys with lesions in inferior parietal cortex (7a and 7b). We find that the parietal animals reach wide of the mark, whereas the cerebellar animals make smaller reaching errors. This shows that what David Marsden said was true of patients was not due to the cerebellar lesions being incomplete.

Glickstein: All of us have some experimental observations that form the core of our belief. My part of the core of my belief was the Myers–Sperry–McCurdy monkeys who had complete cortico-cortical disconnection between visual and motor cortical areas (Myers et al 1962). The animals were competent in reaching at a moving target.

Marsden: It doesn't deny the necessity of the cerebellum. It just shows that patients with cerebellar disease can still use visual information to correct performance, which people with visuomotor apraxia cannot do.

Rizzolatti: I would like to briefly examine how the monkey data relate to ideomotor apraxia. As I described in my paper (Rizzolatti & Fadiga 1998, this volume), in the monkey there are two systems controlling hand movements. One is driven by objects, the other — the mirror system — is related to gesture observations. The mirror system appears to have two functions: that of understanding actions and that of imitating them. In ideomotor apraxic patients, there is no deficit of the first system. Patients are able to reach and grasp objects quite well. The deficit should concern therefore the second system. My guess, however, is that in these apraxic patients the lesion does not destroy primarily the mirror system (typically, ideomotor apraxics recognize actions made by others) but impairs their capacity to use this system for imitating gestures. Thus, although the observed actions are coded by the mirror system, the patients are unable to use this information to produce movements. It is interesting to note that according to most ethologists monkeys are unable to imitate hand actions, the capacity to transform observed and *understood* action in their copies being a late evolutionary acquisition. In this sense all monkeys are ideomotor apraxics.

Thach: With regard to the apraxias and the flow of information from the more ideational/perceptual through to the motor or 'kinetic', Liepmann's interpretation was that of a disconnection of a cortico-cortical pathway. Geschwind provided evidence of such a disconnection in conduction aphasias where the input was intact and the output was intact, but the pathway between was cut and therefore you could not use the perceptual areas to operate the output areas. Is this an analogy to reaching and hand movements? Why then were these preserved after Sperry experiments where deep cuts interrupted the posterior parts from the anterior parts? What *is* the pathway from these posterior areas through to the anterior areas?

Marsden: Geschwind very explicitly described apraxia as an inability for gesture to verbal command, and he associated the failure to reproduce a gesture upon a verbal command to damage to the arcuate fasciculus linking those areas in the superior temporal lobe to frontal regions. In other words, his concept of gesture was based on language-based mechanisms. I tried to illustrate that there is a much wider vista of apraxia which is not language based. Cortico-cortical information from the superior and inferior parietal lobes travels close to the arcuate fasciculus. Thus Geschwind constrained himself to language problems causing defects of gesture reproduction in response to verbal command, but the visual and somaesthetic mechanisms of apraxia are equally if not more important.

Miller: Dick Passingham, I just wanted you to clarify your comment about the comparison between the nuclear and parietal lesioned animals. Specifically, how confident can you be that the parietal lesions didn't interfere with the feedback of visual information through the pons into the cerebellum such that by making that interruptions you have disrupted both systems?

Passingham: I think it is well possible that the parietal lesions produce the bigger impairment because both cortico-cortical and cortico-subcortical routes are compromised.

Jeannerod: We have examined PET activity in normal subjects during tasks involving observation of actions displayed on a TV monitor. When the subjects' task was to observe actions with the instruction to recognize them later on, a strong activation limited to the right parahippocampal gyrus was found. When the instruction was to imitate the observed actions, the activation involved the dorsolateral prefrontal cortex bilaterally and the left anterior SMA. Areas 19 and 7 were also activated in the left hemisphere, whereas area 18 was activated in the right hemisphere.

The content of the observed actions also influenced brain activation. When the observed actions were pantomimes of meaningful gestures, activation was located mainly in the left hemisphere. Activated regions included the left interior frontal gyrus (Ba 45), and the left middle temporal and orbitofrontal gyri. The hippocampal gyrus was bilaterally activated. The medial frontal gyrus was activated in the right hemisphere. By contrast, activations produced by the observation of meaningless gestures were mainly located in the right hemisphere. The right occipito-parietal pathway (Ba 18, 19, 7 and 40) and the right premotor cortex were activated. In the left hemisphere, areas 18 and 7 were also involved (Decety et al 1997).

Marsden: The problem, then, if you accept those data, is that if you accept the clinical observations where classical inability to reproduce gestures is associated with inferior parietal lesions, how do you get the information out of the temporal regions which are activated by the imitated gesture into the inferior parietal regions, which when damaged lead to the inability to reproduce the gesture?

Thier: You mentioned limb-kinetic apraxia and defined this as a loss of the coordination of the melody of movements. This is somehow reminiscent of the usual clinical definition of cerebellar ataxias, although everyday experience tells us that you can easily discriminate cerebellar ataxias from limb-kinetic apraxias. Are you aware of cortical lesions which might mimic limb-kinetic ataxias? Is there a clear-cut difference between limb-kinetic ataxias and limb-kinetic apraxias?

Marsden: I think there are, but I cannot give you hard data. It is a poorly described and worked on field.

Passingham: The problem is that the motor cortex is often included in the infarct, and thus it is the ipsilateral hand that is tested for apraxia. If we impose transcranial magnetic stimulation (TMS) over the left premotor cortex in normal subjects, we can affect the movements on a visuomotor association task (visual choice reaction time) with either hand, whereas if we stimulate over the right premotor cortex we only delay movements with the right hand. So the TMS data on normals support the clinical data on apraxic patients in suggesting that the left hemisphere has a dominant controlling influence over both hands.

Marsden: I would accept that. What is the specific nature of the deficit in the ipsilateral hand?

Passingham: In this case we are using single-pulse TMS and delaying the choice reaction time to visual stimuli.

Marsden: But you're not addressing or speaking to the issue of the nature of the motor deficit of the ipsilateral hand.

Passingham: No.

Lemon: But in those experiments did you find subjects who actually made the wrong choices?

Passingham: We didn't use repetitive TMS; you only get errors with TMS if you use repetitive TMS.

Gibson: Matching two objects in the visual field is very different from using visual information to generate metrics for movement. If you allow people to reach slowly when demonstrating prism adaptation, they often reach accurately on the first trial since they simply match the position of the hand with the position of the target. Patients with disturbed visuomotor integration could still have an accurate final position by using the same strategy.

Andersen: I know you may not usually record eye movements, but I was wondering whether the visuomotor ataxias whether you sometimes see normal eye movements or do you often see both eye and limb movements affected for the same stimulus?

Marsden: The classical Bálint's syndrome did have a gross defect of localization of targets with eye movements. But classical Bálint's syndrome is relatively rare; much more common is isolated visuomotor ataxia. The eye movement disorders and misreaching into space are dissociable.

Jeannerod: In the specific syndromes of ataxia the eye movements have been recorded. Usually, stepwise movements towards the targets are seen.

Thier: One shouldn't forget that these lesions are usually very large so they're probably encompassing eye movement parts of cortex as well as hand movement parts. So the question of whether selective lesions of eye movements can occur as opposed to selective lesions of eye movements hasn't been answered.

Marsden: It is true that you can get selective deficits of hand movements and not eye movements. As you say, I'm unaware of anybody describing selective deficits in eye movements without hand movement deficits.

Georgopoulos: All of these parietal lesions have devastating effects. However, excision of parietal cortex to cure epilepsy seems to be much less incapacitating than lesions due, for example, to stroke. Do you have any thoughts on this? The usual explanation is that in stroke there is damage of the white matter, in addition to that of the grey matter. Could this have something to do with subcortical damage?

Marsden: I'm always wary of deductions from patients who have had excision of cortical areas for epilepsy with no effect, when you would expect them to have an effect based upon the impact of lesions in that area in previously normal people. By definition, you're always removing dysfunctional parts of brain in epilepsy surgery. Patients operated on in this way will have had epilepsy for a long time and therefore will have had a long time to adapt, perhaps using other parts of the brain. The dysfunctional epileptic area may therefore be of no value to the patient whatsoever, except to produce the wretched epilepsy. I don't think epileptic excisions are a robust model for discovering normal brain function.

Georgopoulos: What about 'constructional apraxia'?

Marsden: Is it really an apraxia, if you use the word apraxia to define a difficulty with movement? Do people with so-called 'constructional apraxia' actually have difficulty with movement or is it difficulty with the concept of construction?

Goodale: Richard Andersen raised a point the other day about the patient DF: because she was unable to copy an arrangement of coloured tokens in a proper way he asked whether or not she had constructional apraxia. She doesn't have constructional apraxia from a classical point of view because she has intact mental imagery (Servos & Goodale 1995). If you ask her, for example, to imagine the letter 'D', flip it on its back, and stick it on top of the letter 'V' and then ask her what this looks like, she will say (like most people) that it looks like an ice cream cone. In other words, she can manipulate things in her mind's eye. This is not something that someone with constructional apraxia could manage. Having said that, I would like to re-emphasize a point I made earlier: constructional apraxia is a poorly defined concept. It has been linked to spatial disorientation, spatial inattention, and a variety of other visuospatial deficits.

Georgopoulos: Constructional apraxia has been pretty well established in the literature as a stand-alone disorder even since Kleist's classical work (Kleist 1934) in which he defined it as a disturbance 'in formative activities such as assembling, building and drawing, in which the spatial form of the product proves to be unsuccessful, without there being an apraxia for single movements'. Not only is the disorder established, but its possible hemispheric lateralization has also been debated. Although early studies pointed to a special role of the right cerebral hemisphere in constructional apraxia (Benton 1967, Mack & Levine 1981, Piercy et al 1960), more systematic later work (reviewed in De Renzi 1982, Gainotti 1985) supported the notion that *praxis* is most probably subserved by both hemispheres.

Marsden: The deficit is certainly defined: the problem is the use of the word 'apraxia' which has an the implication that it is primarily a motor deficit.

Georgopoulos: I don't think that constructional apraxia is the consequence of a conceptual defect. For example, a patient can recognize a stick as a stick, and a square as a square, and yet may be unable to construct a square with the sticks.

Thach: The idea that optic apraxia is only an inability to *move* the eyes well is incorrect. Patients are also commonly unable to maintain a gaze on target. Characteristically, they will be talking with you and not foveate you; they'll be looking off to the side, and this is often the way they're recognized clinically. But they will not be aware of that and will say that they are looking at you. This part is the agnosia, the lack of perception of the deficit. Then in tests they will also have errors in visual perception. They have gross gaze deficits and cannot correct them, in contrast to the patient with a cerebellar lesion who will be able to correct and get on target. I believe that the basic defect in cerebellar lesions is in metrics and the inability to combine the appropriate muscle package instantly.

Stein: Do you always have to have bilateral lesions to get optic ataxia? If so, why? Surely you should get optic ataxia in the contralateral field.

Marsden: Many cases have been bilateral lesions, but there are also many unilateral lesions, left or right hemisphere.

References

Benton AL 1967 Constructional apraxia and the minor hemisphere. Confin Neurol 29:1–16

Decety J, Grezes J, Costes N et al 1997 Brain activity during observation of action. Influence of action content and subject's strategy. Brain 120:1763–1777

De Renzi E 1982 Disorders of space exploration and cognition. Wiley, Chichester

Gainotti G 1985 Constructional apraxia. In: Frederiks JAM (ed) Handbook of clinical neurology. Elsevier, Amsterdam, p 491–506

Glickstein M 1994 Cerebellar agenesis. Brain 117:1209–1212

Kleist K 1934 Gehirnpathologie. Barth, Leipzig

Mack JL, Levine RN 1981 The basis of visual constructional disability in patients with unilateral cerebral lesions. Cortex 17:515–532

Myers RE, Sperry RW, McCurdy NM 1962 Neuronal mechanisms in visual guidance of limb movement. Arch Neurol 7:195–202

Piercy M, Hécaen H, Ajuriaguerra J 1960 Constructional apraxia associated with unilateral cerebral lesions. Left and right sided cases compared. Brain 83:225–242

Rizzolatti G, Fadiga L 1998 Grasping objects and grasping object meanings: the dual role of monkey rostroventral premotor cortex (area F5). In: Sensory guidance of movement. Wiley, Chichester (Novartis Found Symp 218) p 81–103

Servos P, Goodale MA 1995 Preserved visual imagery in visual form agnosia. Neuropsychologia 33:1383–1394

Final discussion

Hoffmann: Mitchell Glickstein, why is the human cerebellum wider in the reconstruction you showed than that of a cow?

Glickstein: The simple point is that there is no correlation of vermian size with cerebral cortex, but there's a precise link between the size of cerebral cortex, the pontine nuclei and the lateral nucleus of the cerebellum in different species. Thus whatever the cerebellar hemispheres do, they are doing it in response to what they get from the cerebral cortex.

Hoffmann: I was trying to get to the additional aspects of cerebellar functions which haven't been discussed here. We have only talked about sensory and motor functions, and cognitive functions have been completely excluded in our discussions.

Glickstein: That was by design! I want to make one general point about cognitive functions. A positive claim has lower threshold to be accepted for publication than a negative claim. There are failures to replicate some of the alleged cognitive functions of the cerebellum.

Hoffmann: Definitely our sensory and motor systems aren't better than those of other primates. There must be additional functions, embedded in a relatively much larger cerebellum in humans.

Strick: You've made the point previously that the localization of function in the cerebellum has lagged behind localization of function in the cerebral cortex. There are large regions of the cerebellar cortex that are basically uncharted in terms of their connections and functions. For instance, what are the consequences of removing a part of the hemisphere of cerebellar cortex in the region of crus2? Or ablating portions of the posterior vermis?

Glickstein: Von Koranyi (1890) said that if you cut the corpus callosum of a dog you don't see any effects. In one of those cerebellar series I removed all of crus1 and crus2 on one side. I bought a friend and colleague, who is a vet as well as an anatomist, in to see the animal. He couldn't tell which side I removed. The brain is like a submarine: everything is packed precisely and clearly. If there is a big lateral cerebellar hemisphere, it is there for a purpose — we just haven't figured that purpose out.

Strick: We have the old data from Sperry and Myers that apparently cutting connections between the posterior parietal cortex and the motor areas in the frontal lobe does not abolish the ability of an animal to direct its limb to an object in space. Thus, other circuits are thought to be important in taking visual input and using it to guide limb movement. These other circuits could be the basal ganglia and cerebellar loops with the motor areas of the cerebral cortex. However, in our hands, these circuits don't appear to take information from a one domain (e.g. sensory) and transform it into another (e.g. motor). Thus, we are not left with a good answer to a long-standing question: Is the visual guidance of limb movement directed through cortico-cortical connections or through cerebellar and basal ganglia loops with the cerebral cortex?

Lemon: The reason that we're going around is because we still want to believe that the lesion information tells you what happens in the natural circumstance. We know from the brain imagery studies that there's a nasty mismatch between what you see in the normally behaving brain and what happens in an animal that is forced into using some new or different connections by the lesion that you happen to have made.

Thach: That's a nasty comment about lesions! The problem here in how the cerebral cortical areas are used in guiding movement is that we put the question in an either/or alternative: the control is either cortico-cortical *or* it's cortex–deep structure and back to cortex. Often the resolution of such an argument is that the answer is *both.* You can compensate for the cortico-cortical cut because you have got the other cortex–deep structure–cortex instant action path available. You don't see a loss until you make two lesions.

Marsden: Therefore the crucial question is, what is the special contribution of the two different paths?

Glickstein: I'll synthesize the lesion discussion as follows. An experimental psychologist teaches two monkeys the visual discrimination task. In monkey (a) the left optic nerve is cut, in monkey (b) the right optic nerve is cut. Both retained task performance perfectly. The experimenter concludes the eyes have nothing to do with visual discrimination!

Reference

von Koranyi A 1890 Über die Folge der Durchschneidung des Hirnbalkens. Pflügers Arch Physiol 47:35–42

Index of contributors

Non-participating co-authors are indicated by asterisks. Entries in bold indicate papers; other entries refer to discussion contributions

334

Subject index

A

action recognition 91, 96
action selection 178, 179
action specification 178, 179–180
    dorsal premotor cortex and 182–185
action stream *see* dorsal stream
AIP *see* anterior intraparietal area
akinetic mutism 106
Alzheimer's disease 318
anterior cerebral syndrome 106
anterior intraparietal area (AIP) 88, 98, 110
aphasia 100, 314–315
apraxia 143, 308–331
    aphasia and 314–315
    definition 308–309
    diagnostic tests 319
    isolated limb 318
    lesions 318–319, 325–326, 327
    mapping of cortex 311–313
    neurophysiological concept 321–323
arcuate sulcus 85
area 7 39, 102
    area 7a 123, 124
    area 7b 98
area 46 102
area F4 96, 101
area F5 81–102
    canonical neurons 85–88
    cingulate gyrus and 99
    cingulate sulcus and 99
    evolution of 102
    grasp 82–85
    mirror neurons 88–91
    in monkey 81–102
    motor imagery 95, 101
    motor properties 82–85
    motor schemata 82–84
    neurons 84–85
    projections
        from anterior intraparietal area (AIP)
            98
        from area 46, 102

        from area 7b 98
        to primary motor cortex 98
        from SII 99, 102
        to subcortex 98
        see also dorsal premotor cortex
area MST 123
arm movement
    change in target and 149–152
    cortical control of 176–200
    cortico-motoneuronal influence 206
    degrees of freedom 8
    directional change 164
    directional tuning of cells 148
    discrete movements 147–149
    dorsal paraflocculus 269–270
    feedforward signal 148
    final posture 9–13
    mechanical stiffness 293
    preferred direction 148
    single-cell activity in 148
    in stroke patients 105
    superior colliculus 171
    visual control of 147–170
association 129–146
asterognosis 317
auditory stimuli 118

B

basal ganglia 40, 59, 135, 139, 255–256
    lesion 138, 142
    role in sequential movements 78
    see also subcortex
basis penduculi 255
Betz cell 249
body centric neurons 96
body representation map 65–67
    deep nuclei 224–225
    eye movement fields 78–79
    parallel fibre beam 225
Bolk, Lodewijk 267
braking force
    cell activity 166